A HISTORY OF PLAGUE
IN JAVA, 1911–1942

A HISTORY OF PLAGUE IN JAVA, 1911–1942

MAURITS BASTIAAN MEERWIJK

SOUTHEAST ASIA PROGRAM PUBLICATIONS
AN IMPRINT OF CORNELL UNIVERSITY PRESS
Ithaca and London

Cornell University Press gratefully acknowledges the role
of the Association for Asian Studies First Book Subvention
Program for its support of this book.

First published 2022 by Cornell University Press

Library of Congress Cataloging-in-Publication Data

Names: Meerwijk, Maurits Bastiaan, 1989– author.
Title: A history of plague in Java, 1911–1942 /
    Maurits Bastiaan Meerwijk.
Description: Ithaca, NY : Southeast Asia Program
    Publications, an imprint of Cornell University Press,
    2022. | Includes bibliographical references and index.
Identifiers: LCCN 2022006261 (print) | LCCN 2022006262
    (ebook) | ISBN 9781501766824 (hardcover) |
    ISBN 9781501766831 (paperback) |
    ISBN 9781501766848 (pdf) | ISBN 9781501766855 (epub)
Subjects: LCSH: Public health—Indonesia—Java—
    History—20th century. | Plague—Indonesia—Java—
    History—20thcentury. | Java(Indonesia)—Colonization—
    History—20th century. | Netherlands—Colonies—
    Asia—Social policy. | Netherlands—Colonies—Asia—
    Social conditions—20th century.
Classification: LCC DS646.27 .M44 2022 (print) |
    LCC DS646.27 (ebook) | DDC 614.5/732095982—
    dc23/eng/20220614
LC record available at https://lccn.loc.gov/2022006261
LC ebook record available at https://lccn.loc.gov
    /2022006262

CONTENTS

ACKNOWLEDGMENTS

This book is the product of my involvement with the ERC Starting Grant project "Visual Representations of the Third Plague Pandemic" (336564) in 2018. I owe a debt of gratitude to the project's principal investigator, Christos Lynteris, for his expert guidance and support. His suggestion to consider the focus of Dutch plague photography on "bamboo" has proven fruitful indeed. I gratefully acknowledge financial support for the publication of this book by the Association for Asian Studies and Stichting Historia Medicinae.

I wish to thank Marieke Bloembergen, Robert Peckham, Hans Pols, Susie Protschky, Ria Sinha, and the anonymous reviewers for their comments and suggestions at different stages of writing this book. A special thank you is owed to dear friends who helped to provide access to key sources and offered feedback on challenging sections: Angharad Fletcher, Jack Greatrex, Chi Chi Huang, Nicolo Ludovice, Maria Nicolaou, and Sarah Yu.

The staff at the Nationaal Archief and Koninklijke Bibliotheek in The Hague, the Arsip Nasional and Perpustakaan Nasional in Jakarta, the University of Leiden Library, and the Museum Wereldculturen have been terrific in facilitating my research. Furthermore, the support of my editor Sarah Grossman and her colleagues at Cornell University Press was vital to the completion of this book.

I am deeply grateful for the continued personal and professional encouragement of family, friends, and colleagues around the world. My final thanks are owed to my parents, Paul and Erna, for a lifetime of loving support.

Technical Notes

This book considers the Dutch response to plague in late-colonial Java. While the use of modern Indonesian spelling is generally preferable for scholarship on this region, I have chosen for the sake of clarity and consistency to adopt colonial-era spelling for Indonesian place names throughout (e.g., Soerabaja, Madioen, and Priangan). For the same reasons, most Dutch titles and organizations have been translated into English in the main body of the text with noted exceptions. Where relevant, abbreviations are used based on the original Dutch (e.g., BGD for Burgerlijke Geneeskundige Dienst and DP for Dienst der Pestbestrijding). The words "improved" and "improvement" in relation to the renovation of houses and villages in the name of plague control are used throughout as descriptive (as opposed to qualifying) terms.

The official currency in the Dutch East Indies was the guilder (*f.*). Financial and other numerical data presented in this book are often approximations compiled from multiple sources (see chapter 2).

Through the colonial period, Java was the most tightly controlled island in the Dutch East Indies. It boasted a large and diverse population that grew from approximately 4.5 million in 1815 to over 40 million by 1930. The colonial government was run by a corps of career civil servants: the interior government known as Domestic Governance (Binnenlandsch Bestuur, BB). Administratively, the island was divided into approximately twenty-two *residenties* (residencies) that consisted of several *afdeelingen* (districts) that were led by a *resident* and *assistent-resident*, respectively. These districts tended to overlap with historic *regentschappen* (regencies) that were led by a figurehead *regent* (regent). More locally, Dutch administrators collaborated with the (assistant) *wedono* (district chief) and *loerah* (village chief). The principalities of Djokjakarta and Soerakarta in Central Java remained nominally independent. The central colonial government was based in offices in Batavia (present-day Jakarta), its suburb Weltevreden, and the elevated cities Buitenzorg (Bogor) and Bandoeng. It was led by a governor-general appointed by the Dutch government in The Hague.

This book draws on a large number of visual materials as its historical evidence. Many of these images are available in a database compiled by the ERC-project "Visual Representations of the Third Plague Pandemic" and other digital repositories. I have included a selection of the images most pertinent to the arguments made in this book. Digital object identifiers and permalinks have been provided to access additional visual sources wherever possible.

A HISTORY OF PLAGUE
IN JAVA, 1911–1942

Introduction

Three European men in white attire pose in a partially constructed house in Java around 1919 (figure 0.1). Two have climbed up into the beams, one emerging triumphantly through the skeleton of the roof. Below, two Javanese men in hybrid local and colonial uniform look on. The actual subject of the photograph—the construction—has been captured in its entirety. The roof dominates the image, its latticework contrasting with the sky behind. The structure is placed on a stone foundation and has wooden corner posts and joists. Most of the dwelling is drawn up of a different material, however, cheaper and readily available. Sturdy bamboo poles serve as support posts. The rafters are made of halved or "split" bamboo. The walls are made of a single layer of wicker bamboo mats called *gedek*. More pieces of bamboo are scattered in the foreground, one stalk at the base of the house revealing its hollow interior. The neatly dressed men climbing into the half-finished dwelling have something boyish about them, but the photograph nonetheless conveys a strong message regarding the prevailing race and power dynamics in the Dutch East Indies. To contemporary audiences, this would have been evident not only from the pose and positioning of the human figures, but also from the recognition that this evidently "native" house was no longer fully Javanese. We are witnessing a scene of home improvement in Java: one of the most invasive, sustained, and best-advertised health interventions

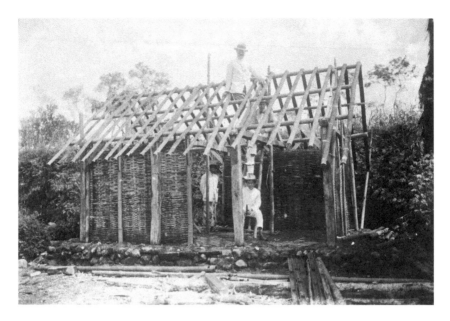

FIGURE 0.1.   Photograph of five individuals at a house being improved at Tjapar, ca. 1919.
G. M. Versteeg, *House at Tjapar with Home Improvement. Kastelijn, Snijders, and Fischmann with Mantri Home Improvement*, ca. 1919, TM-60012999. Courtesy of the Nationaal Museum van Wereldculturen.

of the Dutch colonial period that was implemented in response to the outbreak of plague in 1911.

Plague is a bacterial disease that manifests predominantly in three distinct but equally graphic forms that continue to inform the pandemic imaginary.[1] It is a zoonotic disease, strictly speaking, normally crossing over from animal reservoirs in small mammals to humans by the bite of an infected flea or by the handling of infected animals. In its most common and least deadly bubonic form victims develop acute febrile symptoms and characteristic lymphadenopathy (lymphatic swellings) in the groin, armpit, and neck: buboes. The disease overwhelms the immune system, and patients may ultimately succumb to organ failure. Bubonic plague may progress into septicemic plague, or more rarely victims develop this form through direct contact with an infected source. Here, plague bacilli infect the bloodstream and cause blood clots, tissue death, organ failure, and endotoxic shock. Finally, plague may advance to the lungs, leading to coughing, coughing up blood, and ultimately respiratory failure. This form alone is transmissible directly between humans, by breathing in highly infective particles expelled by patients through coughing or sneezing. Pneumonic plague is invariably fatal without treatment.[2] But as with outbreaks of plague at the turn of the nineteenth and twentieth centuries elsewhere, the disease in Java was less remarkable for its mortality than for the cultural response it provoked.

Between the recognition of plague in March 1911 and its virtual elimination by the time of the Japanese invasion in March 1942, an estimated 215,000 people succumbed to plague: a modest figure that pales in comparison to the 1.5 million deaths attributed in the archipelago to the influenza pandemic of 1918–1919 or the incalculable (and uncalculated) deaths caused by malaria every year.[3] Yet these diseases did not trigger the sweeping countermeasures plague did. After identifying the obligate house rat *Mus rattus* as the principal host or reservoir of plague in Java, increasing the distance between man and rat was presented by health officials as the key to bringing the disease under control. This way, the plague vector—the rat flea, *Xenopsylla cheopis*—was denied access to humans once its preferred host had expired. The traditional Javanese dwelling, drawn up of bamboo and a palm leaf thatch called *atap*, was discovered to offer a multitude of hiding spaces for the rat to live and nest in close proximity to humans without being observed. Consequently, the Dutch labeled the native house "plague dangerous." They imbued historic notions of the "plague house" as a space of transmission with a new, transformed, and *actionable* materiality.[4] In response, over 1.6 million houses were either renovated or rebuilt over the last three decades of Dutch colonial rule in a concerted effort to "build out the rat"—to build out plague (table 1).[5] Millions of houses more were subjected to periodic inspection, and countless Javanese were exposed to a concurrent hygiene campaign striving to ratproof their practices and beliefs along with their homes.[6] Between 1911 and 1942, I estimate that plague control consumed no less than *f.* 85 million and likely more (see chapter 2). Home improvement to counter plague was not unique to Java, but the scale on which it was implemented (insisted Dutch state agents to colonial, domestic, and foreign audiences alike) most certainly was.

This book examines the Dutch response to plague in Java. It stands at the intersection of colonial, medical, and environmental histories of Southeast Asia and traces how plague triggered a tremendous expansion of Dutch state power and cultural influence at a time when—as has been suggested—the "gangrene" had already set its claws into the colonial project.[7] My argument is straightforward: plague prompted a colonial health intervention that was both unprecedented in scale and uniquely invasive in scope. If such a claim is less original to plague studies than to scholarship on colonial Indonesia, a history of plague in Java does make two significant contributions to the formidable body of scholarship on this disease. First, plague has tended to be studied and framed as a "house disease" with a distinct urban preference.[8] In Java, such associations between plague and the built environment were exceptionally strong, but the

Table 1   Plague mortality and home improvement in Java, 1911–1945

	PLAGUE DEATHS	HOUSES IMPROVED
1911	2,155	37,851
1912	2,276	37,851
1913	11,386	37,852
1914	15,756	37,852
1915	6,239	229,601
1916	1,188	141,774
1917	421	76,483
1918	734	47,608
1919	2,954	21,002
1920	9,152	26,705
1921	9,763	42,563
1922	10,956	21,053
1923	8,667	46,874
1924	13,253	50,714
1925	14,484	42,418
1926	7,771	45,291
1927	7,755	42,633
1928	4,600	58,657
1929	4,095	86,852
1930	3,980	67,037
1931	4,539	73,397
1932	6,442	56,987
1933	16,880	28,438
1934	23,239	23,990
1935	12,995	36,572
1936	6,000	53,418
1937	3,814	32,318
1938	2,107	56,265
1939	1,427	54,389
1940	397	39,282
1941	350	–
1942	871	–
1943	1,224	–
1944	242	–
1945	190	–

Sources: *Koloniaal Verslag* (1911–1928) and *Indisch Verslag* (1931–1941), *Mededeelingen van den Burgelijke Geneeskundige Dienst van Nederlandsch-Indië* (1911–1924), *Mededeelingen van den Dienst der Volksgezondheid van Nederlandsch-Indië* (1925–1941), and Dienst der Pestbestrijding, quarterly and annual reports (1915–1921).

outbreak assumed a rural character instead. Home improvement consequently presented a uniquely far-reaching intervention beyond urban enclaves of colonial presence and control. Second, plague scholarship has shown a tendency to focus on epidemic outbreak moments and the immediate responses they triggered—with less attention given to their endemic afterlives.[9] In Java, plague is of interest precisely because of its endemic entrenchment and the remarkably strong and constant health intervention that it (nonetheless) provoked. To explain the importance of this disease to colonial governance despite its modest burden to the Indies death rate, I suggest that plague and plague control in Java offered the Dutch a platform: an epidemic drama against which they could assert themselves locally, nationally, and internationally as an advanced colonial and scientific power. As progressive, ethical, and "modern."[10]

The Third Plague Pandemic

The outbreak of plague in Java took place during a global expansion of this disease known as the third plague pandemic. The origin of this event is often traced back to an outbreak in Yunnan Province in southwest China in 1855 (where plague had in fact been endemic since 1787). Political and economic instability, migration, and urbanization, explains the historian Carol Benedict, helped to carry the disease eastward over the latter half of the nineteenth century. Following an outbreak in Canton (Guangzhou), plague reached the nearby British crown colony of Hong Kong in May 1894.[11] From this key shipping hub on the south coast of the Qing Empire plague attained a global diffusion. In a matter of years, it reached every inhabited continent and established new endemic foci that (as in the case of Madagascar and the United States) exist to this day. By the time the pandemic came to an end in the second half of the twentieth century, plague had claimed an estimated twelve to fifteen million lives—with ten to twelve million deaths in India alone.[12]

The demographic impact of plague was not negligible. Still, the resources mobilized in response to the disease—globally and locally—were certainly "disproportionate to the total number of deaths" when compared to the burden of other infectious disease.[13] The tremendous cultural response to plague was provoked by its high case-fatality rate, on the one hand (ranging from 60 to 100 percent between its bubonic, septicemic, and pneumonic forms), and its cataclysmic history, on the other. The plague that entered Hong Kong in 1894 exhibited "all the symptoms of the true bubonic pest which devastated Europe in the Middle Ages."[14] It was consequently equated with a disease that had been pandemic twice before: the "plague of Justinian" (541–750) and the

Great Plague (peaking in Eurasia between 1346 and 1353), better known as the Black Death. Both events had led to such enormous loss of life and to periods of social instability that "plague" had come to be framed in eschatological terms. It was seen as the disease at the end of human existence.[15] That is to say, when plague became an object of knowledge of European scientific medicine at the turn of the nineteenth and twentieth centuries, physicians and officials seeking to study and control the disease operated "under the bane of its perceived ability to wipe out humanity."[16]

On Hong Kong being declared an "infected" port on May 10, 1894, its colonial government accepted the assistance of a Japanese team of bacteriologists led by Kitasato Shibasaburō—an apprentice of Robert Koch. His arrival was followed shortly after by that of Alexandre Yersin, a product of the school of Louis Pasteur, who worked in nearby Saigon. As representatives of new and rival medical schools that led the way in microbiology, they were on a mission to identify a possible causative organism of the dread disease. The story of their competition has become somewhat legendary. Kitasato was welcomed by the British colonial health service, which furnished him with laboratory space and provided samples from plague corpses for his experiments. Yersin was forced to set up shop in a makeshift bamboo shed and had to procure his samples illicitly.[17] The two scientists identified the plague bacillus within days of one another. Kitasato announced his discovery first and with the backing of the directing health officials in Hong Kong, but his account was contradictory and his samples were polluted.[18] Yersin's later communication accompanied by clear microphotographs was favored, and the bacterium named after his mentor: *Pasteurella pestis.*[19]

The landmark discovery of the plague bacillus may have been equated with the discovery of plague itself as a discrete disease entity, but it did nothing to explain its origin or transmission.[20] Over the following years, plague spread around the world and Hong Kong became implicated as the center of a global pandemic: a plague port. In 1895, the city was free of cases, though plague manifested in the neighboring Portuguese colony Macau. In 1896, plague "came calling again" and would recur annually in Hong Kong until 1929.[21] Also in 1896, the disease broke out in the port city of Bombay, from which it spread across British India. Two years later, plague was introduced into Mauritius and Madagascar and may have "leaked" from Yersin's laboratory in Nha Trang to cause a local outbreak.[22] In 1899, plague outbreaks were reported in Manila, Honolulu, Porto, and Alexandria. San Francisco, Buenos Aires, Rio de Janeiro, and Sydney hosted outbreaks the year after, and in 1901 there was an outbreak in Cape Town. Given the location of the Dutch East Indies at the crossroads of routes of trade and migration between South and East Asia, the Americas, and Australasia, the failure of plague to establish itself in the archipelago about this time was a source of puzzlement. The response to plague, meanwhile, radically differed from place to place: ranging from panic to denial, from lax to outright "draconian" countermeasures, and from the dismissal of "native" hygienic practices to the mockery of modern medical science.[23] Everywhere, the newly established bacterial cause of plague collided with existing theories, assumptions, and prejudices about its nature and transmission to form hybrid etiologies.

In the early years of the pandemic, argues the anthropologist Christos Lynteris, the notion that plague was a "soil disease" built on older suggestions that plague was caused by inhaling telluric gases. These theories now held that bacilli infected the earth, remained dormant within it to start fresh outbreaks at long intervals, and suggested a number of interventions. In Hong Kong, such notions supported the demolition and burning of the Chinese neighborhood Taipingshan.[24] Similarly, in Bombay, health officials demolished buildings in plague-stricken quarters and dug up their earthen floors to "expose" the soil to the perceived disinfecting qualities of sunlight, air, and often fire.[25] In the process, native practices that facilitated contact between humans and soil were dismissed by colonial officials as plague dangerous. Their ire settled, for instance, on the barefoot coolies of Hong Kong or the women of Calcutta who used dirt to clean metal objects.[26] Simultaneously, suggests the medical historian Robert Peckham, health officials were preoccupied with the "infective propensity of Chinese things" that were being stored in and shipped from Hong Kong. Here and elsewhere, the perceived ability of the plague bacillus to hide among a proliferation of "things" rendered plague an exportable commodity, leading to the disinfecting or burning of personal items as well as merchandise.[27]

Then, of course, there were prevalent social and racial associations that cast one group or another such as Chinese, Indians, or *hajjis* as human carriers of plague. In one well-known example, racist sentiment played a part in the burning of Chinatown in Honolulu in 1899.[28] In San Francisco and elsewhere, it led to ineffective quarantines being placed on Chinese neighborhoods. In Brazil, Argentina, and South Africa, white elites similarly implicated poorer, nonwhite communities and sought to push them to the margins of cities.[29] Plague, in short, remained an epistemologically uncertain entity that was easily worked into existing notions and biases on the nature, origin, and transmission of disease. By the time plague arrived in Java, many of these theories persisted and importantly informed early responses to the outbreak. But in the meantime, a radically new theory of plague transmission had also gained traction.

Today, plague is understood as an infectious disease that primarily affects rodents and is most efficiently transmitted by the so-called oriental rat flea. Rats in particular have become central to contemporary narratives of plague transmission. It is our "epidemic villain" of choice.[30] That animals were also affected by plague was a truism by the end of the nineteenth century but, argues the anthropologist Nicholas Evans, while the "modern-day iconography" of plague is "replete with images of rats as plague carriers," the notion that animals played a role in its transmission to or between humans was "unheard of before the turn of the twentieth century."[31] Though even Yersin had pointed to the rat as a *vehicule* of plague, it was only in 1898 that another Pasteurian scientist, Paul-Louis Simond, presented preliminary evidence that plague could be transmitted by the bite of an infected rat flea.[32] His theory was met with skepticism but over the following decade, explains Evans, members of the Second Indian Plague Commission (1905–1917) laboriously supplied the evidence that supported this "rat-flea-man" hypothesis.[33] Other species of rodent such as gerbils, marmots, and tarbagans were subsequently implicated as "sylvatic or wild hosts" of plague. Plague consequently came to be situated at the intersection of human and animal life: helping to lay a foundation for the concept of zoonosis.[34] At the time in British India, however, the theory was rallied once more to reaffirm existing racial and social hierarchies. Europeans concentrated less on the unproblematic agency of the rat itself than on the native customs that fostered "improper" relationships between humans and rats. The "uncovering of rat agency," suggests Evans, ultimately made "native bodies and habits knowable and, crucially, judicable."[35] Similar discrepancies, as I demonstrate over the course of this book, were present in Dutch assumptions on plague and plague transmission in the Indies.

The Dutch East Indies

In a chapter in the incisive series of books *Asia Inside Out*, the historian Eric Tagliacozzo provides a snapshot of the Dutch East Indies in 1910. The Dutch colonial government, he suggests, found itself "close to the apex of its dominion" over the archipelago. Geographically, the colony had grown to its fullest extent. Mapping and surveying missions documented the territory under Dutch rule and the people it contained with ever greater precision. Railroads penetrated the hinterlands of Java and Sumatra. Advances in shipping knitted outlying islands closer together. The number of state agents at the political periphery steadily increased, and the Royal Dutch East India Army (Koninklijk Nederlandsch-Indisch Leger, KNIL) was an increasingly professional military force. Yet the stage was set "for disasters that were just around the bend."[36] Government corruption and maltreatment of the population persisted; discontent was rife. Nationalist forces had been set in motion with the founding of the political organization Boedi Oetomo in 1908 and, as the historian Hans Pols explains from the perspective of Indies physicians, they steadily increased in strength, diversity, and outlook.[37] But if, as Tagliacozzo put it, the gangrene nibbled away at the Dutch colonial project after 1910, why did he not substantiate his metaphor by referencing the pathogenic threat that entered the Indies that very year? Given his emphasis on the figments of colonial rule that exuded confidence, his inattention to healthcare is unsurprising. After all, if many indicators suggested the robustness of the Dutch colonial state at this time, medicine was not among them. The arrival of plague in Java and subsequent measures to contain it, however, would materially expand Dutch dominion for decades to come.

Since 1827, a civil health service had operated in Java as part of a military health service. The health of the Indies population, consequently, was secondary to the care of Dutch military and government personnel. Repeated attempts to separate these branches had failed, while the system was criticized alternately for drawing resources away from the military and for the neglect of civilian health.[38] For most of the nineteenth century, only a handful of larger settlements boasted a municipal or port health officer. Various plantations engaged a physician to look after employees and a small number of private physicians were scattered across Java.[39] In her study on developments in the medical market of the Dutch East Indies over the late nineteenth and early twentieth centuries, the historian Liesbeth Hesselink put the number of European-trained physicians in the Indies in 1850 at less than sixty. By 1900, this figure had risen to 228: a significant increase, but far too low to cover a population of nearly thirty million people in Java alone. The vast majority of the Indies population instead received medical care from the *doekoen*, men and women who tended to specialize in a particular health practice and who gained their knowledge orally and experientially. Their number, estimated Hesselink, was about 33,000 in 1900.[40] Meanwhile, the number of medical institutes (including psychiatric hospitals) stood at around eighty in 1900. They were run primarily by the army and offered about 4,000 beds.[41] A government medical laboratory known as the Geneeskundig Laboratorium was opened in 1888.

The Dutch colonial health service—such as it was—was supported by a small number of Javanese medical assistants. The Batavia Medical College had opened in 1851 and graduated a steady trickle of junior physicians and *vaccinateurs* who, in return for stipends, were obliged to work for the colonial state for a period of ten years.[42] The curriculum steadily expanded in length and complexity, and in 1902 the college was renamed the School for the Education of Native Doctors (School tot Opleiding van Inlandsche Artsen, STOVIA). Nevertheless, it was only in the late 1920s that graduates from STOVIA or its sister college in Soerabaja (which opened in 1913) were placed on a par with European-trained physicians: financially if not socially.[43] By the end of the nineteenth century, there were ninety of these *doctor djawas* in the service of the government. An additional four had taken up private practice. A handful pursued further education in the Netherlands.[44] The *doctor djawa*—a name that stuck even after graduates were awarded the title Inlandsche arts (1902) and Indische arts (1913)—occupied an ambiguous position in colonial society. Often, students enrolled in their early teens and saw their ties to family, local customs, and traditional values severed. Expecting to matriculate into Dutch society upon graduation, Indies physicians were in for a "rude awakening," being denied recognition as full and highly educated colonial citizens. It was this unsatisfactory state of affairs, Pols suggests, that led to their active involvement in nationalist movements.[45]

About 1900, a gear change had taken place in Dutch colonial policy. After decades of public debate, the government in The Hague formally moved away from viewing the Indies as a "colony of extraction" to pursue a new course guided by liberal ideals of "lifting up" local populations in preparation of a distant independence.[46] The so-called *Ethische Politiek* involved a "suite of liberal-developmentalist reforms" and was the Dutch answer to the French *mission civilisatrice* and the Anglo-American "white man's burden."[47] It was, in many ways, an elitist policy, couched in terms of Christian responsibility, haphazardly implemented, full of contradictions—"fragmented"—and perhaps simply a new attempt to justify authoritarian colonialism.[48] The ethical policy sought to square (in name if not in practice) social, political, and cultural violence in the Indies with contemporary discourses on modernity, citizenship, order, and nationhood, both among Dutch colonial and metropolitan populations themselves and among the people "whom they presumed to govern."[49]

While this new government rationale certainly entailed taking responsibility for the health and wellbeing of its colonial subjects, the arena of public health was a striking example of the tension between ethics and economy that emerged under this regime.[50] It would take five years from the announcement that the government intended to fulfil its so-called debt of honor to the Indies population before a committee was formed to arrange a separate civil medical service.[51] It took another five years before this organization came into being. An independent Civil Medical Service (Burgerlijke Geneeskundige Dienst, BGD) was finally created in January 1911, months *after* plague was thought to have entered Java, and months *before* it was recognized.[52] Administratively, the new health service would fall under the Department of Education and Worship. For years, the new organization remained severely understaffed and as late as 1920 not all positions of regional *gouvernements arts* had been filled.[53] Plague control dominated the first years of its existence, necessitating the creation of a separate plague control service (Dienst der Pestbestrijding, DP) that was active between 1915 and 1924. The DP was later reintegrated as a branch of the renamed Department of Public Health (Dienst der Volksgezond-heid, DVG).[54] Outside Java and parts of Sumatra these government bodies held very little sway. Finally, as a further demonstration of its subordinate po-sition, the BGD's *f.* 7.5 million budget for 1914 compared poorly to the funds allocated to other branches of the colonial government, such as the civil ser-vice (*f.* 12.6 million), infrastructure (*f.* 26.0 million), education (*f.* 13.0 million), and the armed forces (*f.* 46.5 million).[55]

And what of the health challenges that faced the young civil medical ser-vice? The archipelago was beset by endemic and epidemic diseases such as hookworm, yaws, dengue fever, beriberi, tuberculosis, typhoid fever, cholera, and smallpox. Vaccination against smallpox was in all likelihood the only area in which real and lasting progress was made. Indeed, smallpox vaccination may well be the principal contender to my argument that plague control was the most invasive public health intervention of the Dutch colonial period.[56] As the historian Peter Boomgaard has shown, by 1850 some 350,000 vaccinations were carried out annually in Java. After 1890, the Landskoepokinrichting opened in Batavia and produced a steady stream of both vaccine and *vaccina-teurs*. After 1895, it operated jointly with a new branch of the Pasteur Insti-tute.[57] By 1934, 1.4 million new vaccinations were being given in Java alone, with an additional 470,000 in the Outer Islands.[58] Leprosy, another disease that caused Dutch colonials great anxiety, was the subject of intense public and sci-entific debate. Unlike plague, however, it failed to become the target of a sustained health intervention. As the historian Leo van Bergen has suggested, the erroneous framing of leprosy as a hereditary disease allowed government officials to disqualify it as a disease control priority.[59]

Even counting the devastating influenza pandemic of 1918–1919, however, there was one health threat that trumped all others.[60] "More than all afore-mentioned diseases together," declared a report by the BGD of 1920, "it is ma-laria that erodes the health and prosperity of the population of the Dutch East Indies."[61] Given that Dutch plantations in Java and Sumatra supplied the bulk of the world's stock of the antimalarial drug quinine (over 90 percent by the time of the Second World War), it was not as if the colonial government was unable to pursue the control of this disease with vigor. It was simply not a priority, and control of this disease hinged on environmental factors also.[62] Meanwhile, the threat of new and deadly diseases looming from abroad was not lost on Indies health officials. Plague scares had been common since the disease first spread from Hong Kong after 1894. Furthermore, the construction of the Panama Canal after 1904, as I have argued elsewhere, raised the specter that another, "American," plague could also be introduced into the Indies: yellow fever.[63] In both cases the Dutch favored a cheaper policy of modest preventive measures to a more sound but expensive precautionary strategy. Consequently, as of January 1911, the vast archipelago counted some 275 ports that received ocean-going steamships and only two quarantine stations: the first at the island Onrust off the coast from Batavia, and a second at the Sumatran port of Belawan outside Medan.[64]

The Dutch emphasis on an infrastructural intervention against plague—home improvement—must be situated within a broader pattern in the colony to pursue building solutions. "Feats of engineering" made for a highly popular visual genre among Dutch colonials. Photographs for instance offered spectacular scenes of infrastructural ingenuity that allowed roads and railways to overcome the dramatic natural obstacles such as mountains, rivers, and ravines that the Indies had to offer.[65] Another example is provided by the Kelud engineering works. When this volcano erupted in East Java in 1919, its large crater lake was responsible for creating especially deadly mudflows. In response, a newly organized volcanological service became responsible for the construction of drainage tunnels that sharply reduced the volume of this lake in an attempt to mitigate the impact of future eruptions.[66] Engineering offered similar solutions to other health challenges. The poor social and hygienic conditions among indentured laborers at the Deli plantations in Sumatra, for instance, became a target of so-called welfare capitalists (who had helped to create these conditions in the first place) at the end of the nineteenth century. The Senembah Company, a subsidiary of the Deli Company, was set up to serve as a model of enlightened management. In 1897, it hired the German physician W. A. P. Schüffner to oversee a thorough hygienic overhaul. A system of hospitals, clinics, and schools emerged in the region, and at Senembah Schüffner piloted the construction of new, model houses and the improvement of water supplies.[67] At the same time, the coolie population was subjected to such strict behavioral regimes that the anthropologist Ann Laura Stoler has referred to them as "virtual laboratories for technical and social experimentation."[68] Meanwhile, the physician originally placed in charge of plague control in Java, Willem Thomas de Vogel, had freshly arrived from Semarang, where he had been a city councilor together with the prominent philanthropist H. F. Tillema. Both were convinced of the health benefits of proper house design and urban planning, and had been instrumental in the development of a new "hygienic" neighborhood.[69] These flagship health interventions certainly inspired the home improvement scheme. Taken together, these policies suggest a quite peculiarly Dutch colonial optimism to "engineer" social and environmental improvements in the Indies that other scholars have also identified.[70] In this regard, one could also point to historical and contemporary initiatives in the Netherlands such as the "colonies of benevolence" and land reclamation in the Zuiderzee. Indeed, both of these initiatives combined an intervention in the natural environment with experiments at social reform.[71]

Images and Epidemics

Images are central to our understanding and experience of disease. Scholars have pointed out the role of the visual in the advent of European scientific medicine (biomedicine) from the nineteenth century as well as the role of images in informing lay ideas about the nature and transmission of disease. Effectively, disease and public health events have become "unimaginable" without a range of images.[72] If a photomicrograph of a pathogen provided an "ontological" representation of disease, as the French physician-philosopher Georges Canguilhem suggested in 1943, and if images of disease hosts and vectors came to represent transmission as well as culpability to render disease actionable, then a range of alternative visualizations sought with less precision but equal conviction to document the relations and conditions underpinning infectious disease incidence.[73] As I have argued elsewhere, through the lens of scientific imagery of the viral disease dengue fever, all such images played a role in articulating cogent disease identities at the turn of the nineteenth and twentieth centuries. And all these images have been crucial in informing our response (or lack thereof) to specific diseases.[74]

By 1894, tables, graphs, and maps had long since become staples of epidemic visualization. But beginning with the outbreak of plague in Hong Kong, a new form of visual representation emerged that Lynteris has called "epidemic photography."[75] This photographic genre constituted a departure from the clinical gaze of older medical photography and its focus on patients and symptoms. Instead, it encompassed "the entirety of social and natural life as theatres of infection and counter-epidemic intervention."[76] The lens was trained on the people, objects, animals, and practices that had become implicated in plague transmission or control—Chinese migrants, burials in Madagascar, personal protection equipment in Harbin, rat dissection in India—and perhaps most importantly on *space*. As the historian Lukas Engelmann put it in reference to plague photography in Honolulu, epidemic photography overwhelmingly reflected the concern of doctors, epidemiologists, and government officials with "the locales, the environment, and the buildings in which plague cases appeared or threatened to arrive. The photographic focus of plague images was emphatically the epidemic's ecology."[77] Plague was the first pandemic to be photographed, and the focus and composition of plague photography has informed the ways in which outbreaks have been represented ever since: from Ebola and Zika to COVID-19.

There is a wealth of visual material related to plague in Java and it forms an important part of the historical evidence of this book. More than illustrations, I show, these images were critical in shifting popular and scientific understandings of the disease. They informed and justified the Dutch response to plague and were presented as visual evidence of the progressive nature of colonial rule in the Indies. Over the course of this research, some 650 unique plague-related photographs have been identified. As per the argument of Lynteris and Engelmann, few of these photographs qualify as "medical" photographs. An initial set of sixty-five photographs contained in the first volume of the government periodical *Mededeelingen van de Burgerlijke Geneeskundige Dienst* have a diverse focus. People (patients, assistants, but not physicians), objects (warning signs, fumigation devices), places (houses, villages, evacuation camps, pawnshops, schools), animals (rats), and practices (trade across a cordon sanitaire, home inspection) are all placed beside one another.[78] In photographs taken in subsequent years, the built environment became the dominant focus: the images feature houses or villages in various stages of being plague dangerous, undergoing improvement, or having been improved. For instance, in a set of 200 photographs obtained from the Museum Wereldculturen, more than half focus on houses, their interior, or the improvement work. Dozens of other photographs—again predominantly focused on the built environment—were found in archival, museum, and university collections. Even in Dutch biomedical publications, photographs of plague patients, hosts, and vectors were fairly rare.

Many of these photographs could also be seen to feed into an important secondary photographic genre, the *camera ethica*, that the historian Susie Protschky has investigated along with other contributors in an edited volume. Protschky suggests that advances in photography, predating plague photography by about a decade, coincided with the advent of the ethical policy about 1900, the two processes resonating with one another by their respective promises of "modernity, progress and civilization."[79] As photography underwent "an early stage of 'democratization,'" a larger cast of nonprofessional individuals were able to produce a more diverse set of photographs that allow historians to "sample" the ways in which "a broader selection of the Indies population . . . selectively engaged at the local level with ethical discourses and articulated diverging visions of the present and future."[80] Many of the photographs documenting plague and plague control in Java could be read along these lines. In the case of figure 0.1, one could argue that it is revealing of social hierarchies in the Indies, and of Dutch colonial self-imagination and representation, but also of how the photographer (a plague physician) and his subjects (two plague physicians, two plague *mantris*, and one civil servant) envisioned a modern, healthy, Indies house: it was a light, airy, and orderly dwelling in which the man seated atop the beams appears to take a considerable degree of pride. Nonetheless, the image worked to assert "racial and civilizational difference," and photographic counterpoints that articulated Javanese perceptions of the home improvement scheme have not been identified.[81] Meanwhile, in this photograph of home improvement, as in others, we might also see a continuation of an older genre of nineteenth-century Indies landscape painting that, as Protschky suggests elsewhere, by its omission of conflict and exploitation "symbolically asserted European sovereignty over Indonesian landscapes."[82] In the case of Dutch plague photography, however, this symbolic visual assertion of sovereignty was at once grounded in a highly material intervention. In fact, these photographs go far beyond the symbolic: they captured supposedly improved landscapes in which European sovereignty *had been* asserted to transform them into something new. The stunning alteration of the built and natural environment that was captured and put on display in this manner has prompted me, in chapter 3, to suggest that photographs of home improvement might be most productively studied as a form of colonial spectacle.

Along with photographs, Dutch health workers produced copious scientific imagery of plague such as maps, graphs, tables, and diagrams, but also a range of materials that specifically targeted a lay Indies audience. Collectively referred to as *medische propaganda*, these materials explained biomedical views on the nature and transmission of plague, argued for the need for home improvement, and urged people to keep their dwellings rat-free. As we shall come to see, all of these materials served more than one purpose and spoke to more than one audience. Quasi-anatomical photographs of the plague house documented the presence of rats and guided countermeasures against plague, but also allowed Dutch physicians to demonstrate their scientific ability by helping to articulate a distinctively Javanese plague ecology or ecosystem (*avant la lettre*) to foreign scientists. The study of plague in Java, consequently, also led to a new (if imperfect) understanding of the complexity of human-animal relations.[83] Health messaging ostensibly sought to instruct the Javanese about plague and its prevention. But photographs of health messaging events, meanwhile, were also presented to colonial, metropolitan, and foreign audiences as demonstrations of "ethical" colonial governance and local acquiescence to European interventions.

The visual culture of plague in Java, in short, served Dutch epidemiological practices, educational objectives, and ethical discourses. It may have also sought to articulate racial and cultural difference between colonizer and colonized, albeit through a focus on the built and natural environment of Java rather than through its people. Throughout this set of Dutch plague photography, moreover, these images appear imbued with a certain nationalist drive to demonstrate scientific and political prowess. Plague had exposed the vulnerability of the Dutch East Indies to disease. Plague *control* offered a route through which to channel Dutch representations of themselves as a political, cultural, and scientific power in the East to local, domestic, and international audiences alike. But importantly, I must stress that home improvement was not just a gimmick. Coupled with the intervention into the daily practices and beliefs of the Javanese, the adjustments wrought in Java's built and natural environment did in fact contribute to the gradual elimination of plague from affected districts. The two-pronged intervention could not keep up with the spread of plague from East to West Java, however, and meanwhile it did so much *more* than simply bring plague to heel.

Organization

In this book, I argue that plague in Java provoked perhaps the most dramatic health intervention of the Dutch colonial period. Plague control would have a lasting impact on Javanese material culture, health practices, and its natural and built environments. The disease and the Dutch colonial response to it facilitated unprecedented governmental oversight and control over the land and its various human and animal inhabitants. Quite likely, it constituted the most far-reaching and durable colonial intrusion into the lives of millions. Each chapter contributes to this overall argument from a particular angle in roughly chronological order. At the same time, these chapters seek to make smaller contributions to the existing scholarship on plague, colonialism, and the environment in late-colonial Asia.

In chapter 1, I look at the initial outbreak of plague in the district Malang in March 1911 as the fulfilment of a period of "anxious suspense" in which physicians and officials feared the introduction of plague into the Dutch East Indies. How, this chapter asks, were existing notions of the role of the house in plague transmission rearticulated to situate the traditional bamboo dwellings of the Javanese at the center of Dutch anxieties for this disease? Having established the role of photography in this process, chapter 2 continues by tracing the early development of what would become the signature response to plague in Java: home improvement. This scheme effectively "colonized the home," I argue, by regulating, restricting, and partially recuperating the use of traditional Javanese building materials and architectural forms. In the process, local populations came more clearly into the purview of the colonial state, while home improvement entailed a dramatic expansion of Dutch influence over the Javanese landscape. It was an intervention that was rivaled only by the vast plantations established here and elsewhere in the Indies. At the same time, home improvement placed increasing pressure on the growth and availability of natural resources—and indeed upon the Javanese ability to pay. The plague control measures, chapter 3 elucidates, were not solely pursued for the benefit of the Javanese. Rather, plague and plague control in Java were broadcast to diverse Dutch and foreign audiences in lectures, photographs, exhibitions, and even tours to articulate Dutch political and cultural superiority, the ethical nature of Dutch colonial rule, and Dutch scientific ability. Scenes of home improvement, I suggest, offered a colonial spectacle through which colonial power relations were reified and the continued need for Dutch colonial rule established.

In chapter 4, I explore how home improvement was in fact insufficient as a response to plague. In a plot twist, it emerges that Dutch health officials had recognized from the start that home improvement was to be accompanied by home inspection and hygiene education to *keep* the improved dwelling rat-free. Home improvement merely served to eliminate various nesting spaces. It was intended to facilitate a regular cleaning of the house that was to become *adat*—a part of local practices and beliefs grounded in Islamic and animist traditions. A range of powerful visual technologies sought to instruct the Javanese in the art of inhabiting the home and to inculcate new hygienic practices and beliefs. If home improvement colonized the Javanese house and by extension the land around it, "plague propaganda" sought to replace existing Javanese ideas of cleanliness and practices of health with European ones. This expansion of Dutch state power and cultural influence through plague control may have been inadvertent at first. However, when home improvement presented new objections in the 1930s and an efficacious vaccine became available, officials stressed the continued need for the two-pronged approach they had refined over the years: home improvement and hygiene education. That being said, the economic downturn of the 1930s had a significant impact on the plague control efforts. Consequently, we see the highest number of plague cases over this later period when plague moved into West Java (see chapter 3, table 4). Chapter 5 explores these problematics. It returns to a theme first addressed in chapter 1, namely the notion of the house as a site of multispecies encounters and the implications thereof on human health. Home improvement, it was grudgingly acknowledged, could very well have constituted the most "permanent" intervention against plague but it was also becoming implicated in fresh "explosions" of malaria by inadvertently creating mosquito breeding sites and just as permanently facilitating human-mosquito contact. As for plague: between vaccination with a locally developed vaccine and a highly systematic home improvement scheme, the number of annual cases was ultimately brought down to the low hundreds by the end of effective Dutch colonial rule in 1942.

CHAPTER 1

Plague, Rats, and the House in Java

> We physicians, who have never seen a plague patient before, ordinarily know little more about plague than what our books and periodicals have taught us.
>
> —Isaac Groneman, *Pestbestrijding Naar Aanleiding van Gesprekken met Dr. Yersin*, 1899

On March 22, 1911, the Danish physician Peter Koefoed, who ran a private medical practice in the resort town Malang in East Java, was called by the *wedono* of Toeren to attend to a close female relative (figure 1.1). *Raden Adjeng* Moerko, a member of the local aristocracy, had recently arrived from the popular hill station at Batoe where her husband worked as an *inlandsche* teacher to visit her family. While staying with relatives at Gadang, she had suddenly fallen sick. Koefoed described the woman as "a severely ill patient." She ran a high temperature, "was depleted of her energy," and displayed a "small but very sensitive glandular swelling in the groin." She died that same day.[1] Moerko's unfamiliar but foreboding symptoms had prompted Koefoed to take a blood sample. Upon returning to his practice, he prepared several glass slides with drops of blood, stained them with methylene blue and Giemsa solution, and placed them beneath the lens of his microscope. Soon, he arrived at a fateful diagnosis and alerted the chief health officer of the district. His samples contained plague bacilli.[2]

Anxious Suspense

According to the distinguished physician Isidore Snapper, writing in 1945, "medical authorities in the Dutch East Indies lived in anxious suspense" of

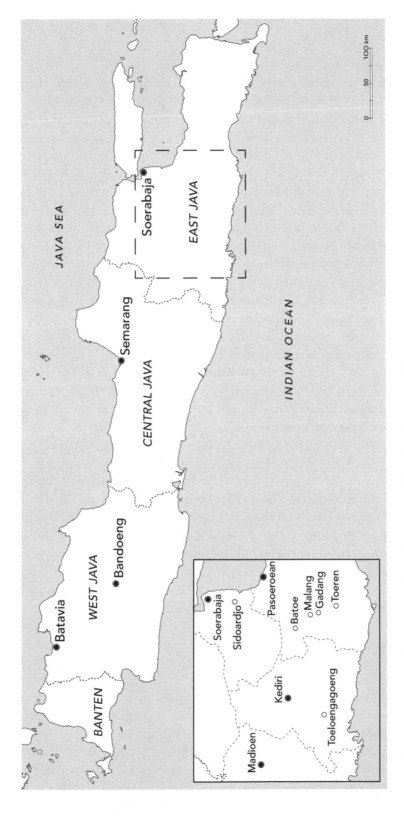

FIGURE 1.1. Map of the island of Java and the vicinity of Malang, 1911–1942. Map by Cartographics.

plague for years before its "inevitable" introduction into Java.[3] Since the onset of the third plague pandemic in 1894 there had indeed been several plague scares. The vast archipelago counted hundreds of ports, several of which stood in direct communication with Hong Kong and subsequent "plague ports" such as Bombay, Honolulu, Sydney, and Rangoon. Few of them boasted any health facilities at all.

In 1899, plague broke out in Penang, a British colony opposite North Sumatra across the Strait of Malacca. The outbreak caused widespread concern both because of its proximity and because it "demonstrated that the climate of the Indies offers no protection against its possible occurrence here, which we had thus far presumed."[4] Indies insurance agencies petitioned the governor-general to take preventive action.[5] The Dutch legation in Paris was "summoned telegraphically" to arrange a delivery of plague serum from the Pasteur Institute, which was sent to the regions deemed most at risk.[6] Local authorities were instructed to improve overall hygienic conditions and "exterminate vermin" recently implicated in plague transmission.[7] Furthermore, an engineer was allegedly sent to the remote Karimon Djawa islands to supervise the construction of a plague barracks to house potential victims or serve as a quarantine site. Years later, as a member of parliament in The Hague, this individual recalled that at the time there had been a shared sense among his colleagues in the civil service that an outbreak was imminent.[8]

In the meantime, plague had been epidemic in the neighboring US-occupied Philippines between 1899 and 1906.[9] More disturbingly, in a somewhat hushed-up incident there had been two cases of locally acquired plague at the port of Belawan in Sumatra in 1905.[10] But somehow, despite being situated at the crossroads of shipping routes between the Indian Ocean and the Western Pacific, and despite being surrounded by plague foci on all sides, the Dutch East Indies avoided being swept up in the first waves of the new pandemic. Given the scarce preventive measures that were in place, most health officials attributed this to luck. Others, as mentioned, were more optimistic. In the fact that plague failed to gain a foothold in the Indies for so long, they saw evidence that the hot climate of the Indies was inhospitable to the disease.[11] Regardless, fears that plague might eventually slip into the colony were pervasive. Over the first months of 1911, this anxiety extended well beyond "medical authorities" and became almost palpable.

Two months before Koefoed identified a case of human plague in the rural interior of East Java, the procurator of trading company Zorab Mesrope at Soerabaja, Vagarshak Apcar, informed the private physician J. W. van der Spek that one of his *mandoers* had died and a second was sick. Earlier, numerous dead rats had been found at one of the company's warehouses in the busy port city. Apcar had previously lived in British India and quickly drew a connection between the dead rats and his suffering employees. Could this, he asked, be plague? On inspecting the corpse, van der Spek identified "no visible symptoms of infectious disease." The sick man was diagnosed with *van der Scheerse koorts*, a painful but normally benign dengue-like disease. The physician was on the alert, however, and two municipal physicians were called to corroborate his findings. They agreed that there were no signs of plague on the corpse and diagnosed the patient with malaria instead.[12] A few weeks later, van der Spek was called to a Chinese patient whom he diagnosed with typhus. The next day, a colleague visited two female servants at the Pasar Pabean Tengah, a local market, who were severely ill. They displayed glandular swellings that, again, raised suspicions of plague. All three patients were removed to the infectious disease hospital, and the two women died some days later. The chief medical officer at Soerabaja, Floris Wijdenes Spaans, ordered blood samples to be taken from these patients and had them sent to the Geneeskundig Laboratorium at Weltevreden (the suburban seat of Dutch imperial power south of Batavia) with a request to screen them for plague bacilli. In the meantime, the houses of these unfortunates were disinfected and the other residents "locked up" for five days. The blood samples returned negative results for plague, but still the neighborhoods in which these cases had occurred were watched for other suspicious cases of disease for a month.[13]

At the start of March, a *doctor djawa* touring the district Goenoeng Kendeng in the residency Soerabaja was informed that a native teacher at Tjankir had been sick for some time. He too was moved to the infectious disease hospital in the city, where he died three days later. He too had displayed glandular swellings. And he too had blood samples taken and sent to Weltevreden that revealed nothing out of the ordinary. The same went for a Chinese man from the neighborhood Kembangdjepoon in central Soerabaja, who was admitted on March 7 and died the following day.[14] Two more samples taken from potential "ancillary" and "femoral" buboes were submitted to the Geneeskundig Laboratorium by unknown physicians from Madioen and Soerabaja respectively. Again, no plague bacilli were found.[15] Meanwhile, at the mental asylum at Lawang, a few kilometers north of Malang, the physician A. Boon was called to see several "fever patients" in the nearby *dessa* Meling. Shortly afterward, a *doctor djawa* by the name of Soemowidigdo was "sent to follow up on these cases." Ominously, he reported that aside from malaria "there was another disease present" in the community. A careful literature review led him to diagnose these patients with *drüsenfieber* (glandular fever).[16]

The lively Indies press had by this time caught wind of these and other mysterious plague-like cases.[17] "Already on December 10," wrote the Dutch nurse

J. Dijkstra later from Malang, "we heard talk of a strange disease. The people came down with severe fevers, sometimes vomited blood, had lumps in the armpit and the groin, and in *most* cases died soon after."[18] At the end of January, a case of plague was said to have occurred aboard a ship at Semarang carrying pilgrims returning from the *Hajj*.[19] An article in *De Preangerbode* on February 28 called attention to the string of suspicious cases of disease in East Java and painted a particularly vivid (not to say prescient) scenario. One of these days, the author wrote, an ordinary train might arrive in Batavia "just like always." Among its various goods it would carry a small package destined for "the men of science at the laboratory." Seemingly innocuous, it could very well contain the bloody evidence that Black Death had found its way into Soerabaja.[20] Rumor concentrated on potential cases in East Java, but a minor plague scare was also reported in West Java when in mid-February a woman died aboard a train (carrying returning *hajjis*) traveling from Krawang to Bandoeng.[21]

Reports of mysterious cases of disease began to cause unease among health officials as well. On March 10, Wijdenes Spaans was said to have issued a decree in Soerabaja calling for the general extermination of plague's suspected host, the rat.[22] Meanwhile, the steady supply of samples arriving from three neighboring residencies in East Java accompanied by the request to screen them for plague bacilli raised suspicion at the Geneeskundig Laboratorium that something was afoot. Its director, J. de Haan, who had studied the plague bacillus at the Pasteur Institute in Paris back in 1900, later recounted his growing disquiet and described the challenges involved in analyzing the materials he received. Blood samples were notoriously difficult to work with in human plague cases to begin with, and some of them had dried up en route or were of insufficient quality to prepare cultures. Samples of liquid taken from patients with suspected buboes had likewise dried up or were found negative. As a result, no action was taken in Batavia.[23]

Finally, on Monday, March 27, an ordinary train arrived in Batavia. It carried an innocuous package forwarded to de Haan's laboratory by the directing health official at Malang. This package contained three glass slides prepared by a local private physician using blood samples taken from a severely ill Javanese woman who had had enlarged lymph nodes in her groin and who had since died. Two slides had previously been stained and revealed "clearly visible diplo-bacilli" that bore a "strong resemblance to plague bacilli." The third sample was "subjected" to Gram-positive staining to no result: supporting de Haan's suspicion that what he was looking at through his microscope was indeed the Gram-negative diplococcus that scientists had since 1894 referred to as *Pasteurella pestis*: the plague bacillus.[24]

Plague in Java

Despite enduring concerns that plague could find its way into the Dutch East Indies, the colonial government and its health services were poorly prepared when the disease was recognized in March 1911. Plague was a predominantly urban disease, and the fact that it had somehow leaped over major port cities and apparently entrenched itself in the rural interior of East Java baffled officials and physicians alike. Malang, the capital of the eponymous district in the residency Pasoeroean, had developed rapidly since the early nineteenth century as a center of the local plantation economy. Its higher elevation and cooler climate had, ironically, lent the region a reputation as a health resort for European colonials.[25] The public health services of Malang had however not kept pace with the construction of neoclassical villas, "Swiss-like chalets," and hotels, allowing the introduction of plague to be overlooked. As discussed in the Introduction, even at major port cities precautionary measures against plague had been minimal. As of 1911, there were barely two functioning quarantine stations in the vast archipelago.[26] Every three months, one newspaper claimed, the government purchased small amounts of plague serum from the Pasteur Institute and distributed it between a select few towns in case of an outbreak. The efficacy of this serum was not beyond doubt, and its supply was certainly inadequate.[27] In fact, the Indies had not possessed a formal civil medical service until January 1911. When the plague bacillus was identified in Malang, this civil medical service (Burgerlijke Geneeskundige Dienst, BGD) was, as Jan de Waal Malefijt, the Dutch minister of colonies, put it, "still in diapers."[28]

First Responders

As elsewhere, the first recognition of plague caused a frenzy, if not quite a panic or denial.[29] But health and government officials were reluctant to declare an outbreak just yet. After confirming Koefoed's diagnosis, de Haan met with the leaders of the BGD. Governor-General Alexander Idenburg was informed. Local health authorities in Malang received a telegram to apprise them of the laboratory results. And the next day, the *sous-chef* of the new health service departed for East Java to "start a local investigation."[30] Willem Thomas de Vogel was a key figure in the development of health policy in the Dutch East Indies. Born in Toeban in 1863, he had pursued medical training in Leiden and Berlin between 1886 and 1895. In 1897, de Vogel returned to the Indies to set up a private medical practice in Semarang, where he became the chief municipal physician two years later and was elected to the local municipal council in 1906. After joining the BGD in 1911, de Vogel became full director at the start of 1913 and was instrumental in moving away from an initial focus on curative medicine toward public health and disease prevention. De Vogel was one of a handful of people who decisively shaped the Dutch response to plague in Java over the following thirty years.

Arriving in Soerabaja on March 29, de Vogel interviewed civil servants and physicians who declared that they had seen suspicious cases of disease since February. Of course, the plague rumors had reached Batavia long before as well and these allegations were hardly news. As de Vogel's wife Suzanna observed in a letter to her mother-in-law:

> Wim had to leave unexpectedly for Soerabaja and Malang the day before yesterday. Several times before suspicious plague-like cases had been reported in the *Oosthoek* and now a real case has been identified in Malang.[31]

The epidemiological intelligence gathered by de Vogel was nonetheless crucial to constructing a timeline of events and helped to determine the geographic reach that the disease had already attained. Correlating the information provided by physicians with rumor and population statistics, de Vogel later speculated that plague had been present in East Java since the final months of 1910.[32] On March 30, he traveled south to the district Malang. At the hill station Batoe, the home of the first identified plague case, de Vogel inspected six corpses and four patients. Since February 18, he learned, thirty-five people had fallen sick in the village and only three of them had recovered.[33] A telegram arrived in Batavia shortly after, belatedly stressing that "the presence of a bacteriologist was desirable."[34] De Haan departed for Malang and set up shop in a "primitive" but practicable laboratory in an outhouse of the local hospital.[35]

Rumor that plague had broken out in Malang now circulated widely in the Indies press, and on April 1 the *Nieuwe Rotterdamsche Courant* broke the story to audiences in the Netherlands. The newspaper published three sensationalist telegrams on its front page, at least two of which were factually wrong. They announced that plague had been brought to Malang by a pilgrim returning from the *Hajj*, that hundreds had died and Europeans had fled the district, and that a government bacteriologist had been sent to investigate.[36] As it happened, Idenburg had not yet chosen to inform his superiors in The Hague of recent developments. Consequently, there was some tension when Minister de Waal Malefijt wrote to him the following day:

> The news of the outbreak of plague in Malang has caused great consternation. Already yesterday, Saturday April 1, the Department was mobbed from all sides following the publication in the *N. R. Ct.* of three telegrams of a worrying nature. I reassured the public that the telegram

I received from you that morning made no mention of plague or even a suspicious case of disease. Nevertheless, I was disturbed and hence signaled for further information—alas, I saw my fear realized today![37]

It was only following this telegraphic prompt that Idenburg informed the Dutch government of the outbreak by the same medium—in the most succinct possible terms: "46 cases of plague at Malang, strict measures have been taken."[38] It would take another three days before de Haan was able to furnish further bacteriological evidence that the outbreak was indeed plague and caused Malang to be officially declared an "infected district."[39] It took several more weeks—as well as a good deal of chance—before he could demonstrate the presence of rat plague in the district as well.[40]

In a letter from Idenburg to de Waal Malefijt dated April 5, the governor-general acknowledged that the presence of plague had been overlooked for at least two months. Possibly expecting a scolding, he defended the oversight of the dread disease by stressing, "One would never have expected her first within the interior!" Now that the disease had been recognized the colonial government took quiet but forceful action. "I assure you that *no* method will be left untried, and no cost be spared."[41] Subsequent written and telegraphic communications stressed how plague's "atypical" character in Java had prevented its early recognition. When de Waal Malefijt's letter of April 2 arrived in Batavia four weeks later, Idenburg responded fiercely:

> I telegraphed you *immediately* when it became clear that the disease was plague. It appears that before this official recognition private telegrams with alarming messages arrived in Europe, but I cannot help that. As [governor-general] I cannot send you old wives' tales. What if it was *not* plague?[42]

The governor-general continued by highlighting the potential economic fallout that ill-founded rumor could have caused, and reiterated his defense of the belated recognition of plague. The symptoms of victims did not correspond to classical plague, and "even after spending several weeks in the midst of the epidemic Dr de Vogel laments that . . . cases of fever that were not diagnosed as plague turned out to be plague after all."[43] This failure to recognize plague early on, stressed de Vogel in the wake of the outbreak, was not at all unique to the Dutch colonial context. Indeed, the time that had elapsed between plague's suspected introduction in October 1910 and its identification at the end of March 1911 five months later "compared favorably" with previous outbreaks in Johannesburg and Bombay.[44]

Countermeasures

The recognition that plague had now been introduced into Java, as had long been feared, prompted a flurry of activity. Strict measures were indeed implemented. Haunted by the millions of lives plague had claimed in India since 1896 and the tens of thousands of deaths caused by a devastating outbreak of pneumonic plague in Manchuria only months earlier—to say nothing of the economic consequences—Idenburg gave de Vogel a free hand to try and contain the outbreak.[45] In a private letter Idenburg recorded his personal recommendation to burn entire *kampongs* if that was what it took.[46] This was indeed the fate of several settlements such as the *dessa* Banjak, where ninety people out of a population of 859 were diagnosed with plague in rapid succession.[47] The residents were moved to an evacuation camp, the houses burned, and the village was reconstructed on a nearby mountain slope. A photograph of the new village shows houses built in neat rows, made of bamboo poles and woven mats and roofed with thatch, with rice paddies and jungle in the background (figure 1.2). The rebuilt village predated the development of a new transmission theory of plague in Java, offering a sharp contrast to subsequently rebuilt houses as we will see. Primarily, however, de Vogel strove to implement the recommendations is-

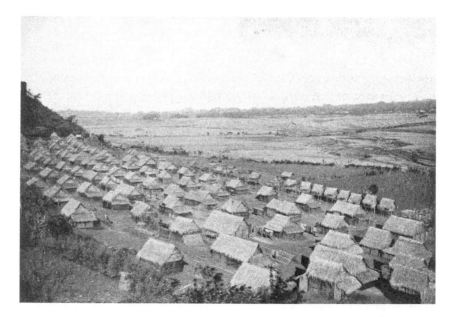

FIGURE 1.2. Photograph of the rebuilt *dessa* Banjak, 1911. Willem Thomas de Vogel, "Uittreksel uit het verslag aan de Regeering over de Pest-Epidemie in de Afdeeling Malang, November 1910–Augustus 1911," *Mededeelingen van den Burgerlijken Geneeskundigen Dienst in Nederlandsch-Indië* 1 (1912): 30–111, fig. 15. Courtesy of the University of Leiden Library.

sued by the Second Indian Plague Commission (1905–1917): focusing on isolation of the victims, evacuation of their families and neighbors, quarantine of pneumonic plague patients and affected areas, and disinfection of "infected" houses and villages.[48] This last objective was pursued through fumigation with sulfuric acid or by unroofing houses to expose the interior to sunlight. Concurrently, rat catching and extermination "began across Java" and in particular within the residencies Pasoeroean and Soerabaja.[49]

Over the first weeks of April 1911, a slew of additional countermeasures was devised, consecrated by gubernatorial decree and communicated to officials and physicians by letter, telegram, and telephone. On April 1, de Vogel sent telegrams requesting local authorities in Malang and neighboring districts to close footpaths leading out of the district through the Ardjoeno mountain range that formed a natural boundary to the north and west of the district. Lodewijk Kreischer, the *resident* of Pasoeroean, was instructed to relocate from Probolinggo to Malang and received telegrams from the colonial government stating that Idenburg "desired energetic control measures against plague" and that "no expense was to be spared."[50] By April 6, four out of eight subdistricts in Malang had been declared infected.[51] On April 7, a telegram instructed the commander of the KNIL to provide soldiers to enforce a full quarantine on Malang, formalizing a request sent two days earlier to "lend as much assistance as possible."[52] Kreischer was instructed the same day to "close major routes of communication" leading out of Malang. He was apparently unwilling to implement this forceful measure, as a note is attached to this message in the archive stating that "the resident does not understand this telegram."[53] A new telegram received two days later could not be evaded, however; it specified that "all traffic along ordinary roads outside of infected areas" was to be halted, that human travel via railway was prohibited, and that goods could be exported via rail only after fumigation of the carriage.[54]

Following the closure of Malang, the next priority was the creation of an effective intelligence service to identify and report new cases within the district (see chapter 4). The information gathered by local informants was collated at the end of each day and exchanged via telephone between the *regenten*, *residenten*, and *assistent-residenten* of the plague-affected districts before being passed on to de Vogel's headquarters.[55] At the end of each week a map was produced that showed plague-affected *kampongs* and indicated the number of cases of both human and rat plague. The maps demonstrated plague's wide distribution over Malang, and worryingly the succession of maps revealed that the spread of the disease was not contiguous. Rather than spreading from one *kampong* to the neighboring one, plague's pattern of diffusion was erratic and would later be characterized by Dutch physicians as "metastatic," a term that likened plague to a tumorous growth.[56] Victims were primarily among the

Javanese and Chinese population, though the (Indo-)European population of
Malang also counted several victims. Two children of a Dutch administrator
at a local tea plantation contracted plague and died.[57] The European daughter
of an administrator at a cinchona plantation, aged nine, had contracted plague
and was being nursed at the home of the *assistent-resident* of Bodjonegoro
(neighboring Malang).[58] Nurse Dijkstra also wrote of a nine-year-old European
girl (possibly the same) who was nursed by her (vegetarian) parents according to their own (natural) healing methods and who was fortunate enough to
survive. With proper care in fact, argued Dijkstra with just a hint of criticism
of the government, many more Javanese victims might survive as well.[59]

At some distance from infected *kampongs* evacuation camps were built. The
camps featured temporary dwellings built in Javanese building styles, made of
bamboo and *atap*. They were slightly elevated above ground and constructed
at a cost of about *f*. 30 each:

> In these the cases of bubonic plague would be housed with their entire
> family, after being furnished with clean clothes and bedding. [Their] in-
> fected house would then be fumigated with a straw fire and sulfur. . . .
> Only when 2×24 hours have elapsed after fumigation the roof will be
> removed, and the inside of the house is exposed to the power of sun and
> fresh air.[60]

The neighbors of these "infected houses" were informed of the danger that
plague-infected rats and fleas might lurk in the vicinity of their abodes. They
were given the choice between moving into the evacuation camp as well and
staying with relatives elsewhere. Their houses were subjected to "prophylactic
treatment."[61] Once in the camp, inmates progressed along a three-tier system
from the sick camp to the observation camp to the inoculation camp—or the
graveyard. In the first stage, families stayed with their diseased relatives. Conveniently, wrote de Vogel, "this compensated for the total absence of a nursing
staff."[62]

After the death or recovery of the plague patient, the family would relocate
to the observation camp for the duration of the incubation period of the disease
to make sure that no further infection had occurred.[63] Finally, in the inoculation
camp, they would receive inoculations with one of two preparations. Neither appeared to afford any protection and the practice was soon abandoned (see chapter 5).[64] Out of concern that some victims might develop highly contagious and
highly fatal pneumonic plague, the evacuation camps were later provided with
small huts for the patient "within calling distance" of the main dwelling. Thus,
a "congregation" of family members would not collect around the patient.[65]
After the plague patient had moved on, their bed was burned and the roofs of

their hut removed "to expose the interior to fierce sunlight." Alternatively, the entire structure would sometimes be burned. In the case of the former, the hut would only be roofed again from sixteen to twenty days later, "to obviate any chance" that fleas infected with the plague bacillus had survived.[66] If a patient was in fact diagnosed with pneumonic plague the victim would be segregated and placed in a dismal hut: surrounded by a double fence of barbed wire and placed on a floor of Portland cement that allowed easy cleansing after the death of its occupant.[67] After observing a Javanese man tending his child who was suffering from pneumonic plague through the "half-opened door" of his house without falling prey to the disease himself, de Vogel later recounted, hatches were installed in the pneumonic plague huts that allowed for this method of nursing.[68] A solitary photograph of Javanese *mantris* carrying a plague corpse out of a pneumonic plague hut while wearing a face mask exists, but sources indicate that such personal protection equipment was generally shunned.[69]

The strategy to evacuate "infected houses" was based on the longstanding assumption that plague was contracted within the house. This theory was commensurate with the more recent rat-flea-man transmission hypothesis. Evacuation was thus seen as the key to halting plague transmission. "Holding that plague is a house infection," wrote A. Deutmann, who had taken charge of plague control in the district Karanglo, the utility of the instruction to leave infected dwellings "is obvious."[70] This more or less compulsory "advice" was "fully understood" by the inhabitants, wrote de Vogel, albeit on spiritual rather than bacteriological grounds. "No resistance was encountered."[71] At the same time, however, many of the countermeasures employed by de Vogel suggest how competing notions of the nature and transmission of plague persisted. The raising of the temporary dwellings above the ground and the placing of pneumonic plague huts on a cement foundation, for instance, suggest that Dutch physicians lend credence to the notion that plague bacilli could infect and endure within the soil.[72]

As for the "infected" plague houses themselves, these were initially "fumigated with sulfur."[73] A Clayton device—"the only one available in Java"—was purchased to make this process more effective but it was so heavy that it could not be moved outside the town of Malang.[74] Indeed, in a photograph, we see the device being dragged through a street in Malang by no less than twenty men.[75] The method proved cumbersome and ineffective, and was quickly abandoned. "Little hovels were always burned," according to Deutmann, as were the houses of all pneumonic plague cases. After all, the native was wont to expectorate, he wrote, and since the floors of even the best houses normally consisted of beaten earth the very ground on which the house stood was "infected" and "polluted" with plague bacilli. Fire was the surest disinfectant.[76]

Whitewashing was applied as well, but primarily the houses of plague victims had their roofs removed to expose their interior to the sun to rid them of rats, fleas, and bacilli. Plague and plague control consequently left a desolate scene in their wake. On walking through the severely affected and abandoned *dessa* Karang Tengah, Deutmann reflected, "here the ruins of a burned house were to be seen, next to this another, there a plague house forlorn and uninhabited, the roof taken away to admit the sun."[77] Despite these interventions, plague continued to spread through Malang. A handful of cases in the neighboring residencies Kediri and Madioen remained localized to their eponymous district capitals for the moment, while a handful of confirmed cases in Soerabaja caused the port city to be declared "infected" in early May.[78] By the end of May, nearly one thousand cases of human plague had been identified (table 2).

Table 2   Bacteriologically confirmed cases of human and rat plague in Malang, 1911

	HUMAN PLAGUE	RAT PLAGUE
March 30, 1911	21	0
April 6, 1911	42	7
April 13, 1911	69	6
April 20, 1911	94	20
April 27, 1911	111	13
May 4, 1911	139	6
May 11, 1911	148	4
May 18, 1911	175	2
May 25, 1911	130	0
June 1, 1911	103	3
June 8, 1911	48	1
June 15, 1911	48	0
June 22, 1911	51	0
June 29, 1911	40	0
July 6, 1911	41	2
July 13, 1911	40	1
July 20, 1911	59	3
July 27, 1911	34	7
August 3, 1911	41	2
August 10, 1911	33	9
August 17, 1911	29	0
August 24, 1911	34	0
August 31, 1911	19	1
	1,549	**87**

Source: Willem Thomas de Vogel, "Uittreksel uit het verslag aan de Regeering over de Pest-Epidemie in de Afdeeling Malang, November 1910–Augustus 1911," *Mededeelingen van den Burgerlijken Geneeskundigen Dienst in Nederlandsch-Indië* 1 (1912): 33–114.

The Matter of Expertise

A key challenge that faced de Vogel in the early days of April was the fact that neither he nor his colleagues had any experience working with plague. Whether as physicians, epidemiologists, or bacteriologists, the Dutch knew little more about plague than what books, periodicals, and photographs might tell them.[79] In a lengthy telegram to The Hague to inform the Dutch government on recent developments, Idenburg explained that bubonic plague had initially been mistaken for tropical malaria, and pneumonic plague for tuberculosis. The oversight, he insisted, was understandable: "No physician had previously seen plague, medical handbooks paint very different image from that seen here . . . even now difficulty with diagnosis."[80] In a letter to de Waal Malefijt, written three weeks earlier, Idenburg made much the same point. Even now, he wrote, de Vogel faced great challenges separating cases of plague from cases of other febrile diseases.[81] Coupled to these diagnostic difficulties were, as mentioned, the persistent epistemic anxieties about where plague might "lurk" and how it might spread.

Soemowidigdo, the *doctor djawa* who had reported malaria and *drüsenfieber* in Meling in early March, was widely blamed for his misdiagnosis. His failure to recognize plague, critics claimed, was responsible for the fact that the disease had already spread far and wide. From a letter by Suzanna de Vogel of May 4 we learn that her husband placed responsibility for the situation elsewhere:

> For [the spread of plague] this *doctor djawa* is blamed heavily, but Willem thought that the officers of health in charge of the civil medical service were much more to blame. They kept reporting high mortality in the kampongs from malaria in a region where malaria is infrequent and never bothered to look themselves.[82]

In his final report on the outbreak at Malang, de Vogel made his defense of Soemowidigdo official. At the same time, he adopted a milder tone toward his colleagues by underscoring their communal lack of experience with plague:

> None of us knew the disease from experience. . . . What medical man without any experience of plague, in a country where plague had never appeared, is willing to certify people with softened and broken-down lymphatic glands . . . as plague patients, thereby bringing upon himself the responsibility for an unnecessary panic and all the consequences thereof?[83]

While Soemowidigdo was thus recuperated and ultimately received a decoration for his contribution to the plague control efforts, the problem of deficient expertise was never truly solved.[84]

Acutely aware of the absence of a plague expert in the Dutch East Indies, de Waal Malefijt sent a telegram to Idenburg the day after he was informed of the outbreak. The Amsterdam bacteriologist Johannes van Loghem, he signaled, "had been found willing" to aid the control efforts at Malang.[85] As a protégé of a prominent professor of hygiene, van Loghem was already on the way to becoming a leading infectious disease researcher in the Netherlands. From 1908 to 1909, just after the identification of two autochthonous plague cases at the port of Belawan, he had served as director of the Pathological Laboratory in Medan. At the time, he and his wife (the entomologist Johanna van Loghem-Pouw) had studied local mosquito and rodent populations to call attention to the looming threat of plague and yellow fever to the Indies.[86] One of these fears had now materialized. As it happened, van Loghem had published a short paper on the nature and transmission of plague in a nursing journal only weeks before the outbreak in Malang was recognized. In it, he suggested that the successful control of this disease ultimately hinged on the control of its host, the rat. In practice, this came down to "the construction of better houses."[87] In a meeting with de Waal Malefijt on April 3, van Loghem agreed to travel to the Indies to assist the control efforts but apparently insisted on a set of conditions that were at first unpalatable to the BGD.[88] With these unclear difficulties smoothed over, Idenburg sent a telegram on April 8 asking van Loghem to bring with him "two compact sets of Laboratory equipment."[89] Crucially, however, van Loghem was no plague expert either. His knowledge of plague was primarily academic. Aside from a study of the rodent population in Sumatra, van Loghem had attended a medical congress in Bombay in 1909 where plague was certainly on the agenda. Afterward, he made a study trip to the Indian Museum in Calcutta to compare Indies and Indian rats.[90] This, it would seem, was the extent of his experience with plague.

In sharp contrast to the British approach when faced with outbreaks of plague in Hong Kong and Bombay, the Dutch colonial government made no identifiable attempt to recruit the assistance of what was by now a veritable corps of foreign plague experts at work closer by in Asia. No Alexandre Yersin or Kitasato Shibasaburō, no Waldemar Haffkine or Wu Lien-teh, nor any lesser-known physician or bacteriologist was invited to aid the control efforts in Java. If anything, Haffkine's plague vaccine was imported from British India.[91] A few years later, members of parliament questioned the government over its inability to recruit Dutch nurses, physicians, and bacteriologists to join the ongoing plague control efforts in Java. The question of one parliamentarian on the matter—"whether anyone considered that aside from Dutch bacteriologists . . . we could also hire foreigners, for example those who led plague control in

Manchuria"—was pointedly ignored in the response by the minister of colonies.[92] Other politicians, meanwhile, voiced their displeasure at the prospect of hiring foreign medical workers if vacancies could not be filled by Dutch ones.[93] Raising the suspicion that national and colonial pride was somehow at stake, the Dutch chose to remain "sovereign" in their handling of the outbreak.[94] What makes this situation especially curious is that the Dutch had historically long relied on foreign (especially German) medical practitioners in the Indies.[95] As a result of this shift in policy, modest expertise in the form of van Loghem arrived in Malang only eight weeks after the plague bacillus was first identified by Koefoed: a Dane, as we recall.

Of Rats and Man

In principle, both de Vogel and van Loghem—the de facto leaders of the plague control work—were converts to the rat-flea-man transmission theory. This theory held that plague was a rat disease transmitted secondarily to humans by the rat flea after the demise of its original host. The specifics of this transmission scheme in Java were of great concern. What rats were involved? Which fleas?[96] The quarantine imposed on Malang, according to de Vogel, was justified in part because "we know almost nothing of the rats within the affected districts."[97] On arriving in Malang on May 16, van Loghem would distinguish between three major varieties of rat in East Java. The prevailing type, *Mus rattus*, divided between a "house," or *dessa*, type and a "field," or *sawah* type. Since the rat-flea-man model required "a very close contact between the sick rat and man" in order for infected fleas to be able to make the species jump, suspicions had settled on the normally ubiquitous house rat as the principal host of plague—which would reaffirm the role of the house as a space in which transmission occurred.[98] The question as to how much field rats might also venture into the vicinity of the house remained unanswered—the local population stated they did—prompting speculation that this species played a role in the dissemination of plague between villages.[99] Meanwhile, the common rat flea *Xenopsylla cheopis*, the principal vector of plague, was certainly abundant in Malang but so were other species. Might other "common parasites" between humans and rats play a role in transmission?[100] And how were humans themselves implicated in the spread of plague?

To answer these and other questions, the Malangese were encouraged by a small fee to catch as many rats as possible and to deliver them to de Haan's improvised laboratory for examination. The precautionary measure to dip caught rats in tar encumbered early bacteriological attempts at determining the presence of rat plague.[101] Thousands of rats were delivered every day, moreover, necessitating the construction of a dedicated "rat furnace" to dispose of the potentially dangerous cadavers.[102] House rats were initially intended to be collected, but the vast majority of rats that arrived at de Haan's laboratory were field rats. Skull measurements conducted by van Loghem subsequently established the kinship of these two types, but they displayed critical biological and behavioral differences that brought the former into much closer contact with humans.[103] Only, where were they? When prompted, wrote de Vogel, the residents of Malang insisted all house rats had already been caught.[104] "The consideration that a people naturally gifted with hunter's instincts as the Javanese, could not trace the house rats, was taken as an additional proof that they were indeed very scarce."[105] In the subdistrict Karanglo, Deutmann likewise stressed that "not a single house rat was found, however much we searched for them."[106] This unexpected scarcity of rats during an outbreak of human plague had previously been observed elsewhere, and caused lingering doubt as to whether rats were the sole *infectionsquelle* (wellspring of infection) of the disease.[107] Adding to this uncertainty, de Haan's bacteriological investigations into rat plague—hampered by tarred and charred specimens—resulted in far too few positive diagnoses to verify the presence of an epizootic, let alone confirm a "rodent link" to human plague.[108] By the beginning of May, barely forty-six cases of rat plague had been identified (see above, table 2). When van Loghem finally arrived in Malang, he agreed that "on superficial examination, there appears to be no connection between human plague and rat plague."[109]

"At the time when the number of plague cases was highest," reflected de Vogel some months later at a meeting of the Far Eastern Association of Tropical Medicine (FEATM) in Hong Kong, "no house rats could be produced by the inhabitants."[110] "We lived in uncertainty," added Deutmann in a report to the government, "and could not prove that in Malang human and rat plague coincided."[111] Nonetheless, the search for rats continued unabated. Men and boys ventured into the fields to dig out the nests of field rats, "easily" catching some 100 rats an hour—mostly very young ones. But the scarcity of house rats remained a source of unease. In a meeting with physicians and officials in early May, the *resident* of Kediri observed:

the Native, it appears, primarily kills field mice. Indeed, the hunt for these is a lot easier than for house rats and mice, that, especially within bamboo dwellings, readily flee along all sorts of stiles and fences onto the roof and can as a matter of fact hide in all sorts of nooks and crannies. And yet, the killing of house rats and mice seemed to me a lot more important than the extermination of field mice.[112]

His statement turned out to be prophetic. And while de Vogel did not disagree, he replied that for the moment the role of all rats remained "an open question." But by June, significant objections had risen against the role of field rats in plague transmission. They were healthy, lived apart from humans, and carried far fewer fleas.[113] The field rat, in short, appeared to play no role in the epidemiology of plague in Java.

If the number of human plague cases had dropped slightly by this time, de Vogel confessed in a letter to his mother of June 7, he could not say whether this improvement was "because of our interventions . . . or because we removed people from their infected houses just in time."[114] Despite the absence of plague-infected house rats (or any house rats), Dutch anxiety lingered on the house (the *Javanese* house) as the primary space of plague infection. But what caused this structure to be "infected" and hence "infective?" As in plague outbreaks elsewhere, their earthen floors, cluttered objects, lack of ventilation, dark spaces, and the hygienic practices of their occupants were all suspect.[115] Such purportedly pathogenic properties were in turn easily layered upon generic colonial disdain for the native house, native hygiene, and the poor state of sanitation in the archipelago as a whole.[116] They could *not*, however, be directly correlated to either the introduction or the spread of plague. With the dismissal of the field rat as a possible source or carrier of plague, the question of the missing house rat from these plague-stricken dwellings assumed new urgency.

Could it be, ventured van Loghem at this time, that the rats that inhabited a plague house had already died inside?[117] This thought "had struck no one before," exclaimed Deutmann, "but where might all these dead rats be?"[118] The investigators now launched a "systematic investigation of the houses where plague had occurred," and soon van Loghem himself uncovered the remains of a rat beneath a slanting ceiling directly above the bed of a Chinese plague victim. "On searching 5 surrounding houses on the same day, one nest with 2 plague rats was laid bare." These specimens were host to several fleas that were found to carry plague bacilli.[119] Elsewhere, de Vogel had the masoned ridge and tiled roof of a plague house removed and uncovered a rat nest "containing the mummified corpse of a rat." Furthermore, upon splitting "the bamboos of the native house" he discovered food remains "that could have only been brought there by rats."[120] House rats and their nests were now found in similar and other hiding spots around the house. Time had been a crucial factor in their earlier failure to confirm the presence of these dead rats within the vicinity of the plague house. In British India, the period that elapsed between the death of the plague rat within a house and the death of a human plague victim had been determined to average around 11.5 days. A series of decomposition studies led by Otto de Raadt demonstrated the rapid demise and/or "mummification" of the rat corpse within this window, provided that it was not consumed by predators first.[121] As a result of these two breakthroughs, the mystery of the missing house rat (dead or alive) from plague-affected dwellings was solved. "Fresh" plague rats were a rarity within the house of a plague victim. By the time human plague had manifested *the rat plague had moved to the neighbors.*"[122]

The Plague House

The systematic search of the plague house initiated by van Loghem was but a first reconnaissance. Encouraged by their breakthroughs, de Vogel organized fifty *woningbrigades* across the district to search the dwellings of new plague victims as soon as they were identified.[123] Now, they had "a chance of finding plague rats and of determining whether human and rat plague coincided or not."[124] This inquest, I have proposed elsewhere, possessed a curious medical character.[125] Like a diseased body dissected by the pathologist, the plague house was opened up to the gaze of Dutch physicians and bacteriologists to expose the rodent infection hidden within. Surgically, the brigades removed the outer layer of tiled or *atap* roofs, peeled apart the double *gedek* walls, carved open decorative wooden doorposts, and took a lancet to the bamboo poles of frame and furniture. Small, previously unnoticed holes in various parts of the construction became markers of the presence of rats and nests within the "dead space" between walls and on the ceiling. Bite marks along natural or man-made openings into bamboo beams suggested they had been widened by rats to gain access into their hollow interior.

> Upon discovering such a bamboo with gnawed joints, the hole c.q. [or else] both holes were closed so that nothing could escape, then the bamboo was loosened from its place in the house, taken away, laid on the ground and split open. Many rat-nests were found this way.[126]

Rapidly, it became evident that the infestation of the traditional Javanese house by the obligate house rat was far more extensive than previously imagined. Early discoveries called attention to the roof as a shelter of the scansorial rat, but the brigades determined "that nests could be found in much closer vicinity to man."[127] Most disturbingly, perhaps, the house rat had a tendency to nest within the bamboo frame of the *balé-balé*: the iconic Javanese bedstead that was the principal item of furniture in a Javanese household, as well as a stock object in Dutch literary and visual representations of the Indies. "One can scarcely imagine a closer contact between man and rat," shuddered de Vogel.[128] On one rat retrieved from a *balé-balé* in Kaproe, van Loghem found twenty-two fleas containing "typical" plague bacilli.[129] In Madioen, he encountered a "fresh plague rat with 35 fleas" insolently lying dead on the bed itself.[130]

This newly identified pathology of the Javanese house warranted careful documentation. The quasi-anatomical / quasi-epidemiological nature of these investigations—conducted by and for physicians—was strikingly evident across a series of visual materials produced in the process. These media were key in rearticulating the relation between plague and the house in Java, and consequently to the formulation of the Dutch response to this disease.[131] They helped frame the house not as a "passive" space in which plague could spread, but as an active participant in its transmission.

Given the evidentiary aura with which they were imbued, photographs were key to situating the traditional bamboo house at the center of an emergent and distinctively Javanese plague ecology.[132] They captured the presence of rat cadavers around the plague house, or homed in on minute details that suggested their presence. On one level, these images merely provided examples of the rat's ability to live "at the edge of sight" of human occupants—or exposed the hitherto unsuspected vitality of what the anthropologists Ann H. Kelly and Almudena Marí Sáez refer to as "shadowlands and dark corners" inside the house.[133] On another level, they constituted unprecedented visual evidence of the *nature* of the plague house. The house was no longer a space in which infection—only recently understood as a process of zoonotic spillover—occurred: it was physically complicit in the process. On a metaphoric plane, finally, one could go so far as to say that the infestation of the house (i.e., the circulation of rats and fleas through the hollow arteries of the bamboo house) mirrored the infection of the human body and the *Pasteurella pestis* bacilli coursing through the veins of the plague patient—and could be seen without the "complicated mediation of the microscope."[134] It is important to draw attention to this metaphor, for the medical gaze evident in early Dutch plague photography would remain strong. The house-as-body motif, as chapter 3 demonstrates, was especially prominent in the large number of photographs of home improvement that would be taken in subsequent years.

The traditional bamboo dwellings of the Javanese consequently became an object of intense medical and colonial scrutiny during the initial outbreak of plague in Malang. In his government report, van Loghem provided a rough description of the "typical" suspect dwelling:

> The outer frame . . . usually consists of strong bamboos, less often of wood, and the vertical main poles (*soko goeroe*) bear horizontal beams (*blandar*). The inner frame also consists of vertical wooden or bamboo supports, which bear horizontal beams (*pengeret*) at right angles to the blandars. Vertical poles (*tiang*) rest on the blandar and pengeret which again support the ridge of the roof (*blandar woewoeng*). The inner frame is generally constructed of bamboos. . . . The inner room of the house very often has a horizontal ceiling (*pyan*) consisting of bamboo matting.[135]

A stylized blueprint accompanied this typology and illustrated what we might think of as the "normal" physiology of the bamboo dwelling. The image illustrates how these various foreign building elements linked up, but it does more than simply depict the base infrastructure of the house. Given the role now attributed to bamboo as a link between rat plague and human plague, and placed beside dozens of photographs documenting the rat-infested pathology of the house, one might ask whether this blueprint did not in fact represent a transmission diagram of sorts. It resembles what the historian Lukas Engelmann has referred to as a "spatial diagram," a hybrid epidemiological diagrammatic image that sought to provide an answer to the question of "how and why epidemics occurred only in some spaces."[136] The lines sketching out the "strong bamboos" of the frame simultaneously captured the vascular network that ran through the Javanese house and circulated rats, fleas, and their germs to human occupants—rendering it innately plague dangerous.

Other scientific imagery also played a role here. The *woningbrigades*, for instance, had gathered valuable information on the preferred nesting spaces of the house rat in Malang.[137] While underscoring the dangerous proximity of human and rodent bamboo dwellers, the tabulated presentation of this data exposed significant differences in their distribution that could be put down to small variations in house design or the use of particular materials (chapter 2, table 3). As the anthropologist Christos Lynteris has suggested, such tables were "entwined in an intricate exchange of opinions, arguments, and judgments" regarding the origin and transmission of plague.[138] Crucially, they also suggested a possible intervention. The *pyan* that yielded 50 percent of nests at Kotta Malang was a stylistic feature encountered primarily in larger towns. The comparatively meager 2.5 percent of nests hidden beneath the roofs of Karanglo were a positive outflow of the fact that "the soil is more suitable for the production of tiles." By implication, the organic *atap* roofs that prevailed elsewhere emerged as another hazardous material in which the rat found shelter. These discrepancies, argued van Loghem, afforded a vital "indication as to how plague may be forestalled."[139] If rat extermination had proven both unfeasible and ineffective, the statistics compiled by the *woningbrigades* suggested a powerful alternative: to increase "the distance between man and rat." "The plague problem in a country where rats have become infected," van Loghem concluded, "thus resolves itself . . . into a question of dwellings."[140] Citing beneficial results with interventions in the built environment "in other countries"—an oblique and euphemistic reference to such events as razing Taipingshan district in Hong Kong, burning Chinatown in Honolulu, and forced evictions and reconstruction in Bombay, but also to housing reform in Taiwan and Brazil—he and de Vogel would now advocate a new approach to plague control in Java: home improvement.[141]

By August 1911, the etiology of plague had thus acquired a unique spatial and material component that rendered the traditional bamboo dwellings of the Javanese physically complicit in plague transmission. Its infective propensity rested within both its materiality and its design, to which would soon be added its defective "inhabitation." Photographs colluded with diagrams and tables to situate the structure at the center of Dutch plague anxieties. These media were instrumental in successfully defending the existence of a nascent Javanese plague ecology and legitimizing the high-handed health intervention it inspired: to colonial, metropolitan, and foreign audiences alike. If plague concerns abroad had settled on the soil, on people, on lack of ventilation, on dark spaces, or on a proliferation of "things," in Java they came to rest on the hollow, tubular bamboo of which the native house was constructed. It is important to point out that Dutch plague anxieties might very well have come to rest on a different material, or on the Javanese plague patient instead. Shipments of rice from China and Burma in October 1910, for instance, were implicated in the introduction of plague into East Java. In later years, the local distribution of *padi* was understood to be the vehicle by means of which infected fleas were transported from one *kampong* to another: helping to explain the "metastatic" diffusion of plague across Java. But as suggested, the focus on the bamboo house fed into longstanding concerns about plague's relation to the built environment, and also linked up with a broader Dutch desire to "engineer" health solutions.[142] Moreover, it conveniently kept the dismal sight of diseased colonial subjects out of the picture—literally.[143] As such, the home substituted for the patient and unlike the latter it was amenable to treatment. Home improvement, furthermore, had a productive quality to it that could be broadcast to diverse audiences as a symbol of good governance. It had already been successfully applied elsewhere, but in the Dutch East Indies it would be pursued with unprecedented vigor.

At the FEATM meeting in Hong Kong in January 1912, de Vogel showed his colleagues a collection of the visual materials described above. His presentation included some nineteen photographs that demonstrated recent Dutch discoveries that rats in Java nested in close proximity to humans: "especially in the bamboo of which Javanese houses in this district are constructed."[144] In particular, the image of a dead rat embedded within a hollow bamboo beam cut open by the investigators would become iconic of the nature of the plague threat in Java (figure 1.3).

The image helped to implicate this natural material as much as the rat as an agent of plague. Other powerful images included photographs of a *balé-balé* featuring long incisions across the top of its bamboo frame through which the trained eye could make out a score of rat nests within, or a series of more suggestive images that captured access and exit points into various parts of the bamboo frame that exposed a hidden network running through the house. While some of these photographs appear staged—such as here, where the front leg of a dead plague rat dangles languidly over the side of a split bamboo beam—their mechanically produced "objective" reputation helped to inform a new understanding of the role of the house in plague transmission. Dutch scientists would successfully defend this view to foreign scientists in

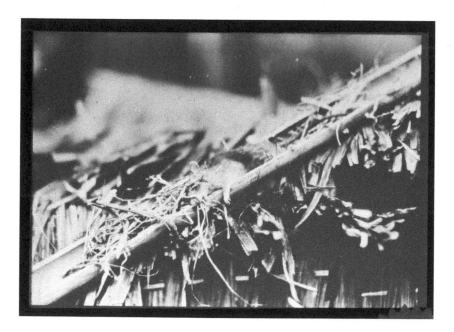

FIGURE 1.3.   Glass plate negative of a rat cadaver inside a hollow bamboo beam, date unknown. Paul Christiaan Flu, glass negative, slide cabinet, drawer 22, slide 24. Courtesy of the University of Leiden Library.

years to come.[145] Shown within the context of his lecture on the connection of man and rat in the plague outbreak in Malang, de Vogel was able to deploy these images in such a way as to argue that this connection rested in the very materiality of the Javanese house. In other words: they allowed him to insert a new bamboo link in plague's putative rat-flea-man transmission chain.

Conclusion

At the beginning of 1911, longstanding anxieties that plague might enter the Dutch East Indies were realized. When the disease was recognized at the end of March in the rural interior of East Java, the colonial health services responded forcefully, though in a manner that betrayed enduring uncertainties in their understanding of the nature and transmission of plague. The initial difficulty in confirming rats as the animal host of plague was resolved over the months of June and July by a "systematic" investigation of the houses of human plague victims that revealed an unsuspected proximity between human and rodent "bamboo dwellers." Photographs, tables, and diagrams mapped out the presence of the house rat within the traditional Javanese dwelling, and were rallied to formulate a nascent (and distinctively Javanese) plague ecology. This protoecology concentrated on the traditional Javanese house and settled on the use of "native" construction materials as well as building designs that were seen to actively facilitate human-rat contact and thereby allow infected rat fleas to cross the species boundary. These first months of investigation consequently established the house as both a space and a *vehicle* of plague transmission, but simultaneously as the weakest link in a reformulated rat-flea-house-man transmission scheme. This framing laid a foundation for one of the most far-reaching and invasive health interventions of the Dutch colonial period.

CHAPTER 2

Colonizing the Home with Bamboo, Tiles, and Timber

> It was already dusk under the heavy trees, the bananas
> lifted the cool, green paddles of their leaves, and beneath
> the stately canopy of the coco-palms sheltered the little
> bamboo houses, poetically Oriental, idyllic, with their
> *atap* roofs, their doors often already closed or, if open,
> framing a little black inward vista, with the vague outline
> of a *baleh-baleh*, on which squatted a dark figure.
>
> —Louis Couperus, *De stille kracht*, 1900

Ten years before plague broke out in Malang, the celebrated Dutch author Louis Couperus toured the region while visiting his brother-in-law, the *resident* of Pasoeroean.[1] Drawing on the experience to create the fictional setting for his novel *De stille kracht*, he painted an evocative image of the native house in East Java.[2] Little did Couperus suspect that the "poetically Oriental" dwellings he conjured would become the object of such intense colonial scrutiny a mere decade later—or did he perhaps recognize their subversive potential? In his novel, Couperus pitches his European protagonists against an indefinable "hidden" or "silent" force that permeates the Dutch East Indies and that is at once cultural, natural, and supernatural. The "little bamboo house" epitomizes this resistance to foreign intrusion. Nestled beneath a verdant jungle canopy, it merges into Java's majestic landscape to "shelter" its occupants from colonial oversight.

In the previous chapter, I suggested how plague offered Dutch state agents an opportunity to subject these "idyllic" dwellings to a thorough quasi-medical examination. The subsequent framing of the Javanese house as a link in the transmission chain of plague from rat to human on account of its very materiality and design provoked an unparalleled intervention in the built environment of Java. Between 1911 and 1942, some 1.6 million houses in East and Central Java in particular were either renovated or rebuilt according to increasingly precise standards in an attempt to make life for the obligate house rat inside "unbearable."[3] This public health intervention quite literally bulldozed over much of Java's cultural diversity and largely severed the historic interdependence that had grown between bamboo and the Javanese. Moreover, "home improvement" brought both the structure and its inhabitants under much closer government supervision.

This chapter explores the evolution of home improvement over the first decade of plague in Java. In this formative period, the scheme became increasingly systematic. The use of bamboo in home construction—Java's principal building material—was at first regulated, then banned, before being partially recuperated. I venture that this dramatic intervention against plague not only sought to make the traditional bamboo-*atap* house "rat-proof" but draw on a well-known phrase by the historian David Arnold to suggest that home improvement effectively "colonized" the house, its inhabitants, and the very landscape in which it stood.[4]

Bamboo

To appreciate the impact of the reconfiguration of bamboo as a link between rat plague and human plague, and the public health response it supported, it is necessary to reflect on the significance of this material about 1900. The *Bambuseae* are a tribe of fast-growing perennial grasses encompassing over 1,200 species that had long since enmeshed themselves into the cultural fabric of Southeast Asia.[5] As a dominant feature of (sub)tropical vegetation that could grow up to 30 meters in height, bamboo was used in all sorts of products and, consequently, it also became central to European imaginations and representations of the tropics. Bamboo was a key marker of that "potent and prevalent form of othering" referred to by Arnold elsewhere as "tropicality."[6] This iconic "skyscraper with hollow stems" was used across Asia to build dams, irrigation works, and dwellings, or was processed into food, utensils, and decoration.[7] "The bamboo is one of the most wonderful and most beautiful productions of the tropics," exulted the famed naturalist Alfred Russell Wallace in his book *The Malay Archipelago* of 1869, "and one of nature's most valuable gifts to uncivilized man."[8] More dynamically, we might draw on the historian Timothy LeCain's recent neo-materialist argument—that human societies are shaped to a high degree by their interaction with the things and nonhuman animals around them—to suggest that the peoples of Southeast Asia struck an "alliance" with this versatile product of nature.[9] Bamboo allowed them to negotiate the region's volatile typhoons, earthquakes, heat, and monsoon rains. The semipermanent bamboo structure was light and airy, easily destroyed, quickly rebuilt, and highly economical.

In the Dutch East Indies, the use of bamboo was so ubiquitous in every facet of life, commented the scholar J. A. Loebèr in 1909, that one could say the archipelago was stuck in a "Bamboo Age."[10] In Java specifically, bamboo utensils served both everyday and ritual purposes. For instance, the use of bamboo knives by the *dukun* to cut the umbilical cord or perform circumcision was frequently commented on.[11] Bamboo weaponry such as the *runcing* spear was used in both real and ceremonial fights and often constituted the only defense against Dutch colonial forces.[12] In the early nineteenth century, the Swiss author Pfijffer zu Neueck had extolled bamboo for "combining all the advantages of strength and elasticity." On its use in house construction, he wrote:

> To build their *pandoks* [sic] (homes or huts) the Javanese employ the bamboo, which is strong and easy to manipulate. For a home of four to six rooms one requires about seven or eight hundred pieces of bamboo. One piece from 20 to 50 feet costs 3 or 4 *duiten* or 2 cents. The tools are similarly made from bamboo. Four good craftsmen are able, within a week, to make a firm and strong home.[13]

Neueck's emphasis on affordability was not incidental. With wild and cultivated groves proliferating across Java, the practical and economic value of bamboo—layered upon its spiritual and medical significances—was difficult to overstate. Indeed, from the annually published *Koloniaal Verslag* we learn that the sufficient planting of this "highly useful" material for the benefit of local populations was in fact a concern of the Dutch colonial government well into the twentieth century.[14]

Toward the turn of the nineteenth century, European colonials in Southeast Asia adopted more ambiguous attitudes toward bamboo. While the material itself continued to be praised for its strength and adaptability, the manifold bamboo houses encountered within the region were variously recast as dark, permeable, and primitive, qualities that were in turn associated with poverty, disorder, immorality, and disease. In Hong Kong, writes the historian Robert Peckham, bamboo dwellings were vilified by British colonials as "makeshift" squatter abodes rank with disease and immorality, before being recuperated after 1894 as "organic" and "well-ventilated" structures that compared favorably with the overcrowded, plague-infested tenements of Taipingshan.[15] Meanwhile in Hanoi, the French colonial government considered the bamboo *paillote* a fire hazard and began regulating their construction in the city from 1892 onward. A contemporary author pertinently pointed out in 1900 that, inside, vermin was "assurrée d'une hospitalité permanente."[16] In the Dutch East Indies, the pharmacist, entrepreneur, and philanthropist H. F. Tillema launched a vehement critique of housing conditions in the colony in a series of heavily illustrated books published through the 1910s and 1920s. Rarely did the Javanese *not* inhabit a bamboo house, he claimed, while his tone betrayed his dismay over this state of affairs.[17] Photographs of various specimens were adorned with fragmented captions that revealed Tillema's concern with the perceived darkness, permeability, and impermanence of these structures and the impact these qualities had on human health and morality.[18]

These generic, place-specific considerations echoed contemporary discussions on housing in Europe and North America, and reflected both novel biomedical concerns and a good dose of classical nineteenth-century moral anxiety. They reframed bamboo structures as undesirable even when colonials relied on them as much as local populations. Indeed, when Alexandre Yersin identified the plague bacillus in Hong Kong he did so in a "matshed" laboratory erected on the grounds of the Alice Memorial Hospital.[19] In the US-occupied Philippines, during an outbreak of malaria in 1906, soldiers were evacuated from their garrison at Camp Stotsenberg to a hastily constructed bamboo barracks (which proved unhelpfully conducive to mosquito breeding).[20] And during an outbreak of plague in East Java in 1911, residents of affected villages were moved into temporary bamboo *pondoks* while their houses were being disinfected. Over the following months, however, the "rat census" in Malang prompted a conceptual shift toward the bamboo house as a site of multispecies encounters, in which the tubular bamboo facilitated the transmission of zoonotic disease. In other words, in the Dutch East Indies bamboo became potentially pathogenic.

Home Improvement

The identification of bamboo as a material link that connected rat plague to human plague prompted the question of how this chain might be broken. Vaccination and fumigation had generated discouraging results. Rat extermination was a futile endeavor. Rather, argued Willem de Vogel and Johannes van Loghem, the key to plague control rested in widening the distance between man and rat. By "building out" the rat, the rat flea that transmitted the plague bacillus would have no access to human hosts.[21] Home improvement had previously been deployed with favorable results in Rio de Janeiro in Brazil and Taihoku (Taipei) in Japanese-ruled Taiwan.[22] But only in the Dutch East Indies, insisted Dutch state agents over the following decades, had this strategy been fully recognized as the most permanent intervention against plague. In Java, home improvement would be implemented with unrivalled zeal.[23]

The *woningbrigades* described in chapter 1 that established how rats could live and nest in hiding spaces throughout the house also offered a first indication of

Table 3   Location of rat nests in the houses of five plague-stricken *dessas* in Malang in 1911 as a percentage of a total of 2,500 nests

	KOTTA MALANG	KARANGLO	PENANGOENGAN	NGANTANG	TOEREN
Roof					
Atap (thatch)	0	2.5	13	19.3	2.2
Ridge	3.9	7	3.2	12	12.3
Oesoek (diagonal bamboo)	3.3	0	0	0	1.3
Pyan (ceiling)	50	1.5	2.3	0.5	11
Frame					
Soko (vertical bamboo)	1.7	1.6	0	1.5	0.3
Blandar (horizontal bamboo)	20	44	26.2	23	14
Pengeret (inner bamboo beam)	2.2	13.5	10.4	14.7	8
Wood (rotten)	0	0.5	4	1.4	1.3
Wall					
Gedek (woven bamboo mat) and plinth	9.4	7.4	14	10	12
Door	0	7.5	1.7	0.9	1.3
Floor	3.9	0.5	2.2	1.2	5
Pogo (storage space hanging from roof)	1.7	1.7	3.5	4.6	1
Balé-balé (bedstead)	2.9	9	11.6	6.6	28
Stable	0.6	3.5	6.7	4.1	1.3

Source: J. J. van Loghem, "De Pest op Java," *Nederlands Tijdschrift voor Geneeskunde* 56 (1912): 200–234.

how to remove them (table 3). Their tabulated data identified the horizontal bamboo *blandar* as the most popular nesting space of the rat by far: yielding a full quarter of all nests found. In response, de Vogel had the ends of these "dangerous bamboos" sealed off with cement or covered with sheet metal.[24] The *balé-balé* with its frame of large bamboos contained anywhere between 2.9 and 28 percent of rat nests between different districts. Existing specimens were similarly closed off, and a contest was held to design a new "ratproof" model.[25] The vacant spaces beneath the roof were more challenging. Replacing *atap* with tiles was a good start, but "great financial difficulties were involved in introducing tiled roofs all at once in the whole district of Malang."[26] Other rat-prone features of the house, as chapter 4 explores in more detail, required not just a physical intervention but also a behavioral one. For instance, the installation of a "movable" inner wall provided access to the "dead space" between the customary double *gedek* walls (chapter 4, figure 4.1). Likewise, a hatch in the *pyan* allowed access to the ceiling. Both adaptations were moot, however, if the previously oc-cluded spaces they provided access to were not regularly inspected for the presence of rats or nests.

From September 1911 onward, the Dutch limited their response to plague to the evacuation of the inhabitants of affected houses and villages, followed by their "improvement." In November, van Loghem returned to the Netherlands to lead the Department of Tropical Hygiene at the new Koloniaal Instituut in Amsterdam. Meanwhile, de Vogel began a regular commute between Weltevre-den and Malang. For the moment, the number of new plague cases was falling. But home improvement was inherently reactive, and new plague cases contin-ued to be identified. One newspaper likened the disease to an elusive South American guerilla soldier: striking now here, then there.[27] Still, government sources indicate that through 1912 plague remained "localized" to parts of the residency Pasoeroean. Individual cases occurred in the capital towns of the resi-dencies and districts Soerabaja, Kediri, Madioen, and Toeloengagoeng. Control measures that year consisted of "evacuation, rat extermination, inspection of traffic out of infected districts, and home improvement."[28] Though cases began to rise again toward the end of 1912, health officials promoted home improve-ment in various publications as an intervention that offered a permanent solu-tion to the plague threat: breaking the chain of transmission.[29] That being said, the implementation of the scheme was inconsistent, and its efficacy was not beyond doubt.

It is noteworthy that bamboo continued to be widely used through the first years of home improvement. The material had been implicated in the trans-mission of plague, but physicians regarded its hazards as navigable. Nothing "of importance" was reported on bamboo in the *Koloniaal Verslag* of 1912 and 1913. But by 1914, the pressures that home improvement placed on the avail-ability of this construction material became evident. "In some parts of the dis-trict Malang in the residency Pasoeroean," stated the *Koloniaal Verslag* of 1914, "bamboo scarcity prevails despite the increased growth of this product, since extraordinary quantities are required for new dwellings."[30] The follow-ing year, approximately 875 *bouw* were "planted with different kinds of bam-boo to support home improvement in the service of plague control." Large quantities of bamboo were transported across Java at a cost for the state, again in support of counterplague construction works.[31]

Colonizing the Home (I)

In November 1912, de Vogel returned to East Java to inspect the ongoing plague control efforts in Soerabaja, Pasoeroean, Kediri, and Madioen. The port of

Soerabaja had been declared infected for a second time, and Nicholaas Swellengrebel—who had succeeded van Loghem as chief bacteriologist—had written of mishaps in the execution of the home improvement scheme. After countering local attempts to circumvent quarantine regulations in Soerabaja, de Vogel traveled on to Madioen where he identified potentially lethal oversights in the houses that had already been improved. The devil was in the detail, he observed, providing pen sketches on the margins of his report to illustrate common mistakes. For instance, the holes cut into the horizontal bamboo *blandar* (beams) that allowed them to be pierced by the vertical bamboo *soko* (posts) were often too wide and not properly sealed. Another mistake was that pieces of bamboo placed diagonally between *blandar* and *soko* to increase stability were now made of "split" bamboo but installed convex (with the hollow part upward) and thereby created a comfortable nesting space for house rats that did not mind an incline. The *soko* itself was frequently sealed at the lower end but not at the top. Finally, the installation of the aforementioned moveable inner walls and ceiling hatches presented myriad difficulties that left the dead space they concealed uninspected. While some residents had come up with ingenious solutions, these spaces had largely been reinfested by rats. In Kediri and Toeloengagoeng, wrote de Vogel, these deficiencies were compounded by a lack of conviction among the directing health officials in home improvement as an efficient counterplague measure.[32]

When he finally returned to the district Malang, de Vogel was glad to see that home improvement in the first affected *kampongs* had been nearly completed. The mistakes seen in neighboring districts had been avoided.[33] The tide of plague had turned—for now. But at what cost? Plague and plague control, de Vogel observed not without pride, had warranted a strong public health intervention that was strikingly evident in the local terrain:

> Driving westward along the road to Ngantang, I was struck by the changed appearance of the landscape that extends itself along the west slopes of the Ardjoeno up to Gabes near Patjet. Everywhere the red roofs of the homes in the various *dessas* contrasted markedly with the green background, giving a somewhat European impression, and at the same time an impression of the wealth of population in the district, while in the past the *atap*-covered homes concealed the population density. The whole area was hit hard by plague last year. Now cases here are rare.[34]

Home improvement had not just made the Javanese house ratproof (if that), it had effectively taken possession of the dwelling and—by extension—its occupants and the land around it. Where the traditional bamboo-*atap* dwellings had merged into the "green background" and concealed the populace from colonial oversight, the red-tiled roofs of "improved" houses stood out clearly and revealed "the wealth of population" that had come into the purview of the colonial government. The scene witnessed by de Vogel might resemble that seen in a photograph of "a newly built village near Batoe" (figure 2.1).[35] Neatly tiled roofs top wooden-beamed structures, nearly uniform in shape and size, and laid out in an orderly pattern, interspersed with separate rice storage sheds. The village forms a stark contrast to Couperus's character sketch of the Javanese house in East Java. As it turns out, it is the village of Banjak once again. This village had previously been rebuilt using native construction materials, before van Loghem's epiphany regarding the presence of rats inside the house (chapter 1, figure 1.2). In both cases, the government-enforced improvement is evident by the spatial ordering of the village (i.e., the grid pattern). Unlike before, however, the village now forms a stark contrast with the surrounding landscape: exuding, in the words of de Vogel, "a somewhat European impression" amid the *sawah* and tropical foliage.

As the number of plague cases began to rise toward the end of 1912, their distribution at first appeared to support the efficacy of home improvement.

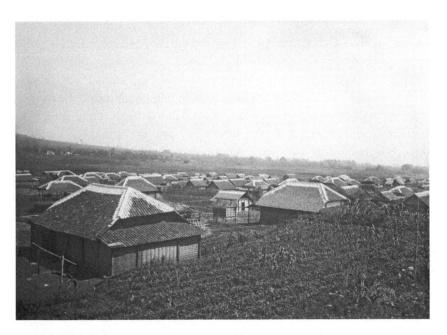

FIGURE 2.1. Glass plate positive of the improved *dessa* Banjak, ca. 1912. Unknown, *Plague Resistant Houses in a Recently Founded Village near Batoe*, ca. 1912, TM-10024151. Courtesy of the Nationaal Museum van Wereldculturen.

In a letter to Governor-General Alexander Idenburg discussing de Vogel's report, the outgoing director of the BGD observed:

> While its [incidence] . . . is noticeably higher in Kediri and Madioen than last year, so that the peak of cases for 1912 far exceeds that of the previous year, the peak of cases in Malang was not half as high in 1912 as it was in 1911. In this I see—together with Dr. de Vogel—a beneficial result of the only in Malang methodically implemented home improvement.[36]

This euphoria was tempered, no doubt, by a rapid increase in cases over 1913 and 1914 in Malang and adjacent districts. Home improvement nonetheless continued to be implemented and was steadily placed on a more solid financial and legal footing. In July 1912, for instance, the *assistent-resident* of Malang had prepared a sizeable budget of f. 1,000,000 to be spent on home improvement over the next four years. To this amount the BGD added another f. 250,000. Between July 1912 and June 1913, 10,268 houses in the district were said to have been improved. Another 17,776 still awaited renovation. The implementation of the program was inconsistent, however, and expenses had already exceeded the budget for the first year by more than f. 16,000.[37] In the district Kediri "all those houses that qualified" had been improved by August 1913 using tiles instead of *atap*, but here too there was a resurgence of plague.[38] If home improvement was indeed efficacious against the disease, a more systematic implementation was required. Consequently, in July 1914, following two visits to the plague-affected districts, Idenburg signed a plague ordinance that gave the "improvement and demolishment of plague dangerous buildings" by state agents a legal basis and paved the way for a more comprehensive intervention.[39] Shortly before stepping down in 1916, Idenburg appears to have made a final intervention that scaled up the reach of plague control, instructing that the renovation works should target blocks of houses all at once instead of the houses of individual plague victims only.[40]

Soerabaja

Over the first weeks of the outbreak of plague back in 1911, the port city of Soerabaja emerged as a likely candidate as the original point of entry of the disease into Java. In September and October 1910, large quantities of rice had been imported through the city, presumably carrying infected rats and fleas from Burma or China. Rail transports had subsequently carried the disease into the interior, but surprisingly (given its reputation as an urban disease) plague failed to get a hold on the human population of Soerabaja itself. An epizootic, however, would explain reports of unusual mortality among the rats of Soerabaja and nearby Sidoardjo, as well as the mysterious plague-like cases of disease described in chapter 1. In early April, several cases of rat plague in the city were bacteriologically confirmed in samples of *Mus rattus* (of the "house rat" variety) as well as *Mus decumanus* (the common brown rat).[41] Fifty professional rat catchers were hired to mitigate the chance of an outbreak. They received a commission of 2.5 cents per rat, "but," reflected the *resident* of Soerabaja, "there are easier ways to earn more money" and the yield was unsatisfactory.[42] Likewise, de Vogel was not impressed by the overall attitude of the urban population toward the dread disease and its prevention: characterizing it as passive and indeed "lax."[43]

Plague did not pass the city by entirely, however, and in the evening of May 3 three cases were bacteriologically confirmed. In response, Soerabaja was declared an "infected" port in accordance with Article 7 of the Sanitary Convention of 1903.[44] As a leading economic center of the Dutch East Indies, the consequences of this event were severe.[45] Every day, estimated the *resident*, 10,000 people departed the city via road or rail, small sailing craft or oceangoing vessel. Every year, hundreds of millions of guilders worth of goods were shipped from its port, the largest in the colony.[46] Immediately after Soerabaja was declared an official plague port, major shipping companies such as the Koninklijke Paketvaart-Maatschappij and Lloyd refused to take on passengers or freight for fear that their ships would be quarantined at their destinations. Local traders complained loudly.[47] The quarantine enforced on Malang was not extended to Soerabaja, however, and the transport of goods and people overland (including to another port city such as Semarang) was not prohibited.[48] Civil servants sought to work out a solution, and in a telegram of May 10 Idenburg informed the Dutch government that overseas passengers were allowed to depart from Soerabaja again after medical examination and disinfection of their luggage.[49] By May 16, another three cases had been reported but here the disease came to a halt and after three weeks Soerabaja's status as an "infected" port was revoked.[50] By then, mercantile elites had suffered sufficient financial losses to prompt a more proactive response. As the epidemic in Malang continued unabated, they recognized that the threat of reinfection hung over the city like the sword of Damocles. At a meeting with representatives of trade and industry, health officials further fostered their sense of civic responsibility by observing the financial damage that could be done to the owner of a well-stocked warehouse by the discovery of even a single plague rat.[51]

In response, reflected the *resident* in a report to Idenburg the following September, "the residents realized the looming danger of the presence of plague-infected rats, and sought to embark on a battle against the rat."[52] As in Malang, the house was seen as an important battleground between man and rat—even before van Loghem's epiphany regarding the nesting habits of the house rat. By early June, citizens of Soerabaja had formed the Soerabaja General Health Committee (Algemeen Soerabaisch Gezondheidscomité, ASGC) under the leadership of the president of the local chamber of commerce. The private health committee set itself the aim of improving living and hygienic conditions in the city through a program of rat catching, home improvement, and the destruction of slums.[53] Within days, the ASGC collected f. 98,750 in donations from local and international companies based in Soerabaja.[54] "Partially we pursued the reduction of rats present by catching and killing them," reported the physician and committee member Johannes Terburgh later, "while inspection of the salubrity of houses and commons was intended to prevent their inhabitation by the rat as much as possible." By October 14 the ASGC had collected and spent well over f. 134,000 and had renovated an estimated 2,690 houses. An additional 859 houses had been renovated at the expense of residents themselves. "Home improvement conducted in the first phase," had however "not yet been in accordance with the requirements that would later be demanded."[55] But on the bright side, the *resident* of Soerabaja reported that the "native population, who usually view the instructions of the government in their interest with some suspicion, have curiously supported the measures of the committee with complete confidence"—despite the European encroachments into their "intimate existence."[56]

Already in September 1911, the new health committee found itself in financial difficulty. In a letter to Idenburg, the *resident* wrote that the citizens wished to organize a lottery to further finance the "plague free making and keeping" of the municipality, but their request was denied.[57] When funds threatened to run out at the end of the month—just before a visit by Idenburg to the plague-stricken districts—the municipal government made f. 30,000 available to carry on the home improvement work for another two weeks. These figures suggest that between the initial f. 98,000 pledged in June and the end of September, just f. 6,000 more had been collected in private donations. Nevertheless, the work done by the committee was viewed favorably by the government. De Vogel, for one, described its organization as "masterly."[58] The committee certainly sought to broadcast its achievements, and a number of "before and after" photographs of dwellings renovated under its leadership (marked with flags carrying its acronym) were produced (see chapter 3). A source dating back to early September 1911 states that the ASGC was awarded another f. 100,000 in government funding to continue its work.[59] I have been unable to confirm this, but at any rate the ASGC would be reorganized into a quasi-governmental organization in the wake of Idenburg's visit.[60] In this second phase of its existence, half of the cost of home improvement conducted in Soerabaja was funded by the municipal government. Homeowners were required to cover the remaining half themselves, presumably by means of advance loans—as would become the rule for home improvement elsewhere.[61]

By early 1912, the ASGC claimed to have renovated a quarter of all houses within the municipality of Soerabaja. Preliminary measures (of an unclear nature) had "already been taken for another few thousand." Before the end of the year, wrote Terburgh, the entire city could be "improved."[62] The Chinese neighborhood had been purposely left alone for the moment, and a narrative of Chinese intransigence to European public health measures followed.[63] Attempts to have the Chinese population renovate their own homes or collect the funds to do so had failed and proper legislation was required to "force their cooperation."[64] Rat catching (at an increased premium of 5 cents per rat) had by that time been altogether abolished.[65] Meanwhile, physicians had been hired on a temporary basis to conduct health checks at the port.[66] As mentioned, home improvement efforts up until October 1911 had not yet taken full cognizance of the intimate cohabitation of humans and rats that had been identified in Malang. Thus, homes that had previously been "improved" required further corrections. Over the remaining two years of the existence of the ASGC, reflected Terburgh, another four distinct phases could be determined in the method of home improvement that corresponded to progressive insights on human-rat cohabitation.[67] When the ASGC was disbanded in June 1913, all *atap*-covered houses within Soerabaja had reportedly been replaced with tiled specimens. The organization proved unable to build out plague entirely, however. In September and October 1912, cases of human and rat plague had again been confirmed. By November 1912, Soerabaja had been declared an infected port once more. This status was revoked on December 13, only to be reinstated four days later.[68] In response, one newspaper criticized that "the money spent on home improvement in Soerabaja can be considered lost" as inspection and cleaning efforts had quickly been neglected in improved neighborhoods.[69]

Over the following years, a curious situation developed around plague in Soerabaja. While the incidence of human plague cases was very low, the city and its surrounding residency reported dozens (sometimes hundreds) of plague cases through the 1910s.[70] Plague remained epizootic among the rodent population and was implicated as the source of new outbreaks across East Java in districts from which the disease had one stage or another been cleared. A health official of the League of Nations who toured through Java in 1923 observed:

> The only district that has reported plague deaths in each one of the twelve years is Soerabaya. There is reason to believe that infection among the rats of the town of Soerabaya has been continuously present since 1910.[71]

Plague in Java may have been a distinctly rural affair, but cities such as Soerabaja and, later, Semarang were nonetheless seen to play a crucial role. They were regarded as incubators of the disease, places where plague could persist and from which it could periodically surge. The importance of plague *to* Soerabaja waned, meanwhile, and there were said to be "no real anti-plague measures" in place by 1923. Home improvement had apparently been completed, and the focus now rested on the destruction of rats on the crafts supplying oceangoing vessels.[72]

The Plague Service

The calamity of plague in Java had demanded the full attention of the recently organized BGD and caused its uneven development over the 1910s. Chronically understaffed, the health organization was unable to address the myriad health challenges facing the archipelago.[73] The forceful response to plague in 1911 followed by its apparent containment over 1912 gave the impression that this disease, at least, was coming under control. In both years, the total number of reported deaths hovered around 2,200. But over the next two years the number of cases rose quickly (introduction, table 1). In 1913, over 11,000 cases of plague were reported, jumping to nearly 16,000 in 1914. The situation in Malang, where home improvement had advanced furthest, was of particular concern. Here alone, plague deaths rose from 1,503 in 1912 to 6,918 in 1913.[74] As plague resurged with a vengeance, an independent plague control service (Dienst der Pestbestrijding, DP) was created in January 1915 to relieve the BGD and unify the Dutch response to plague.

Given that plague had returned to Malang, the efficacy of home improvement was in doubt. Back in the Netherlands, politicians questioned the wisdom of having abandoned alternative control methods early on.[75] Renewed experiments with fumigating infected dwellings in 1913 were stepped up in the wake of a second visit by Idenburg to the plague-stricken districts in February 1914.[76] Over the first months of its existence, however, the head of the DP, Wilhelm van Gorkom, quickly denounced fumigation as nothing more than a costly, unreliable, and laborious ally of home improvement. In many instances, his team maintained, live fleas had been found even after fumigation, and experiments had further demonstrated the tenacity of fleas in the face of chemical eradication methods. The *assistent-resident* of Malang voiced a string of other objections in a letter of March 17, 1915. As a preventive strategy, fumigation was of no use, he wrote, and like home improvement it was slow. It did not replace the need to evacuate people from their homes for extended periods of time, and the method required considerable manpower that *dessa* residents had to provide without pay. The cost and difficulty of fumigation during the west monsoon were prohibitive. The method damaged buildings and goods. In sum, the cleaning, improvement, and subsequent inspection of houses would cost hundreds of thousands of guilders—but not the millions required for fumigation. Ultimately, fumigation simply did nothing to address the underlying problem: human-rat cohabitation.[77] By April 1915, the DP had returned its focus to home improvement and formulated a mission statement that would frequently be reiterated: "To build or renovate houses in such a way that rats *cannot, or cannot unnoticeably*, nest inside."[78]

With this goal in mind, the plague service began to systematize the home improvement scheme. It issued strict guidelines on the use of bamboo and outright banned the use of *atap*. As before, any "dead space" had to be made accessible to inspection or sealed off completely. Perhaps the most invasive intervention, as discussed below, was the DP's attempt to ratproof Java's distinctive roof designs. The plague service identified the houses in need of improvement and implemented emergency interventions, while the actual renovations fell under the authority of the interior civil service (Binnenlandsch Bestuur, BB). After its completion, the DP took over these houses to approve the corrections and conduct regular inspections. The total number of houses that had already been improved in the name of plague control up to 1915 was unclear as the figures provided across multiple reports often did not correlate. The DP put the figure at roughly 151,000 houses across the residencies Pasoeroean, Madioen, and Kediri—but noted that the district Malang alone boasted some 15,000 improved dwellings that required further corrections.[79] The financial cost of this "colonization of the home" had initially been covered by the Dutch government. The DP now introduced a new system in which this burden was increasingly placed upon the Javanese population itself. The DP identified the dwellings in need of improvement, trained *mantri* inspectors and technicians, and guided building policies. BB provided material, labor, and monetary advances to homeowners with which to pay for the improvements. These loans had to be repaid in eight interest-free half-yearly instalments.[80] The new plague service, consequently, may have been led by physicians but at heart it was a technical rather than a medical service. Care of the sick was absent from its reports and remained the responsibility of the BGD, relatives, and four "plague ambulances" sent to the Indies by the Dutch Red Cross in 1914.

Dessa Cleaning

If home improvement was "the most successful prophylactic" against plague, it was also hopelessly slow as an immediate intervention. Even in his first quarterly report, van Gorkom noted a considerable backlog and by April 1916 the tally stood at 112,315 houses awaiting permanent improvement.[81] Three months later, this figure had been reduced to about 91,154 houses, but as plague spread, more and more houses were added to the list.[82] Naturally, fresh outbreaks required a more rapid response. The original solution—the wholesale evacuation of affected villages—was highly unpopular with local populations. The DP found a solution in the so-called *dessa schoonmaak*, which it described as "acute" home improvement followed by regular inspection:

> This cleaning aims to remove all rats and rat nests from dwellings. . . . During this initial cleaning the roof will be removed and the wooden or bamboo frame inspected and restored. . . . The replacement of *atap* by tiles, precursor of the subsequent home improvement, will be financed by the owner.[83]

Over the course of this cleaning, the house was left open to the elements for a period of ten days in an attempt to kill any fleas and plague bacilli that might have survived the initial rat purge. During this time, the population lived in bamboo *pondoks* in the village commons. When this emergency intervention had been completed, the DP instructed, "a weekly cleaning is implemented that is supervised by a *mantri*" until such time as the permanent improvement scheme caught up.[84] The furniture would be carried outside and the house cleaned and searched in an attempt to make life for the house rat inside "unbearable."[85] After a while, gushed the *assistent-resident* of Malang, the *dessa schoonmaak* no longer required supervision by technical personnel. "The Native starts to take pleasure in his neat environment. Something permanent is achieved through this method."[86] In a similarly laudatory tone, van Gorkom stressed that this process was "much cheaper than evacuation" and generated less resistance from local populations.[87] Such caveats appear frequently across various reports, hinting that plague control was not always uncontested.

It is telling of the priority that plague assumed in the Dutch East Indies despite its comparatively low mortality that van Gorkom stressed that home improvement could target *only* this disease. Given its emergency character, the DP had set a minimum standard that improved homes had to conform to in order to bring plague to heel:

> As general hygienists we would gladly demand more than this minimum and . . . think at the same time about the dangers of malaria, cholera, tuberculosis, typhus, and dysentery. As interested citizens of the State we would support it if home improvement against plague could at the

same time be rallied to improve the solidity and durability of the dessa house. This is however not allowed to us.[88]

The plague service, wrote van Gorkom, "would not settle for less" than breaking human-rat cohabitation. But: "we are not at liberty . . . to set *higher* requirements than those to check rats and rat nests."[89] This approach attracted substantial criticism from public commentators such as Tillema, as well as from government officials and physicians. Nevertheless, many observers would comment over the years on the overall improvement in living standards that the *dessa schoonmaak*, home improvement scheme, and subsequent home inspection conferred with regard to other facets of public health.[90] But such appearances, as I discuss in chapter 5, were deceptive.

Colonizing the Home (II)

According to the anthropologist Sylvia Gooswit, traditional Javanese housing knew very little variation in its basic floor plan. The rank, class, and social relations of its inhabitants were apparent in the size of the house and in the construction materials used. Primarily, they manifested in the shape and style of the roof.[91] While health officials had been concerned since 1911 with the ability of the scansorial house rat to nest inside the *atap* cover, as far as I can tell roof design had not been a specific concern when plague control was organized by the BGD. But from its first quarterly report in April 1915 onward, the DP expressed its fear that specific roof designs were conducive to rat nesting and hence plague transmission. Criss-crossed by wooden and bamboo beams, the upper regions of the inside of the roof were often too dark and too high to be easily searched. If a plague rat died there, its fleas could effortlessly drop onto human victims. Thus, dictated van Gorkom, "the roof construction must be as simple as possible."[92] Diagrams and sketches of desirable and undesirable roof designs featured frequently in the DP's reports, and regulations (such as those for the type of roof tile used) tightened over time.

Hipped roofs such as the *joglo* designated the inhabitants of a dwelling as members of the Javanese aristocracy. The shape was forbidden in new buildings in plague-affected districts, as was the use of *atap* or other plant material. The same went for the similar *pendopo* form used in governmental buildings, and *rampasan* shield roofs. Existing roofs in these shapes were ideally replaced but could be retained if they were roofed with tiles: "the use of natural materials as roof cover is forbidden."[93] The iconic *limasan* design that sheltered more prosperous citizens was simply not allowed. All of these designs had to be substituted with the uniform gable roof: locally known as the *kampung*-style used by ordinary citizens.[94] Home improvement thus cut through existing social structures. If local elites resented this symbolic demotion, their remonstrations were not recorded in government reports. Still, as the well-known Dutch architect Henri Maclaine Pont pointed out in 1923:

> What these prohibitions mean to the sensibilities of the traditionally minded Javanese would be understood by anyone familiar with how distinctions are expressed by fine nuances in the aforementioned roof shapes—with height: the pride of the prosperous; in the number of layers of the lower wooden frame as well as by its decorations and additions: rank and position of the inhabitant and their gender. One could demolish it all, but it appears to be an enforced revolution.[95]

In this respect, too, home improvement enforced a leveling uniformity upon the house as well as its occupants. If this constituted a revolution, it was a cultural as much as a social one that admirers of Javanese arts and crafts would decry.[96] As Gooswit points out, these instructions not only impacted on the houses directly but also effected a demise in the skills and knowledge of local craftsmen such as the *tukang kayu*. Furthermore, many Javanese who had supplemented their income by preparing separate housing elements such as *gedek* walls or simple roof tiles were put out of business.[97]

The transformation of the traditional "plague-dangerous" roof into an improved "plague-resistant" one was captured in numerous photographs. The "before and after" genre was especially popular (see chapter 3, figures 3.1 and 3.2). Here, we may briefly consider another, more narrative sequence of photographs contained in a report by Louis Otten, the last leader of the independent DP, in 1923.[98] The first image shows a house from the front beneath an impressive *"tikelan-(djoglo)"* roof covered with *atap*. The frame of the house appears to have been made of wood, leaving the roof as its principal feature to require "improvement." In the second photograph, the square dome of the *joglo* has been cut off, as it were. The skeleton of the original roof has been retained (as indicated by the remnants of *atap* that still cover the edges). A new hipped roof, described by Otten as a *doro-gepak* or *sinoem* shape, executed in tiles, is being built on top of it. The shape of the roof skeleton and its new cover appear ill-matched as they leave a significant amount of empty space between them, but a final photograph indicates that the former was gradually adjusted to match the latter. This last image shows how, in the end, two sides of the original hipped shape were removed to create a saddle shape instead, with the original roof frame hidden behind (or replaced by) a gable. Often, it is worth pointing out, home improvement came down to demolition and the construction of entirely new houses.

Tiles and Timber

The supply of building materials with which to execute the home improvement scheme was an ongoing struggle. Bamboo—no longer as readily available as it had been at the start of the outbreak—was regarded with growing suspicion after the resurgence of plague in previously improved villages. Dismissing the option of renovating the Javanese house with reinforced concrete instead, the DP turned to timber as the most viable alternative. In Kediri, for instance, the plague service began to exploit new forests to support the scheme in December 1914.[99] But wood, "especially good wood," was far more expensive than bamboo.[100] Furthermore, if renovation in wood had always been preferable, Idenburg had already decreed in November 1914 that homeowners could not be obligated to pay for improvements in wood when the risks of using bamboo could be overcome.[101] The first set of building regulations issued by the DP sought to navigate these various concerns by subjecting the use of bamboo to strict conditions.

Previously, pieces of bamboo had long slits called *trontong* cut into them to make them undesirable as a nesting space for rats. This intervention did not have the desired effect and was now forbidden. Instead, the use of "full" bamboo in newly built houses and houses being renovated in plague-stricken districts was—in principle—prohibited altogether. If the use of bamboo was a necessity, it was to be used only for certain parts of the construction such as the *soko* and *blandar* after closing off its hollow interior with sheet metal or cement. The natural outer glazing of pieces of bamboo was usually sufficient to protect them from rats gnawing through, but parts that had deteriorated had to also be covered with sheet metal. These pieces were never allowed to stand directly in the ground but had to be positioned on a stone foundation. Split bamboo had to be installed without the hollow part being at any point closed off by other parts of the construction. These regulations applied primarily to home improvement in the countryside, as renovations using bamboo in district and residency capitals were forbidden. Even the *balé-balé* was not neglected in these instructions, with an updated building code later mandating that this item of furniture should be made only using laths and split pieces of bamboo installed with the hollow part facing downward. As for the roof cover: *atap*, *alang-alang*, *kadjang*, *klakah*, and other native organic materials were banned as plague dangerous. They were to be replaced with roof tiles—though what kind? Flemish and Javanese designs were prohibited as they could be lifted up by rats to gain entry into the house, while the Malacca type (used in Sumatra) was prohibited because it formed a trench on the upper side where a rat might easily build a nest.[102]

In the port city of Semarang, where there were several victims of plague in 1916, city councillors proposed an ambitious scheme to improve over 24,000 houses against plague.[103] They railed against the standards set by the plague service, however, hoping to exceed the minimum (or maximum) requirements set by van Gorkom. Rather, they hoped to use the opportunity to pursue a more thorough (and costly) form of home improvement that would elevate housing conditions across the board.[104] The cost and supply of wood for this project were topics of debate, and some advocated for a return to the use of bamboo. If this were to be allowed, city councillors stressed it ought not to be done out of frugality. "If we conduct things here in the same cheap way as elsewhere, with poor quality wood," argued one councillor, "the improvement will not be enough and after 4 years we can start anew. If we do it better and more expensively. . . ."[105] Neither the acting director of the plague service, K. van Roon, nor his superior, the director of the Department of Education and Worship (Departement van Onderwijs en Eeredienst), were impressed by this attitude. Not following the national line "slavishly," grumbled the latter, was an undesirable result of too advanced decentralization.[106] The proposal by the city council was rejected by the central government and home improvement took place in the usual manner.

It appears that the concerns of Semarang's city council over the quality of home improvement were not entirely unfounded. As time wore on, the availability of suitable timber diminished. In a letter to the governor-general of June 1917, van Roon observed that the use of wood had "assumed such large dimensions that we can no longer suffice with using the cheaper kinds." Later, in parts of the district Temanggoeng, the poor quality of wood used for the renovations meant that the whole process had to be redone.[107] More expensive wood consequently had to be used, which considerably pushed up the cost of home improvement to both homeowners and the government. In response to rising costs, delays in the supply of building materials, and the still increasing number of houses requiring improvement, the incoming director of the plague service, Otten, wrote to the governor-general in February 1919 on the desirability of a return to the regulated use of bamboo. He observed that efforts to persuade homeowners to invest in renovation in wood had become increasingly forceful. Effectively, people had been forced to opt for renovations in wood without taking into consideration their ability to repay the advances.[108] Afterward, it seems that the use of wood and bamboo in home improvement differed from place to place depending on local availability. In practice, a compromise was often struck that was apparent in the photograph in the introduction (figure 0.1), with the main posts and beams made of timber, and smaller support posts and beams made of bamboo.

But if ratproofing or replacing the bamboo frame of the Javanese house was ultimately straightforward, the roof was a different matter. The rat could scarcely be denied access to the roof, leaving it a major vulnerability.[109] Replacing *atap* with tiles significantly reduced the number of nests within and beneath the roof, but producing and transporting the tiles was the Achilles' heel of the home improvement scheme. In Malang, the 1912 budget for home improvement had been vastly exceeded by providing advances for tile production (which nonetheless failed to keep up with demand).[110] Local production required a large number of workers, furthermore, but labor was also required for other aspects of antiplague work. Consequently, when Idenburg enquired into the pressures that home improvement placed on the local population in July 1912, the *assistent-resident* of Malang replied indirectly by stating that tile production "for cost of the state" would constitute by far the most desirable form of assistance.[111] And while the colonial government would apparently shoulder this burden, as late as March 1915 a communiqué on plague control in Malang implied the continued scarcity of tiles by noting that wherever tiles were unavailable the roofs of houses still awaiting "permanent" improvement were covered by canvas previously used for fumigation.[112] In its search for a viable alternative to both *atap* and tiles, the DP experimented with other forms of organic material: going so far as to import a particular kind of *kadjang* from Borneo.[113]

Wherever plague spread, the DP was faced with the task of establishing potteries to supply roof tiles and sawmills to prepare timber.[114] In Soerakarta, in 1916, the service ran up against the banal challenge that there were no suitable lots available to set up such industries.[115] Elsewhere, there were more fundamental issues with the quality of the soil or the availability of suitable trees.[116] The quality of tiles was another issue. Previously, tile production was a sporadic activity to supplement the income of local populations. The DP, however, required a dedicated industry to supply approved tiles by the million.[117] When Otten took control in 1919, he lamented that tile production remained "as agonizingly slow as before in Malang."[118] The shortage rapidly increased as plague exploded in Central Java after 1920 and the number of dwellings slated for improvement blithely increased. And as plague expanded into this more mountainous terrain, transportation emerged as another obstacle. Millions of tiles now had to be transported to districts that were neither accessible nor suitable for local production—again at great cost.[119] After eight years of plague control, consequently, the cost and availability of timber combined with a persistent shortage of roof tiles to force through a reevaluation of Java's hazardous "native" building materials.

The Cost of Home Improvement

What did home improvement cost and who paid for it? The answer to this question is not readily clear. Between 1911 and 1942, the expenditure on plague was erratically recorded across different government sources. Figures do not necessarily link up and budgets did not correspond to real expenditure. The chief difficulty is that it is frequently unclear whether the figures provided encompass both the "ordinary" funds for plague control (such as personnel, travel expenses, office space, and laboratory equipment) and the "extraordinary" funds to provide homeowners with monetary advances to finance the renovation of their homes—and if repayment was included. Furthermore, it appears that some costs were also covered by other branches of the colonial state. The exact role and expenditure of BB in plague control remain particularly vague in this regard. And finally, the cost of transporting materials and various irregular expenses was occasionally described as having been "for the state."[120] But what these costs amounted to and which department ultimately footed the bill are not always clear.

By reading across multiple sources, we learn that the overall cost of plague control to the colonial state was estimated at about f. 5 million a year in the 1910s and f. 2 million a year through the 1920s.[121] It is unclear whether these amounts covered state expenditure alone or included the contributions of homeowners via the repayment of monetary advances, though for the 1930s I calculated an average expenditure of f. 1.8 million a year *after* the provision and partial repayment of these loans.[122] Together, these estimates would add up to an expenditure of around f. 85 million over thirty years. The budget for plague control was dominated by home improvement, and the budget for home improvement would in turn consist primarily of monetary advances. In 1930, for instance, the loans to homeowners amounted to f. 1.5 million on a total budget for plague control of f. 2.4 million. Salaries across the plague service accounted for another f. 783,870—half of which was for personnel charged with home inspection after the renovations were complete.[123] The extent to which the advances were repaid varied considerably over time and large sums ultimately had to be written off. For example, in 1924, the amount that had to be repaid was f. 600,343 and the actual amount collected was f. 553,664.[124] In the 1930s, economic hardship dramatically reduced the ability of homeowners to pay. Some f. 790,000 was offered in advances in 1933 but only f. 90,461 was recovered.[125] The following year, repayments dropped to just f. 47,413 while a debt of f. 1.4 million was said to be outstanding.[126] There were also considerable differences between regions. For example, in 1927 the departing *resident* of

Soerakarta informed his successor that while the population of the principality of Mangoenegaran had quickly repaid the advances, their neighbors in the principality of Soerakarta still had *f.* 1.1 million in debt outstanding ten years after the renovations were complete.[127]

The cost of home improvement to Javanese homeowners, meanwhile, was (as time went on) estimated at *f.* 10, *f.* 20, or *f.* 40 per house.[128] Additional costs were theoretically covered by the state, though again there was no unity in this regard. In 1917, for instance, the *resident* of Soerakarta claimed that the recent pressure on homeowners to renovate their houses in wood had pushed the average cost in some districts up to as much as *f.* 125 per house.[129] Shortly after, Otten called attention to the disproportion between the cost of producing roof tiles (*f.* 10 per 1,000) and transporting them (*f.* 28 per 1,000) in the more mountainous terrain of Central Java. This cost placed them far beyond the reach of ordinary Javanese, prompting Otten to ask the governor-general to charge homeowners no more than the original *f.* 10.[130] After 1921, it appears that the amount that homeowners were expected to repay was determined with greater consideration of their financial resources—but no doubt the loans constituted a significant financial burden for most families.[131] Indeed, as the head of the department of plague control observed as late as 1937: "The burden of home improvement can lead to money shortages in the dessa and negatively impact on the expenditure for provisions . . . leading to a danger of malnutrition and a reduced ability to withstand infections among the population."[132] Meanwhile, colonial officials would at times maintain that homeowners "preferred to use more expensive materials than strictly necessary" and thereby plunged themselves into financial difficulty.[133] The above cost estimates per house multiplied by 1.6 million dwellings improved would suggest an added financial burden on the population of plague-stricken districts of somewhere between *f.* 16 million and *f.* 64 million.

Finally, the population of districts being renovated were expected to provide a certain amount of labor. The exact form thereof is not entirely clear and likely differed between districts. Java had a long history of forced labor (such as corvée demanded by local elites and through the cultivation system of the colonial state), as well as a tradition of mutual cooperation toward communal projects (*sambat sinambat, gotong royong*).[134] According to the *Koloniaal Verslag* of 1920, home improvement through *sambat* services alone was not possible, but neither could homeowners afford the cost of renovations by means of paid labor. Preferably, it suggested, part of the work should be completed through mandatory *heerendienst* (corvée) of the population, for which they also would receive a minimum wage—though I have found no evidence that this system was widely implemented.[135] The cost of home improvement and other facets of plague control was consequently covered by the colonial state, by homeowners themselves, and by an uncertain amount of unpaid labor. It could consequently not be measured in financial expenditure alone, but also had to account for lost labor to homeowners. All in all, a ballpark estimate that plague control consumed around f. 100 million over a period of thirty years is not extravagant.

The Model House

As early as 1911, de Vogel and van Loghem had "attempted to build a native house of indigenous materials, in which the rat will find it hard to settle." The appeal of such a structure lay in the fact that it could be made with cheap and locally available construction materials, with minimal infringement on local Javanese building practices. Preoccupied by their recent discovery that the house rat lived and nested inside the hollow bamboo frame of the native house, their model structure consisted entirely of split or halved bamboo stalks that were "fastened together with the convex sides against each other." They turned the structure inside out, as it were. Two photographs showcasing their design found their way into de Vogel's government report of the outbreak in Malang, but the model cannot be said to exude an air of great stability. No indigenous alternative was suggested for the rat-prone *atap* roofs. "Whether this method of building provides a practical solution," admitted de Vogel, "remains for the future to decide."[136] Their model failed to gain traction, but more conventional ratproof house models were placed with the headmen of villages affected by plague.[137] These structures demonstrated the aforementioned interventions, such as movable inner walls, closed-off bamboo poles and beams, and roofs covered with tiles. In a pamphlet of 1912 explaining home improvement, the physician Otto de Raadt argued that these models also served to instruct Javanese about how to *keep* the improved dwelling rat-free.[138]

Over the years, more model houses made of indigenous building materials were designed and constructed. According to a pamphlet of the Colonial Exhibition held in Semarang in 1914, for instance, the BGD provided a plague exhibit in the "native" section of the fair. It had constructed a "ratproof bamboo building" that visitors could enter. Inside, they could inspect two scale models of plague-resistant houses. These models featured a bamboo frame, conventional but single walls of *gedek*, and a saddle-shaped roof covered with native tiles. In the first scale model, open spaces in the roof had been filled with brickwork. It featured a ceiling also made of *gedek*, divided into six squares that could be individually removed. The full bamboos of the frame were sealed with concrete and sheet metal, and the poles were placed on a brick foundation. The second scale model was made of halved bamboo, like the original model made by de Vogel and van Loghem. It too featured single walls made of *gedek*, this time covered in a plaster made of cow or buffalo manure, clay, and rice hulls.[139] Whether or not these models were constructed on a large scale remains unclear. They do underscore a preference for the regulated use of bamboo through the early years of the home improvement scheme—contrasting with the "model kampong" built by the DP after 1915 to train its inspectors, which instead featured specimens of wood.[140]

Through the 1910s, the BGD and DP repeatedly expressed the need for independent architectural counsel: an "expert adviser" to lead a comprehensive investigation into native house designs and guide the home improvement efforts. After all, the people who led the plague control work were physicians, not architects or engineers. As the scheme steadily expanded, became more complex, and placed increasing pressure on the availability of construction materials as well as the Javanese ability to pay for them, the matter of professional expertise became more urgent. But here the BGD ran up against the Department of Public Works (Departement der Burgerlijke Openbare Werken). The director of this organization resisted the hiring of an *inspecteur-technicus* by the plague service, and was less than pleased with the fact that the health services were now issuing building codes. The matter became a point of debate even at parliament in The Hague.[141] In a letter to the governor-general of January 1918, de Vogel argued:

> There is at present a wealth of material in the archive at Headquarters collected from across the Archipelago of the different homes of different tribes, water supply, waste management, etc., with clear blueprints, drawings, photographs, and descriptions, which could be processed to design a common model of a home that is comfortable to *Inlanders*, economically viable, and healthy. This collection . . . is still being added to. All this material now remains in the archive deprived of interest.[142]

Having collected this visual record, de Vogel hoped to use these materials to design a model native house that straddled the divide between European principles of hygiene and Javanese building practices. I should point out that his suggestion of this ideal type covered not just plague (like the regulations issued by van Gorkom) but also other diseases that might be checked within the house. The director of public works for his part argued that instead of sidelining his department, de Vogel might profitably consider handing over this archive to "where it more properly belongs."[143]

Exactly *why* the hiring of a single architectural adviser was so contentious when the plague service already employed thousands of laborers is unclear.

The Department of Public Works was deeply involved in other facets of domestic reform in urban areas, however, and may have had a reputation to uphold.[144] Other architects and engineers were also critical of home improvement by the BGD. Articles in the Dutch professional journal *De Ingenieur* contained occasional gibes, for instance, and at a meeting of Indies engineers in 1918 participants spoke of the "horrid things" that plague physicians had done to building codes by their "too detailed interference."[145] Ultimately, the perseverance of de Vogel was rewarded. On January 30, 1919, the governor-general approved the hiring of this *inspecteur-technicus* for the BGD. Soon after, the young architect Henri Maclaine Pont (incidentally a nephew of de Vogel) joined the plague control work.[146] Well known for blending Javanese and art deco styles in his designs, Maclaine Pont traveled widely across Java to investigate various local housing styles and develop strategies to protect them from infiltration by the rat. In lectures, he suggested that it was necessary to instill in the Javanese a *desire* for home improvement, a desire that could be fostered by designing homes according to European hygienic standards but constructing them with native designs and materials.[147] City and *kampong* planning likewise ought to take cognizance of traditional Javanese values, such as a desire to reside near one's parents.[148] In contrast to his uncle's praise of the quasi-European landscapes that home improvement left in its wake, Maclaine Pont was critical of the ways in which the Dutch had eroded Javanese architecture. Instead, he romanticized the indigenous dwelling for attaining "perfect harmony between building shape and landscape."[149] With regard to plague, Maclaine Pont's concern was less with bamboo itself than with the way it was used.

When the FEATM met in Batavia in 1921, Maclaine Pont lectured at length on the "anti-plague bamboo constructions" he had designed over the last two years. Delegates later visited the ongoing home improvement work near Wonosobo. Committed to recuperating the bamboo house, Maclaine Pont lavished praise on this "most surprising material in the world." To those "who do not know how to handle it" bamboo could be a "disappointing" building material, but the bamboo-literate societies of Southeast Asia "cannot do without it." In the last ten years, he reminisced, plague had elicited new objections against the use of "our" material. Diverse methods to ratproof the traditional Javanese house using bamboo had been dismissed as ineffective, laborious, or too damaging to preserve the integrity of the material. Was it truly impossible to have European standards of hygiene converge with Javanese material culture? Maclaine Pont emphatically denied this. His various adaptations were demonstrated in "a little house" that delegates could inspect outside the conference venue. From the outside, the structure had the appearance of a spacious bungalow, covered by a heavy-looking *joglo*-shaped roof covered with tiles. A photograph taken from the inside, meanwhile, reveals a startlingly complex support frame of intertwining straight and curved bamboo laths.[150] Mesmerizing, artistic, and perhaps even ratproof, we may readily assume that the structure did not live up to the more practical requirements of the DP.[151] In fact, at the first Volkshuisvestingscongres in Semarang in 1922, Maclaine Pont had a public disagreement with Otten over whether houses could be made ratproof while retaining the Javanese *limasan* roof.[152]

After being let go by the BGD at the end of 1923, Maclaine Pont continued his defense of traditional Javanese house designs and materials. Indeed, he went so far as to construct a model bamboo house in his own backyard in Batavia. While his grander designs would not be adopted, some of his more practical contributions apparently did come into use. For one, he designed a nail with a flat point that did less damage to bamboo poles and reduced the chance of creating new openings for rats to gain entry into their hollow interior.[153] He also adopted the Javanese practice of impregnating bamboo in seawater, which he claimed would increase its lifespan.[154] A more modest ratproofed bamboo model house designed by Maclaine Pont featured prominently at the second Volkshuisvestingscongres in Semarang in 1925. And perhaps the most powerful vindication of the bamboo house by this architect was the specially designed neighborhood Sawahan in Soerabaja, built for employees of the Semarang-Cheribon Steam Tram Company. Its fifty "rat-free" homes were constructed almost entirely out of bamboo and roofed with a mixture of bark and plaster that resembled *atap*. Their roof design was downright edgy, the shape being somewhere between that of a *limasan* and an anvil.[155]

The design of a ratproof house made of "indigenous" materials remained an ambition of the plague service after its reintegration with the BGD in 1924. Following the departure of Maclaine Pont, further experiments with model houses were continued once more by physicians instead of engineers. For instance, at the next meeting of the FEATM in Singapore, H. Vervoort spoke about his efforts to construct a ratproof dwelling in Medan after a small outbreak of plague in Sumatra. The goal, stressed this physician, was to come up with a design that "disturbed as little as possible the uses and customs of the native population." Though he admitted that home improvement was somewhat antithetical to this principle, it was evidently a "splendid" control method against plague. The principal objection among the population to overcome, acknowledged Vervoort, was "the change in the form of the house, i.e., the prescription of a saddle-shaped roof covered with tiles." To meet this concern, his efforts had concentrated on designing a house with a hipped roof covered with *atap* that had been made ratproof by lining the edges with zinc alongside other interventions—and featuring a wooden frame.[156]

No less than twenty-one photographs and figures of Vervoort's design accompanied his paper. Strikingly, he included a series of images of house models built to scale. As with some of the photographs discussed in chapter 1, it feels as if these houses have been subjected to a clinical or anatomical gaze. Set against a black background, the photographer has either adopted a wide angle to capture these models as a whole or zoomed in on a particular feature such as the roof construction or its cover. Previously, photographs had helped to identify what made the traditional bamboo house "plague dangerous"; others such as these emphasized the interventions that rendered them "plague resistant"— their healthy anatomy, so to speak. A similar argument could be made for some of the photographs of home improvement taken by the physician G. M. Versteeg, which I discuss further in the next chapter.[157] Likewise, their quasi-anatomical focus on "infected" or renovated building parts reflected the trained gaze of their producers and sought to convey a sense of objectivity and professionalism. They demonstrated expertise and, in the case of Maclaine Pont and Vervoort, also sought to reflect an ethical approach by displaying Dutch consideration for local practices. For all of the models discussed here, however, the question remains how many of them were ultimately built.

Conclusion

In the decade following the outbreak of plague in East Java, Dutch health officials fine-tuned their response to the disease. Other control measures were abandoned in favor of home improvement that sought to increase the distance between the plague host—the house rat—and humans. The scale and scope of this intervention gradually increased, however, as plague expanded westward. In response, plague control was placed in the hands of a dedicated organization that concentrated on the identification, renovation, and inspection of plague-dangerous dwellings. While the BGD had continued to rely on the regulated use of bamboo for the improvement work, the DP all but prohibited its use. The *atap* roof cover was likewise prohibited. The replacement of these ubiquitous construction materials placed new pressures on the availability of timber and more especially of tiles: requiring the creation of new industries wherever plague reared its head. These challenges became increasingly acute when the disease reached Central Java, prompting a desire to return to the regulated use of native construction materials while adhering to the goal of breaking human-rat cohabitation.

The impact of plague control on the Javanese landscape and Javanese material culture was tremendous. The "idyllic" bamboo house that seamlessly merged into its environment had disappeared from plague-stricken districts and had been replaced by a uniform, red-tiled structure that stood out clearly from the landscape and fell firmly within the purview of the colonial state. Home improvement not only eliminated unique Javanese roof designs wherever it went but also struck a blow to traditional crafts and woodwork practices. "Plague control," lamented one author, "was almost as bad for Javanese art as the disease is for humans." Carved wooden doorframes, posts, and walls were demolished, while "truckloads" of ornamental objects ended as firewood and had to be replaced with "inferior factory goods."[158] Almost on a side note, the *Koloniaal Verslag* of 1917 reported that the outbreak of plague in the historic city of Soerakarta "had necessitated the reconstruction of the vast majority of this city of 130,000 souls."[159] And what of the social impact? Given the increasingly strict regulations for house construction, the *tukang kayu* who designed and built Java's iconic roofs could no longer practice their trade. Traditional markers of rank, class, status, and gender were removed. Opportunities for less financially solvent members of the community to supplement their income by preparing woven bamboo mats or baking roof tiles were diminished. Hundreds of thousands of homeowners were forced into debts they could ill afford to repay. Finally, home construction had previously been a communal affair that relied on neighborship and local materials. The plague regulations eroded such conventions and relations, and placed new financial and regulatory pressures on the population.[160]

Crucially, it became recognized that permanent home improvement was less important to plague control than altering the behavior of the inhabitants. Even homes that only received acute improvement would remain free of plague if the residents could be induced to inspect their homes for the presence of rats and nests in a weekly cleaning. This social or behavioral facet of plague control was perhaps as invasive as the intervention in the built environment itself. Plague propaganda seeking to instruct the Javanese on "how to inhabit the home" is explored in chapter 4. But first, I turn to an examination of how the spectacle of home improvement was sold to local, metropolitan, and foreign audiences as an outflow of magnanimous colonial rule.

CHAPTER 3

The Spectacle of Home Improvement

> We stopped to visit many villages on our return
> journey. The stupendous undertaking of rebuilding
> many towns is indeed impressive, but I cannot help but
> feel that the Dutch have not shown that foresight and
> intelligence with which they have so successfully
> attacked other problems.
>
> —Victor Heiser, diary, 1926

Plague control made a profound impression on
the built and natural environment of Java. Between 1911 and 1942, some 1.6
million houses were renovated or rebuilt. It was an operation that required
tens of thousands of laborers, overseers, and inspectors. Home improvement
demanded the cultivation of large quantities of wood and bamboo, and the
creation of new industries such as sawmills and potteries to produce uncounted
tons of timber and millions—billions—of roof tiles. The entire process must
have been a sight to behold, and accordingly it was extensively documented.
This chapter explores how home improvement was represented and to whom
it was displayed, both photographically and in person.

The previous chapters have discussed two photographs of Javanese landscapes featuring houses that had been "improved" in the name of plague control. The burned *dessa* Banjak had been rebuilt before the epiphany regarding
human-rat cohabitation within the traditional bamboo house had occurred
(chapter 1, figure 1.2). It was consequently rebuilt using customary native building materials and designs. What gives the village away as having been improved
at all is the orderly grid pattern in which it was laid out. Soon, these houses
would have been regarded as "plague dangerous" once more. The subsequently
improved village Banjak, on the other hand, featured houses that had been made
explicitly "rat proof" (chapter 2, figure 2.1). They were built primarily of wood
and roofed with red tiles, to exude a quasi-European atmosphere.

When photographs of traditional and improved dwellings were placed beside one another they created a powerful contrast, a contrast that to European contemporaries signaled the difference between poverty or prosperity, immorality or vice, and disease or health. The sight of traditional houses or indeed villages undergoing this transformation thus served as a visual affirmation of the new "ethical" course in Dutch colonial governance—even as it reminded the viewer of the continued need thereof. Home improvement thus served functions beyond mere plague control. The intervention constituted a performance of Dutch cultural superiority, scientific acumen, and colonial ability, as well as a government commitment to its young civilizing mission. Its audience was lay and professional, Javanese, Dutch, and international. Photographs and tours (for select audiences) of sites that had been subjected to "improvement" conveyed a compelling vision of Dutch colonial modernity. Home improvement, in short, was quite a spectacle.

Ethics, Epidemics, Spectacle

Over the course of writing this book, I have identified approximately 650 unique photographs of plague and plague control in Java. Of these, 350 contain a reference to the built environment in one way or another—and nearly 300 document home improvement directly. These photographs were taken by a cast of Dutch and Indies individuals, of whom Gerard Martinus Versteeg was by far the most prolific. As a physician with the plague service (DP) between 1919 and 1931 (and director of plague control for Central Java after 1928) he took over 150 photographs of houses, landscapes, and building features before, during, and after improvement.[1]

As part of the larger collection of plague photographs, the images of home improvement fall within the remit of a visual genre that the anthropologist Christos Lynteris calls "epidemic photography."[2] These photographs encompass the entirety of social and natural life that surrounds an outbreak of infectious disease, and in Java specifically reveal a vivid concern with the role of the built environment in the epidemiology of plague.[3] In a similar vein, several of these photographs appear a continuation of the quasi-anatomical photographs that first implicated the traditional bamboo dwelling in plague transmission back in 1911 (chapter 1, figure 1.3). They bear a resemblance to photographs that belong to the older genre of medical photography that documented patients or their symptoms. In this case, however, the plague house was substituted for the plague patient (who remained visually marginalized in Java) to cast *it* as the pathogenic body in need of treatment.

Alternatively, it could be argued that this subset belongs to another photographic genre entirely. The *camera ethica* proposed by the historian Susie Protschky refers to a diverse group of photographs that captured how the Dutch colonial reform period after 1900—sweepingly referred to as the *ethische politiek*—"was photographically envisioned." These photographs captured the various and sometimes competing ways in which local state agents sought to implement or represent ethical policies "on the ground," and the ways in which a broader segment of the Indies population used photography to portray its own ideas about "modernity" and "prospects for social change."[4] From this perspective, photographs of home improvement are sources that shed light on Dutch professional visions in rural Java of what the historian Ruth Rogaski might refer to as "hygienic modernity."[5]

Both of these analytical prisms yield key insights into the production and consumption of scenes of home improvement, but neither appears to capture their significance in full. If this collection is read purely as epidemic photography, the pervasive colonial overtones remain neglected. These photographs did more than rearticulate the role of the house in plague transmission or evince the existence of a peculiarly Javanese plague ecology. Arguably, they had already achieved this by 1912. Examined through the lens of the *camera ethica*, meanwhile, these images are certainly revealing of local visions of modern and responsible governance. But photographs of home improvement do not just provide more or less accidental insights into how state agents negotiated ethical ideals in practice. Rather, they were part of a targeted and sustained campaign to promote home improvement to diverse lay and specialist audiences. Above all, I suggest, scenes of home improvement ought to be studied as a form of Dutch self-representation of colonial and scientific ability in the modern age.

A more suitable analytic frame that puts the performative quality of home improvement at its center derives from the study of colonial spectacle. In particular, one might draw on scholarship on the world fairs and colonial exhibitions that were popular at the turn of the nineteenth and twentieth centuries. These events, after all, were all about self-representation.[6] The historian Marieke Bloembergen has aptly referred to the Dutch contribution to such exhibitions as a *koloniale vertoning*, a double entendre that translates as a "colonial display" or "presentation," with overtones of being staged, dramatic, or exaggerated. Indeed, the Dutch participation in these events was a *vertoning* in itself. Indies exhibitions—within the Netherlands and abroad—created a mirage of imperial significance that could endure only thanks to the tolerance of its competitors. Nonetheless, argues Bloembergen, these events are revealing of the tensions and shifting objectives within ongoing debates about the nature of Dutch colonial rule. The questions she asks about their purpose hold similar relevance for the widely disseminated scenes of home improvement in Java. Were they really "about the Indies, about colonial relations, or about the Netherlands" itself?[7]

The colonial spectacle—whether it was a *vertoning* or not—may be defined as a performance or display of imperial power toward one or multiple audiences, in which cultural and racial hierarchies between colonizer and colonized are visually established within a single moment or frame.[8] Events such as the Delhi Durbar, where Indian princes paid homage to a British monarch, or a "native" performance at a European exhibition, "set the world up like a picture" and invited the viewer to study it as a symbolic representation of the world's "cultural and colonial order."[9] Colonial spectacles informed a process of exoticizing or otherwise articulating "difference."[10] They shocked and beguiled its consumers. In other words, they helped to establish new conventions of seeing by offering a "calculated realism" in which "the gaze renders the other distinct and separate from the self."[11] Photographs helped to entrench such conventions: practically (by reproducing spectacle for audiences elsewhere) and conceptually (through its persistent claims to provide objective representations of the real).[12] Scholars have on occasion argued for the agency of indigenous participants in their own (re)presentation, though the finer nuances of their performance may have been lost on colonial and metropolitan populations immersed in narratives of racial and cultural hierarchy.[13] And if colonial relations of power were indeed visually established in scenes of home improvement in Java, it is important to emphasize that this spectacle was far from illusory. On the contrary: it was grounded in a very real and very *material* expansion of Dutch colonial power and cultural influence.

In this chapter, I argue that home improvement was to a significant extent not about plague control at all. Rather, home improvement offered Dutch health actors an opportunity to "perform colonial modernity" by putting this health intervention on display to an obliging audience of lay countrymen and foreign specialists.[14] Home improvement offered a highly visible intervention against a historically loaded disease. And though slow, it was also effective. But just as importantly, home improvement helped to reaffirm both cultural hierarchies in Java and the international political order by demonstrating Dutch colonial ability and scientific acumen in the context of a new (and poorly defined) civilizing mission.[15]

Photographs of Home Improvement

Photographs of home improvement in Java are themselves far from uniform. They document houses, streets, or villages, include people or not, are candid or staged, and document houses in various stages of (de)construction. A house "laid open" with its roof removed was a particularly popular theme.[16] Here, however, I explore two types of images that stand out for their more explicitly performative qualities: the "before and after" shot and the "tableau vivant."

Before and After

In the hundreds of photographs related to plague in Java, the patient is remarkably absent. There may be all of a dozen photographs of visibly sick individuals. This was unlike other diseases. Patients with leprosy or yaws were readily photographed, for instance, often in various stages of the disease, or over the course of receiving treatment. But medical science needs medical bodies, and in both visual and textual sources on plague in Java it is as though the house was effectively substituted for the patient. *It* was sick. Photography, as I previously argued, successfully documented its pathology and helped to rearticulate its role in plague transmission. And unlike the human plague patient, the house was amenable to treatment. The traditional bamboo dwelling could be subjected to a visibly efficacious curative as well as prophylactic operation that effectively removed its pathogenicity—in the form of rats and nests—to human occupants.

From the outset, photographs of this operation—home improvement—adopted a before-and-after format that contrasted the "plague-dangerous" with the "plague-resistant" house. Already in the first Dutch plague reports published in the *Mededeelingen van den Burgerlijken Geneeskundigen Dienst in Nederlandsch-Indië* (*Mededeelingen*) of 1912, photographs of rat-infested building features were placed beside images of the interventions that rendered them ratproof. Alternatively, we recognize this contrast in photographs of the burned, rebuilt, and improved *dessa* Banjak.[17] The deployment of this genre is not surprising. In his captivating book, *The Afterlife of Images*, Ari Larissa Heinrich observed its utility to medical missionaries in nineteenth-century China who sought to demonstrate the superiority of European scientific medicine (or demonstrate the potential of their labors to audiences back home)—and we encounter it in other colonial contexts too.[18] Photographs of "natives" with grotesque tumors, advanced filariasis, or unsightly yaws *before* treatment were powerfully contrasted with happy, healthy, and productive "individuals" *after* surgery or medication.[19]

These before-and-after shots not only reaffirmed racial and cultural difference but also rendered such difference amenable to treatment.[20] A sanitized, hygienic, and at times quasi-European subject replaced the native.[21] The genre was used in Europe itself too, for instance as evidence of how philanthropic initiatives could transform "vagrants" into "workmen."[22] These powerful visual contrasts, and the uses to which they could be put, would have been familiar to Dutch physicians in the Indies. Building on my previous analysis of the anatomic photography of the plague house, I suggest that the analogy of the house-as-body—or: the medicalization of the traditional Javanese house—persisted in subsequent photographs of home improvement. That is to say, after first diagnosing the ills of the house, photographs next documented its treatment.

SOERABAJA (I)

The earliest before-and-after photographs of home improvement come from Soerabaja. They are part of a group of seven photographs in the Arsip Nasional in Jakarta that can be identified as "plague photographs" by the presence (in three of them) of a flag embossed with the initials of the ASGC. Two were reproduced in a volume of *Kromoblanda* by the philanthropist H. F. Tillema, who credited them to Johannes Terburgh, involved with this organization.[23] As a public/private home improvement initiative active between 1911 and 1913, it is conceivable that these photographs were taken with an eye toward fostering civic pride—but perhaps more likely they accompanied repeated requests for financial support to the colonial government. Four photographs contain traditional houses in a poor state of repair. They fail to make a specific connection to plague or rat breeding and instead emphasize their overall unsanitary state. The occupants are seated or crouched in front of their dwellings in poses that apparently seek to convey a sense of resignation. One photograph discussed below captures a flurry of reconstruction work. The remaining two document the same house: before and after the ASGC came along.

The first image shows a house in a fairly spacious neighborhood (figure 3.1). It is built of bamboo poles, woven bamboo mats, wood, roof tiles, and *atap*. The bricolage of building materials does the structure few favors. Evidently, it has seen better days. The tiled part of the roof is uneven. The *gedek* has holes in it, and parts have become undone. Indeed, at the center of the image one mat has given way entirely to reveal a mixture of building materials crisscrossing behind it. The occupants, presumably a Javanese woman and her son, are seated on the doorstep. The grounds around the house are crowded with objects. An old *balé-balé*, a large water jar, a cup on a bamboo stick, baskets, and cooking utensils are scattered in the foreground. In the background we see more of the same, and all the way at the back there is a fence sagging dangerously toward the side. The scene may remind us of the observation that, in Hong Kong, plague was seen to exist in relation to a host of "indescribable" Chinese objects that "troubled colonial administrators as a source of likely infection."[24] Despite advances in understanding the nature and etiology of plague since 1894, the

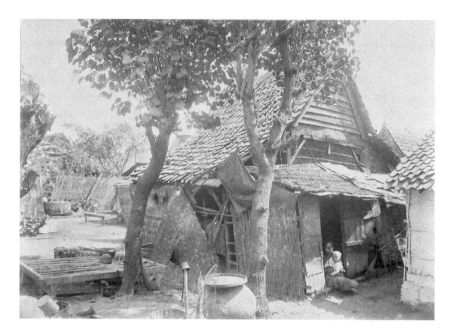

FIGURE 3.1.   Photograph of a house before improvement in Soerabaja, ca. 1911–1913.
Courtesy of ANRI.

emphasis in this image on "junk" tied in to enduring European associations between clutter, disorder, immorality, poverty, and disease.

At a glance, the "after" photograph reveals that the ASGC did not limit its antiplague intervention to the house alone (figure 3.2). Yes, the building has been thoroughly renovated. The roof has been repaired and the *atap* part replaced with tiles. The front door has been moved. New, neatly painted double walls of bamboo matting have been installed, with shutters that allow the outer layer to be opened for ventilation while maintaining privacy. Even the ASGC flag has been improved. It is no longer a monochrome limply draped over the side of the house, but a tricolor gently waving from a corner of the house. The woman and her child are seated directly underneath it, in a symbolic gesture of guardianship that is difficult to imagine as accidental. The pair appear to be wearing better-quality clothing, and in particular the boy's cap stands out. The grounds have been cleared, only the water jar remains. Curiously, its lid has been removed, making it amenable to mosquito breeding. The set consequently sends a conflicted message about public health, one in which evident neatness to counter plague was apparently worth emphasizing more than water storage discipline to counter malaria. The point is worth dwelling on, as home improvement was later recognized as facilitating malaria transmission (chapter 5). For

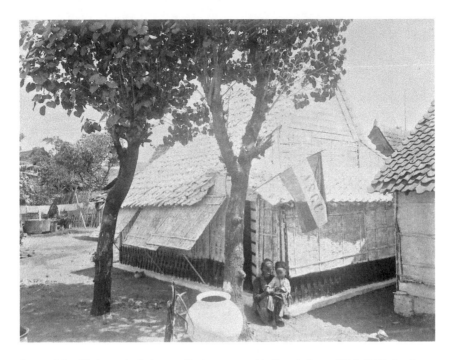

FIGURE 3.2. Photograph of a house after improvement in Soerabaja, ca. 1911–1913. Courtesy of ANRI.

now, we may conclude by observing that in the background of this "after" shot the fence in the background has been provided with an additional—bamboo—support post, while freshly laundered clothes have been put out to dry.

Health, neatness, morality, domesticity: these are themes that pervade this set of images. A direct reference to plague is absent. While subsequent photographs of home improvement tended to have an implicit focus on wood, bamboo, or *atap* to remind the viewer of the assumptions that underpinned the mass renovations, such cues are not readily apparent here. Instead, their creator rehearsed a familiar theme of nineteenth-century public health and urban philanthropy transposed to a Javanese context. They present disease, poverty, and vice (in the form of dirt, clutter, and porosity), and health, wealth, and virtue (in the form of order and cleanliness) as cyclical, mutually reinforcing principles. The "communicative elegance" of the before-and-after shot rested in such contrasts, which testified to the importance of the work done by the ASGC off camera.[25] The medical gaze is present too, not in pathologizing the house directly as a vehicle of plague but in offering an outmoded perspective on the cause and control of disease. Here, hygienic esthetics trump scientific medicine.

KALIKADJAR

Several photographs of home improvement sought to capture the contrast between the traditional and the improved dwelling in a single shot. One such
photograph dates back to 1919, for instance, when the DP was operating at full
capacity.[26] Two houses stand beside each other, and two European officials pose
in front of the house on the left: an impressive display of Javanese design and
craftmanship. The thatched roof, crowned with a metal ornament, towers above
them. To the left, in the shadow of the front gallery, stand three Javanese assistants and/or residents. Unlike in the previous set, this traditional house is in
good condition: sturdy, with an even roof cover, intact *gedek*, and a roof supported by wooden posts. It is only to the trained eye of contemporaries that the
dwelling was a harbinger of plague. The shape and material of the roof had long
since been implicated as conducive to rat breeding. On closer inspection, we
notice that the inner frame is made of bamboo—and if anyone needed remind-
ing of the potential of this material to shelter rats, they only had to look at the
hollow opening of two imposing pieces that happen to be present in the foreground of the image. Finally, a doorway reveals a dark interior. But to the right
of this structure stands its "improved" counterpart. It is smaller, featuring a tiled
saddle-shaped roof, no longer adorned with Javanese metalwork. Through the
front door we look inside and see a window in the back. We notice its solid
wooden frame, the smaller pieces of sealed-off bamboo that support a single
layer of matted walls. The open space above the doorway is presumably intended for better ventilation and the removal of smoke.

The photograph was taken by Gerard Martinus Versteeg—physician, photographer, and prolific diarist active with the DP between 1919 and 1931—at
Kalikadjar in Central Java and had a significant afterlife. It was part of an album
by Versteeg accompanied by the description: "Tikelan at Kalikadjar covered
with *idoek*. Assistent-Resident Kastelijn and Dr. Fischmann." The photograph
was subsequently reproduced in an unidentified album with the caption "Unimproved Javanese kampong house (plague control)."[27] It featured in a third album
as part of a photographic collage offered to League of Nations health officials
who met in Bandoeng in 1930, with the English-language caption: "(Left) an old
plague dangerous house and (right) a rat proof house."[28] Furthermore, a glass
positive slide found its way into the collection of Paul Christiaan Flu, a professor
of hygiene at the University of Leiden, who catalogued it simply as "unimproved
and improved house."[29] Each of these descriptions left things unsaid but also
help to identify an expanding audience. Versteeg describes his photograph in
specialist terms by referring to the technical aspects of the house. The *tikelan*
was a variety of *joglo* roof shape that was explicitly banned. *Idoek* referred to

an organic roof cover made of woven strands of plant fiber. Its more generic descriptions elsewhere suggest how the image came to serve other purposes. Flu would have used it to instruct medical students and civil servants bound for the Indies. The English-captioned collage presented Dutch plague control to an audience of foreign medical experts. Other captions suggest how the image was used to woo a broader audience with the need for home improvement by comparing the monumental (old, unimproved, dangerous) building on the left, with the more modest (new, ratproof) dwelling on the right.

The contrast captured by Versteeg created a more nuanced spectacle than the previous set. It is less moralistic and more in tune with the medico-scientific rationale for home improvement. The house on the left retained a certain ethnographic grandeur that was—tragically—pathological. The house on the right displayed the tremendous but necessary and ethical intervention by Dutch state agents in the name of plague control. The spectacular nature of this intervention was enhanced by the comparisons. In the collage in particular, this photograph functioned as a centerpiece: offset by photographs of houses before improvement, "work in progress" scenes, and allegedly unimprovable "mud houses." The collage as a whole conveys something of the process and complexity of the home improvement scheme, while this image specifically demonstrated its tremendous impact. In one shot, it captures not only the contrast between the traditional and the modern, the ethnic and the European, and the violence done by the latter to the former in the name of health, but also the social, racial, and cultural hierarchies seen (or desired to be seen) to exist between them.

Tableau Vivant

The composed and static before-and-after photographs of home improvement find their counterpart in the messier, active genre of the tableau vivant or "living picture." The photographs I collected under this label stand out for their supposedly candid displays of activity. Some contain just a handful of people; others evoke the grand scale at which home improvement was pursued. At the same time, they appear to convey an esthetic of labor: of productivity in the face of pathogenic adversity, or of a Protestant work ethic (not unlike that on display in the famous *Men at Work* series by Lewis Hine) set in the tropics.[30] Any thoughts of plague proper are pushed away by the sight of people participating in the act of "inspecting spaces" or "building things." The omnipresent white-clad colonial official in this genre conveys his own message: that the Javanese could not be trusted to execute this scheme without European training or oversight. Consequently, civilizational hierarchies are again in evidence, though overall these tableaux appear to foreground "collaboration" rather than "surveillance."

SOERABAJA (II)

The earliest photograph that captured these dynamics was again produced in Soerabaja (figure 3.3). It shows a street with several houses that are all reno- vated at once. A *mantri* inspector poses at the center, standing amid various articles of furniture. But before we set eyes on him, our gaze is drawn toward two men that stand directly overhead on the frame of a stripped-down house. They appear to hold in place a central support post, while one of them looks over his shoulder toward the photographer. Just to their left, a man seated on the beams is manipulating a flag of the ASGC (see chapter 2). Behind them, no fewer than five people inspect the roofs of houses deeper inside the neighbor- hood. Two have shielded their eyes and peer at the roof cover, while the figure furthest to the right again looks toward the photographer over his shoulder. Left of center, the upper half of the image features more houses in the distance that are having work done on their roofs, with one more laborer or resident standing on the roof of a house from which several tiles have been removed.

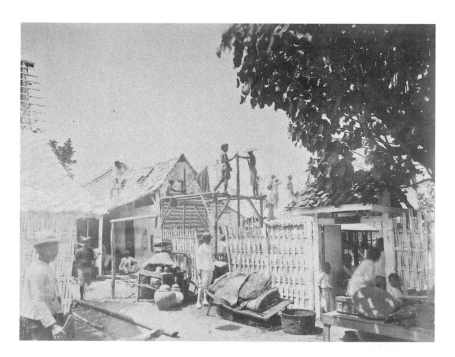

FIGURE 3.3. Photograph of home improvement in Soerabaja, ca. 1911–1913. Courtesy of ANRI.

In the street below, there is a small crowd of people who are mostly blurred. In the corner on the right, women and children are looking at the photographer. People moving in between them appear to be carrying household items outside. On the left, toward the back, we see a man seated inside the front gallery of a house and observing the street scene. Closer toward us, a man has just appeared around the corner of the house. Despite the blur, we can make out that he is carrying a pole of some sort over his left shoulder. As with the photographs from Soerabaja previously discussed, there appear to be few references to plague directly. Without the flag, we would not know the context of these renovations. Then again, there appear to be some other telltale features that might date this photograph to after the identification of the role of the house in plague transmission. Beside the *mantri* stands the potentially hazardous *balé-balé*. In front of him lies a large bamboo beam with the hollow part facing us. And finally, there is the strong visual emphasis on the roofs— which had been implicated as a likely space of rat nesting early on.

Was the scene staged? Perhaps, or perhaps in part. The white-clad *mantri* at the center is the only figure obviously posing. The blurred people at street level would suggest a candid snapshot. From left to right, however, the people on the roofs are all in remarkably sharp focus given that their poses suggest movement. Regardless, it appears the photograph may have circulated and survived in part because of what it could be understood to convey: industry and civic harmony in response to a serious threat to health and economy in Java's largest port city. As mentioned in chapter 2, the ASGC quickly ran out of funds and submitted requests for assistance to the central government. Photographs such as these may have accompanied them. The initial quarantine imposed on Soerabaja in May 1911 had prompted government officials, mercantile elites, and private individuals to join hands in an attempt to improve housing conditions across the city—with visible result. It was a shame, really, that it took an outbreak of plague to achieve it.

Temanggoeng

The photograph that suggested the label of the "living picture" dates to February 1930 (figure 3.4). It depicts a group of white-clad health officials standing in the middle of a large construction site. These European men are busy conferring and gesturing—frozen in movement, except for the blur around the hands of the man in the grey suit. Javanese laborers move in the foreground and inside the construction on the right, while several local women are standing at the back. For a moment it seems as though one is watching the opening scene of a play. The stage is set, the actors are in place, the curtain rises, the tableau is

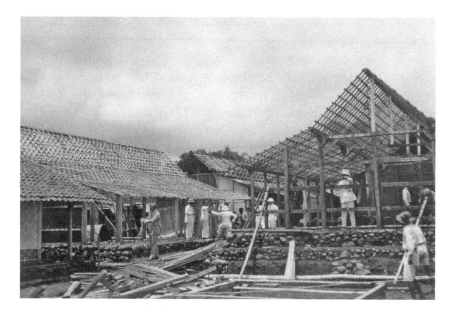

FIGURE 3.4.   Photograph of members of the League of Nations' Advisory Council to the Eastern Bureau inspecting home improvement in Temanggoeng, 1930. TM-60041409. Courtesy of the Nationaal Museum van Wereldculturen.

revealed, and presently all may burst into motion. This theatrical illusion is heightened by the layering of the set, if you will, with the center still unoccupied for a protagonist to enter. A similar atmosphere permeates a second photograph of slightly lesser quality documenting the same scene from a different angle, now featuring workmen climbing ladders, working on a roof, and preparing building materials.[31] It is an illusion, of course, though one that underscores the performative quality of the home improvement scheme as a whole. In fact, the men at the center may have been less inclined toward any such posturing than others. The men in this photograph are members of the Advisory Council to the Eastern Bureau, a regional health organization of the League of Nations. Following the above-mentioned meeting in Bandoeng, the DVG took delegates on a tour along sanitary institutions in Java. Here, they have arrived in the district Temanggoeng to examine home improvement in practice.[32]

The photograph—which appears candid—again conveys an esthetic of productivity: a vision of industry to counter the threat of plague that could, furthermore, be confidently displayed "in the flesh" to a foreign specialist audience. The scale of this particular site is impressive, as an entire village appears to be in the process of improvement all at once. Once again there is little to remind us of plague directly, except for the designs and the construction materials used. On the other hand, the prominent League of Nations health official Frederick

Norman White had already declared that home improvement and plague control were "synonymous" in Java as early as 1923.[33] And likewise, as I demonstrate below, Dutch contemporaries were frequently exposed to the scene of houses in various stages of reconstruction in response to plague. In effect, the renovations themselves were reference enough to plague.

These and other tableaux documenting plague control conveyed the tremendous scale and complexity of the home improvement scheme. They alternatively focused on the identification of plague-dangerous housing elements, the renovations themselves, or for instance the subsequent cleaning and inspection of improved villages.[34] They tell little about what happened outside the frame of the photograph, however, and excluded the opposition to this intervention that textual sources occasionally hint at. Rather, scenes such as these from Soerabaja around 1912 and Temanggoeng in 1930 foregrounded a modern and efficient government service endowed with comprehensive oversight of the people and places it needed to rule. They were scenes of a government capable of organizing a systematic intervention in the built and natural environment of Java on a grand scale. Spectacular scenes. Scenes that demanded an audience.

Audiences of Home Improvement

Home improvement grew into the signature health intervention of the Dutch colonial period. From its inception in 1911, the scheme was broadcast to national and international audiences as the most permanent response to plague in Java. The Dutch may have been late to the party in terms of plague research but, as one physician put it, theirs would be the only country "in which the consequences of the rat-flea-man transmission system were accepted in their entirety" and were translated in a systematic attempt to widen the distance between humans and rats.[35] In the realm of plague control, Dutch health officials fancied, they came out on top. Photographs of home improvement found their way into lectures, fairs, and exhibitions that targeted lay and specialist audiences alike. And, as we have seen, they went beyond mere representation by taking foreign visitors on tour to see home improvement in action. Home improvement was the poster child of colonial healthcare in the Dutch reform period.

Audiences in the Netherlands

How was the Dutch public first acquainted with home improvement in Java? The method had a longer history in plague control elsewhere. In fact, Johannes van Loghem had supported this intervention in a paper published mere weeks before the disease was recognized in Malang in March 1911:

> The battle against plague must in the first place be a battle against the rat. He who has observed how closely, in the tropics, the native and the rat cohabitate will be convinced of the hopelessness of such an endeavor. The house rat finds in the unevenly built, poorly closed-off house, surrounded by waste materials, a safe and rich existence. If one wants to push out the rat, one has to build better homes.[36]

This would remain van Loghem's view for the rest of his life. The subsequent outbreak of plague in Java was feverishly reported on in the Dutch press, which began to expound on the role of the house in plague transmission from about October onward.[37] Home improvement was formally endorsed by colonial health officials with the publication of a series of plague reports in the *Mededeelingen* in 1912. But prior to this, a wider lay audience had already been introduced to the scheme. Soon after returning to the Netherlands, van Loghem embarked on a charm offensive of sorts to clarify to the Dutch public this approach to plague control.[38] Over the years, other physicians took up the cause, resulting in a uniquely sustained and multimediated advertisement campaign for this colonial health intervention.

Lectures

On January 25, 1912, van Loghem gave his first lecture on plague in Java at the Society for Public Welfare (Maatschappij tot Nut van 't Algemeen) in Amsterdam. His audience was primarily lay, but also included health officials and the prominent professor of public health Rudolph Saltet. Extensive press coverage informs us that van Loghem's lecture was accompanied by no fewer than a hundred lantern slides "for clarification." These images were not described, but it seems safe to assume they overlapped with those published in the *Mededeelingen* shortly after. Following remarks on plague's history, nature, and transmission, van Loghem turned to the role of the Javanese house rat. He concluded:

> The transmission of the disease from rat to man is only preventable by home improvement: this is currently implemented in Java at a large scale; it aims to prevent the nesting of the house rat inside the bamboo, behind wall coverings, in the dead space of the roof, and inside the baleh-baleh . . . which can be achieved by this method.[39]

Plague, according to van Loghem, could be prevented *only* by home improvement. The discovery of house rats inside the bamboo dwelling, he henceforth insisted, had reduced "the plague question" to "a question of housing."[40]

About the same time, van Loghem addressed more professional audiences. Early in January, he discussed the situation in Java with members of the Dutch Society of Tropical Medicine (Nederlandsche Vereeniging voor Tropische Geneeskunde).[41] In April, he addressed an international audience at a tropical medicine conference in Hamburg. His invitation to be the opening speaker, according to one newspaper, was "proof that interest in the things he can say about plague in Java is very great among German colleagues." Again, van Loghem explained how humans and rats cohabitated inside the traditional Javanese house: using many "excellent" photographs to illustrate his case. "Now," he was quoted as saying, plague could be fought "rationally" by improving houses "in such a way that no rat could live inside."[42] More lectures and publications in this vein followed, often framing home improvement as the more proper form of plague control—drawing a contrast to presumably inferior strategies pursued elsewhere. "In British India," for instance, van Loghem wrote in 1914, "one must in many regions, out of powerlessness to improve the [loam] dwellings, resort to the less efficacious method of vaccination."[43]

The centrality of images to these outputs was evident. In a lecture at the physics society Diligentia in 1915, van Loghem again used numerous photographs to support his argument on the role of the bamboo house in plague transmission:

> In a series of new lantern slides, the speaker showed us how the polluted condition of the Javanese dwelling and their curious bamboo constructions facilitate infection. The rat makes her entrance along the bamboo posts, gnaws . . . through the bamboo pole . . . until it is completely filled with rat nests where the young rats proliferate and multiply. . . . Curious were in particular the images of the native dwellings, where the speaker pointed out the holes gnawed by rats in bamboo poles, and even the wall next to the bed.[44]

The most direct control measures, van Loghem was paraphrased as saying, were evacuation, fumigation, and the construction of new dwellings designed to counter the presence of rats. Soon after, van Loghem spoke on plague for students affiliated with the society *Oost en West* at the University of Leiden. "Drawing on a long string of lantern slides," he argued that educating the population about plague transmission alone could not hope to hold the disease in check. Since the disease was now endemic among the rodent population of

Java, plague had become impossible to eradicate. The key to its control was to intervene in the conditions that allowed the disease to cross from rats to humans.[45]

Over the following decades, van Loghem maintained his defense of home improvement. A pamphlet on questions of Indies hygiene of 1920 reiterated his views and called on the "better organized" parts of the colony to enforce stricter building regulations even in the absence of plague.[46] Other promotional activities described below took place through the 1920s. And as late as 1937, van Loghem gave a keynote lecture at a joint meeting of the Royal Dutch Geographical Society (Koninklijk Nederlands Aardrijkskundig Genootschap), the Koloniaal Instituut, and Diligentia. Home improvement, he repeated, and in particular the substituting of bamboo building elements for wood, remained the surest way to break human-rat cohabitation in Java and disrupt the chain of plague transmission. Dwelling briefly on recent advances in vaccination, which reinforced the arsenal of short-term control methods, van Loghem concluded his talk "by once more stressing that improvement of the level of housing is a factor of the greatest importance."[47]

Over this thirty-year period, audiences in the Netherlands were treated to lectures on plague control by numerous other individuals. The primacy and efficacy of home improvement was rarely in question. In a lecture early in 1914, the Indies physician Tjipto Mangoenkoesoemo discussed plague control at the *Indische Vereeniging*. Having previously assisted the plague control work in Malang, Tjipto had subsequently been exiled to the Netherlands for his role in an Indies nationalist movement. Despite this experience, he praised home improvement as a plague control method in principle. It was its execution that he took issue with. The population resented the practice of evacuation, he said, while significant parts of the work had to be done by the population "in unpaid service," in addition to extra costs being placed on homeowners. Meanwhile, "nursing and treatment . . . are completely neglected."[48] At a seminar at the *Indisch Genootschap* in April 1915, speakers including Tillema argued that the high mortality figures in the Indies were grounded in poor housing conditions. Plague was a prominent example, and lantern slides demonstrated how rats infested "the common Javanese bamboo house." Sadly, they reflected, plague was the only health threat to prompt a concerted government response that focused on the house.[49] A year later, M. Hijmans, a physician attached to one of four Red Cross ambulances that were sent to Java in 1914 (see chapter 5), lectured on plague in Java at the Hygienic Society (*Hygienisch Genootschap*) before an audience of about eighty physicians. He too praised home improvement as one of the few interventions that might hold the disease in check. For the moment, Hijmans admitted, there was a considerable backlog of houses requiring improvement, forcing the DP to "take refuge in acute home and dessa cleaning."[50] In a two-part essay on the Red Cross mission accompanied by twenty-three photographs published in 1917, Hijmans again emphasized the durable outcomes of the home improvement scheme.[51]

A final example is provided by the Indies physician H. F. Lumentut, who spoke of plague control at the *Indisch Genootschap* in November 1921. His saccharine lecture was certainly more revealing of how Dutch and Indies health officials viewed their own labors—or how they sought to portray them—than of conditions on the ground. He began:

> While in Europe the Great War raged and its peoples tried to destroy each other, one had long since started a battle in Java against plague, an even more dangerous, callous foe than he who possesses hand grenades and artillery. . . . While at different fronts [in Europe], tough young men were killed by the thousands, [in Java] every means was used to return individual, moribund plague victims back to life. What a sharp contrast in our regard to the value of human life![52]

The remainder of his talk was just as romantic (not to say misleading) and lavished praise on the colonial health service. Eloquently, Lumentut took his audience on a tour of a plague-stricken district, describing picturesque landscapes, industrious assistants, and grateful, childlike villagers. The success of home improvement, naturally, was stressed throughout.

Exhibitions

From their number, distribution, and coverage in the press, it is clear that lectures on plague in Java were broadly popular in the Netherlands. The use of photographs and lantern slides said to clarify or illustrate the Dutch response to plague made these events accessible to a wider public. After 1920, the profile of home improvement steadily increased through a medium that hinged on the use of such and other visual materials, the exhibition. Through the 1910s, plague control had already featured at fairs in Java. Now, similar materials would be presented to Dutch audiences at hygiene fairs and Indies exhibitions in the Netherlands that capitalized on the success of the Dresden Hygiene Fair (1911) and the popularity of colonial exhibitions across Europe.[53] The ostensible purpose of these events was to disseminate knowledge about medicine and empire. Simultaneously, they were spaces where developments in these domains could be showcased to foreign audiences and foster national pride.

In 1921, the Dutch Red Cross organized an International Hygiene Exhibition (Internationale Hygiëne Tentoonstelling Amsterdam, IHTA) at the majestic

Palace of People's Industry (Paleis voor Volksvlijt) in Amsterdam.[54] The event sought to educate "the great masses" in the advances of scientific medicine by means of visual materials and prompt more hygienic behavior. The IHTA covered numerous health-related topics, with contributions from international partners that included the British War Office, the US Department of Health, and the Dresden Hygiene Museum.[55] The Koloniaal Instituut also contributed a display, curated by van Loghem, on the subject of tropical hygiene. It offered a snapshot of the most prominent diseases in the Dutch East Indies "with malaria at its center," and the methods by which they could be controlled. Plague—"the most formidable disease"—was naturally present. A reporter for *Algemeen Handelsblad* noted that lantern slides showing "rat nests in the most unlikely spaces of the dwelling" were "once again" present and especially noteworthy.[56] The method of plague and malaria control, reported another newspaper, "is impressed on visitors through photographs and exhibition objects."[57] These included mounted rats, depictions of pathogens, "the stereoscopic images that Professor van Loghem made on his last study tour through the Dutch East Indies," and a "model bacteriological laboratory."[58] The IHTA received a strong endorsement through a visit by the popular queen mother, Emma, who was said to be "particularly interested in the control of tuberculosis, tropical hygiene, and all other noteworthy displays."[59]

Afterward, the Red Cross converted the IHTA into the Traveling Hygiene Exhibition (Reizende Hygiëne-Tentoonstelling, RHT) to promote the insights of modern medicine to a larger (and ideally rural) audience. At a first trial exhibition, it became clear that many of the displays had been altered, condensed, or supplemented. But, reported one journalist:

> At a glance, we found ourselves in the company of familiar submissions. In the first place, there was the Tropical Hygiene section . . . introduced by van Loghem. . . . It offers a range of information on malaria, intestinal disease, plague, worm disease, yaws, leprosy, beriberi, smallpox, etc. One will see diagrams on spread and containment, cultures of plague, cholera, and other bacilli, preparations of diseased organs, fleas, rats, worms, photographs of patients, mosquitoes, hospitals, and last but not least the medicines, sera, and vaccines. A demonstration cabinet with stereoscopic photographs of plague, malaria, leprosy, smallpox, etc. that attracted so many visitors at the IHTA was again present.[60]

There is no specific mention of home improvement in this eclectic presentation. Given the strong visual focus of plague photography on the house, its centrality to plague control in Java, and the discursive emphasis on this intervention, however, images of home improvement were undoubtedly included.

The RHT reopened to the public in Amsterdam in March 1922. It was then moved to The Hague, where Queen Wilhelmina had offered the historic Gothic Hall (Gotische Zaal) as an exhibition space. The event was opened by the prince-consort, Hendrik, and subsequently awarded another visit by Emma. Over the next two years, the exhibition opened in Rotterdam, Tiel, Breda, Roosendaal, Assen, Maastricht, Alkmaar, Groningen, Dordrecht, Leiden, Vlissingen, Eindhoven, Leeuwarden, Den Helder, Utrecht, and Zaandam.[61] Little archival material of this tour remains, but judged by its prominent audience, geographic reach, and period of operation (all as reported in the press), the RHT was moderately successful in achieving its stated aims. In passing, a large Dutch audience became acquainted with some of the health work done in Java, including plague control.

Already in September 1923, the Dutch public had another opportunity to familiarize itself with health conditions in the Indies. In celebration of Wilhelmina's twenty-five-year regnal jubilee, the Koloniaal Instituut ran a special exhibition in its monumental new main building in Amsterdam.[62] A section on tropical hygiene was included in a large hall on the first floor. Several displays informed visitors about "the nature, spread, and control" of the leading diseases that haunted the colony. As for plague, a catalog informs us:

> Plague. (derives from the house rat; control by increasing distance between rat and man = "home improvement"). Diagrams; photographs; rats, etc.[63]

It is a marvelous fragment: the equals sign effectively reducing plague control to home improvement. To the Dutch, they were synonymous indeed. In another display, the curator highlighted the importance of housing to health more broadly. Its focus was on the Indies, but the theme would have resonated with visitors as cities in the Netherlands faced considerable housing shortages. Slum clearance and public housing initiatives were only just getting off the ground (and they were the subject of another section in this exhibition).[64] The display sought to stress that proper housing could tackle multiple health challenges at once:

> Home. (good living conditions counter leprosy, tuberculosis, pneumonia, encephalitis, eye diseases, venereal diseases, skin diseases, worm disease, and plague). Photographs and maps.[65]

This catalog entry, however, is problematic. Not only are we left to wonder about the exact mechanism by which proper housing countered venereal disease, but since housing reform was not pursued outside a handful of cities or beyond plague control, the suggestion thereof was, perhaps, disingenuous.[66]

Indeed, we may recall how the DP had explicitly *rejected* the suggestion of improving houses with an eye to diseases other than plague. Finally, a third display contained photographs and statistics related to the activities of the BGD that pertained to the control of "plague, yaws, smallpox, malaria, etc.," accompanied by a set of unspecified health education materials produced in the Indies.[67] The Jubilee Exhibition had wide popular appeal and reportedly drew 255,000 paying visitors.[68] As for Wilhelmina herself, she managed to crunch in a visit during a formal jubilee celebration in the capital—between the nautical pageant and the gala concert.[69]

I have identified no subsequent exhibitions in which plague and tropical hygiene occupied such a central position. Nevertheless, they were a recurring theme at various events. The Indies Exhibition in Arnhem of 1928, for instance, featured a small section on health and disease control. It contained a large poster explaining the rat-flea-man transmission scheme and photographs of rats' nests inside the traditional Javanese house that dated back to 1911.[70] The Indies Exhibition in The Hague of 1932 featured numerous materials that the Koloniaal Instituut had previously provided for the Paris Colonial Exposition of 1931. Included was a large section on tropical hygiene that paid special attention to leading diseases, such as malaria, smallpox, yaws, and of course plague. The materials taken over included diagrams and photographs that reportedly explained how plague control in the Indies focused on "widening the distance between man and rat."[71] Also on display were "giant model[s] of the malaria mosquito and the plague flea."[72] Meanwhile, a permanent exhibition on tropical hygiene curated by Flu had opened at the University of Leiden in 1931. Among other things, it informed visitors of "the improvements that must be made in house construction, in relation to the control of [plague]."[73] Finally, as one of the three constitutive branches of the Koloniaal Instituut, tropical hygiene was part of the permanent exhibition in its museum. In a photograph of this section from 1936, we see a large display case with five enlarged plague photographs that again dated back to the original outbreak in Malang in 1911. There is the rebuilt *dessa* Banjak, an evacuation camp, a *mantri* sorting rat skulls, an isolation barracks for pneumonic plague patients, and finally the "rat furnace" at the plague laboratory in Malang. Two displays further back, there is a large photograph of a Javanese house with a *joglo* roof—part, perhaps, of a section on home improvement?[74] Remarkably, even in the midst of World War II, the Instituut put on an exhibition on social care in the Dutch East Indies. In a photograph of the display on healthcare we notice that plague remained a prominent topic. To the right, we see a large photograph of a bamboo beam containing a rat nest. Beneath it, visitors could inspect two "improved" house models. The accompanying sign read, "Plague control, home improvement"—once more equating the two.[75]

FILM

If lectures, traveling exhibitions, museums, and newspapers failed to reach some audiences, then perhaps parts of Dutch society would finally learn about plague and plague control in the Indies through a medium with true mass appeal, film. Late in 1926, the physician J. J. van Lonkhuyzen, leader of the DVG, asked the well-known filmmaker Willy Muellens to produce what would become known as *the* plague film. The seventy-minute-long, three-part assemblage that resulted from this collaboration stands out as one of only a handful of films on plague among an otherwise vast visual archive.[76] It is a silent black-and-white film interspersed with Dutch and Malay subtitles. The film includes live-action shots, animated sequences, and various bits of static and animated scientific imagery. These elements conspire to explain the nature, transmission, and control of plague in Java since 1911. As a whole, however, *De pest op Java* is a curious blend of the ethnographic and the educational—as was observed when it came out.[77]

The plague film captured home improvement in motion pictures for the first and possibly last time. It contains long shots documenting various stages of the process. First comes the methodological dissection of the traditional Javanese house, which leads to the discovery of rats and nests hidden inside the bamboo beams and *atap* roofs. Next, the structure is unroofed, renovated, and finally inspected. Wide-angle shots of villages before improvement ("blending into the green background," as Willem de Vogel might put it) are contrasted with neatly tiled houses having undergone improvement. A Dutch newspaper commented:

> It is made clear, that the chief cause [of plague] rests within the defective housing conditions of the Javanese, as each house offers accessible nesting spaces for rats, the spreaders of the epidemic. Everywhere, where more modern houses arise, the disease reduces in intensity before our eyes.[78]

The natural history of plague, bacteriological investigations, medical treatment, and the role of rice in the "metastatic" spread of plague are all covered. A significant part of the film is devoted to teasing out the role of the house in plague transmission—and the interventions designed to counter it. Still, van Loghem commented that the process could have been documented "with more precision."[79] Newspapers were generally positive, with one reporting patriotically, "The film is, in our view, a convincing argument in favor of the strong work of our plague control workers."[80]

Originally, the film was intended for an Indies audience, but it received generous attention in the Netherlands as well. Its production was closely followed in the press, with one reporter writing about their "sneak peek" in March 1927.[81] When completed, the film was first screened before a select audience in The Hague that included van Lonkhuyzen (on furlough) and the minister of colonies. It was subsequently shown around the country, often accompanied by a lecture. In November 1928, for instance, Flu introduced the film during an "Indies Week" organized by students at the University of Leiden.[82] In March 1929, E. F. Hermans of the Institute of Tropical Medicine Leiden-Rotterdam gave two lectures on plague control in the Indies before an audience of German "professors, physicians, medical students, and members of the local medical mission" in Cologne and Aachen, followed by a screening.[83] He repeated this performance before a lay audience in Breda in February 1930.[84] The film was also shown at an exhibition of medical missionary activities in Tilburg in August 1930.[85] By 1933, however, health officials wrote that the plague film had become dated and screenings apparently came to a halt.[86]

Audiences Abroad

The previous sections already indicate that Dutch health workers did not limit their promotion of home improvement to domestic audiences alone. There were lectures in Hamburg, Aachen, and Cologne. The IHTA explicitly targeted an international audience. Indies exhibitions appealed to broader foreign audiences also.[87] Meanwhile, the international medical community in Asia was introduced to the Dutch approach to plague control as early as January 1912 in a lecture by de Vogel at a meeting of the FEATM in Hong Kong. Like van Loghem, he presented home improvement as the surest way to control plague in the long term and illustrated this argument with photographs. Dutch plague research published in the *Mededeelingen* was frequently translated into English or German. In the Indies itself, events such as the Colonial Exhibition in Semarang (1914) or the Pasar Gambir held annually in Batavia through the 1920s and 1930s certainly attracted foreign expatriates and habitually included displays on Dutch health work in the colony. Furthermore, sources suggest that the Koloniaal Instituut contributed displays on tropical hygiene to Dutch exhibitions in Copenhagen (1922) and Brussels (1923), and at the Dutch pavilion at the Paris Colonial exhibition (1931). These were curated by van Loghem and offered "a rich collection" of photographs from which plague control could scarcely have been absent.[88] Another source claims that home improvement was included in an Indies diorama by the *mooi Indië* painter Leo Eland at the 1939 World Fair in New York.[89] But the evidence for a sustained promotion campaign of plague control to lay foreign audiences is sparse. In this section, we may more profitably explore the ways in which the Dutch broadcasted the spectacle of home improvement to visiting specialist audiences instead. After 1920, a steady trickle of foreign physicians and officials visiting Java would be taken on tours of the plague-stricken districts to view home improvement in practice. Often, they were taken into the thick of it, visiting villages where plague had recently broken out or where houses were still undergoing improvement. Though these were not Potemkin villages exactly (as one commentator had suggested after a tour by the governor-general in 1914), there was some degree of selection in what visitors were shown.[90] Areas that had been improved at an earlier stage, for instance, were often skipped: leaving the condition of improved villages after some time had passed in the middle. Instead, officials brought out charts, graphs, and maps to point out the dramatic reduction of plague incidence in districts where home improvement had already been completed (table 4). Nevertheless, these tours were carefully orchestrated.

The Far Eastern Association of Tropical Medicine

In August 1921, the Dutch East Indies hosted a diverse company of medical experts and health officials from South, East, and Southeast Asia at the fourth meeting of the FEATM. This important intercolonial event served at once as a specialist conference where medical knowledge was exchanged and as a diplomatic forum where regional health regulations were drawn up. Meetings of the FEATM, furthermore, became "a great showcase for host governments to demonstrate their good health governance through . . . organized excursions to their prized modern hospitals, laboratories, and quarantine systems."[91] The 1921 edition included a visit to all such venues and concluded by taking a smaller number of "official delegates and their ladies" on a field trip into the heart of Java. First, the route passed through "some of the most beautiful countryside" to reach the archeological site at Borobudur. From here, the party of thirty-five continued to the *kraton* of the Sultan of Djokjakarta, "where Javanese princesses will perform a native dance." Finally, delegates traveled on to inspect plague control work in the regency Wonosobo.[92] In short, the company of foreign health officials was presented with all the natural, oriental, and biomedical spectacle that Java had to offer.

On arriving in Wonosobo, delegates were given a lecture on plague and plague control in Java by Louis Otten, the bacteriologist and final leader of the independent plague service. Along with de Vogel and van Loghem, Otten would decisively shape the development of plague control in the Dutch East Indies. Indeed, his medical career was tied to this disease. Only weeks after the outbreak in Malang in 1911, Otten volunteered to join the plague service.

Table 4   Plague deaths per year in East, Central, and West Java, 1911–1940

	EAST JAVA	CENTRAL JAVA	WEST JAVA	TOTAL
1911	2,114	41	0	2,155
1912	2,128	148	0	2,276
1913	10,384	1,038	0	11,386
1914	14,435	1,321	0	15,756
1915	4,753	1,484	0	6,239
1916	549	639	0	1,188
1917	137	284	0	421
1918	182	552	0	734
1919	169	2,785	0	2,954
1920	244	8,895	13	9,152
1921	257	9,501	5	9,763
1922	137	10,819	0	10,956
1923	73	8,323	271	8,667
1924	157	12,547	549	13,253
1925	250	12,959	1,275	14,484
1926	70	6,830	871	7,771
1927	219	6,364	1,172	7,755
1928	35	3,741	824	4,600
1929	73	2,210	1,812	4,095
1930	3	2,282	1,695	3,980
1931	30	3,031	1,478	4,539
1932	5	2,071	4,366	6,442
1933	8	1,685	15,188	16,880
1934	2	2,668	20,569	23,239
1935	1	2,687	10,307	12,995
1936	4	1,693	4,490	6,190
1937	44	1,150	2,620	3,814
1938	20	616	1,447	2,083
1939	15	403	1,123	1,541
1940	2	141	253	396
Total	**36,464**	**108,908**	**70,128**	**215,500**

Source: *Indisch Verslag* (1941): 90.

He obtained his doctoral degree in Amsterdam two years later with a study on plague transmission, quickly rose through the ranks of the plague service, and served as its director between 1919 and 1924. As described in chapter 5, Otten later developed an efficacious live vaccine against plague that achieved a spectacular decline in plague mortality. For the moment, however, and indeed even after introduction of his vaccine, Otten remained a faithful supporter of the home improvement scheme. As he told the delegates of the

FEATM, the key to bringing plague under control ultimately hinged on the control of rats:

> But whereas the direct war on the rat and its extinction by mechanical, chemical or bacterial means offers no chance of success, the only way left is to break this contact by indirect means, i.e., by depriving the rat of its living and nestling places indoors, and so the whole plague-problem is reduced to a housing question.[93]

In other words, Otten reiterated the argument developed by van Loghem and de Vogel that since plague hinged on human-rat contact, the key to its control rested within the house. The Dutch were late contributors to plague research, Otten admitted, but over the course of the last decade he claimed they had perfected its method of control in the form of home improvement. There had been "countless difficulties and disappointments" as the scheme developed, he told his audience, but ultimately Dutch health workers had succeeded "by means of reconstructing the existing houses" to suppress and indeed stamp out the disease. In passing, Otten alluded to the important caveat that an improved house was only ratproof in so far as the house was regularly cleaned and inspected—but it was home improvement itself that was on display. Following a lecture filled with photographs of "native houses and their construction," as well as the Dutch "mode of house improvement and village disinfection," delegates were allowed to visit several nearby villages undergoing improvement.

THE HEALTH SECTION OF THE LEAGUE OF NATIONS

In 1922, Java was visited by another foreign health official. Frederick Norman White, an epidemiologist and former member of the Second Indian Plague Commission, was conducting a study tour of East and Southeast Asia on behalf of the Health Section of the recently established League of Nations. His reports provided an inventory of regional health challenges, disease control methods, and medical education systems that formed a basis for the creation of an Eastern Bureau in Singapore in 1925. This regional health organization was largely funded by the Rockefeller Foundation and was the center of an "epidemiological intelligence service" that exchanged information on the incidence of infectious disease between member states.[94] Cholera, plague, and smallpox featured prominently in White's report, as these diseases could cause ships and harbors to be quarantined. Malaria and hookworm surveys were also included, being prevalent parasitic diseases that had been prioritized by local Rockefeller operatives.[95] Special attention was paid to the incidence of the *Aedes aegypti* mosquito on account of ongoing concern for the introduction of yellow fever into Asia, for which this mosquito serves as a vector.[96] In Java, however, White's travel diaries reveal a particular interest in plague and plague control.

After arriving in Batavia in January 1923, White traveled to Bandoeng in the company of van Lonkhuyzen to inspect the palatial new laboratories of the Pasteur Institute and Landskoepokinrichting. On January 5, he reported:

> We left Bandoeng by the 5.30 a.m. train. . . . We were joined by Dr. Ver-steeg, the medical officer at present in charge of the special plague department of Java. I was anxious to see as much as possible of the country where plague has been especially prevalent in recent years and of the anti-plague measures; thither we were bound.[97]

The company followed roughly the same itinerary as before. They arrived in Djokjakarta, visited the historic temple complex at Borobudur, and "hurried away" at 5 o'clock to Wonosobo. "We motored fast," he narrated, "only stopping to see a few things of 'plague interest.'" The next day,

> we had a fairly full programme to work through . . . chiefly concerned with plague. I motored to see infected villages and the improvements made in the dwellings of the villager as an anti-plague measure. . . . I learnt much in little time. We finished up in a small town called Garoeng, westward of Wonosobo. . . . The afternoon I spent with Dr. Versteeg, with figures, charts and maps of plague incidence.[98]

White observed that he had taken several photographs of the renovations but that these turned out to have been underexposed. It is a shame indeed, for it would be pertinent to see how a foreign official chose to document the scheme. Nevertheless, the tour continued and on Sunday:

> van Lonkhuyzen, Versteeg, and I started motoring to Semarang. There was much to see en route, plague villages, plague improvement schemes, a plague "laboratory" &c and yet more wonderful scenery. . . . We visited Ambarawa, a town with an interesting plague history.[99]

What made this history of particular note remains unspecified, but the centrality of plague to White's tour of Java was becoming apparent.[100] On arriving in Soerabaja two days later, White's interest in plague control was demonstrated once more by his request "to see the houses in which the last cases of plague had occurred, (awful houses they were)." On a slightly critical note, White observed that rat plague had persisted in Soerabaja since 1911 and that efforts to control it were sparse. Home improvement had been completed, and the focus of local officials rested on fumigating the barges that supplied oceangoing vessels to kill stowaway rats and fleas.

In White's final report to the Health Section on Java, plague remained a prominent subject. He described in detail the operating of a plague intelligence service, the keeping of records on the disease, and its history and epidemiology since 1911. Certainly, there was room for improvement. The plague mortality figures all added up to 100 percent, he reported, indicating that the Dutch methods were "inadequate for the detection of other than fatal cases."[101] A full page devoted to home improvement, however, was more positive. It began:

> Many measures have been tried, found wanting, and rejected. I do not think it an exaggeration to state that at the present time house improvement and plague prevention are synonymous terms in Java.[102]

Following a familiar narrative of how rats found unlimited shelter inside the traditional bamboo house, White claimed that some 750,000 houses had been renovated. He ended by observing the curiously poor results that had been achieved with vaccination, but not before lavishing further praise on the organization and efficacy of home improvement:

> The success that appears to have attended these measures is most encouraging. In this way the severely infected districts in East Java were cleared of plague and have remained plague free for a considerable number of years. . . . I was privileged to see a good deal of this house improvement work and was favourably impressed. It is effective, it is permanent but it is slow and costly.[103]

The permanence of home improvement was a favorite claim of Dutch health officials as well, who used it to argue in favor of the scheme even after an efficacious vaccine had become available in 1935. The visit by White, meanwhile, was fondly remembered by them. In particular, they appreciated an outcry of admiration attributed to him, namely "that only an obstinate Dutchman would not shrink" from the daunting task they had set themselves by opting for home improvement.[104] As for White himself, his inspection tour made a lasting impression. Thirty years later, in his presidential address to the Royal Society of Tropical Medicine and Hygiene in the United Kingdom, he reflected warmly on his visit and once more lauded Dutch health work in what was, by then, their former colony.[105]

THE ROCKEFELLER FOUNDATION

Perhaps the most critical foreign visitor that Dutch colonial health officials entertained was Victor G. Heiser. This colorful American physician served as Director for the East of the International Health Division of the Rockefeller

Foundation. In this role, he conducted surveys of health challenges in individual countries, pursued opportunities to demonstrate the Rockefeller's signature health interventions, sought to sway officials and physicians toward the Rockefeller's vision of improving health, and inspected the results.[106] This philanthropic organization pursued the control of leading endemic diseases and argued this would ultimately pay for itself by increasing economic productivity. Its initial focus was on hookworm but quickly expanded to malaria and other health threats.[107] From his successive travel diaries, it seems that Heiser had mixed feelings about the Dutch East Indies. In his first tour of Java in 1915, he was generally positive about the availability and organization of health services in the colony. His collaboration with de Vogel seemed promising but no Rockefeller program got off the ground until 1924. Moreover, de Vogel's successor, van Lonkhuyzen, was less enamored with Rockefeller initiatives and required considerable persuasion to lend his support.[108]

On a visit in January 1926, Heiser was not impressed. He was disgruntled not to receive special treatment at customs and his subsequent diary entries alternate between effusive praise for Dutch control over the population and repeated barbs at people, places, and policies. While the purpose of his visit was to survey a hookworm control demonstration, van Lonkhuyzen also took Heiser on a tour of the ongoing plague control work in Wonosobo and Banjoemas.[109] Later, at a meeting with various health officials, Heiser recounted how he was pressed "to express a frank opinion of their plague measures." He obliged:

> I told them I considered them wrong in principle; that if plague was to be controlled by their methods unthinkable sums would have to be provided; that since they had only 2 or 3 million guilders to spend, the method they were pursuing could not accomplish control. It is now their practice to wait until plague appears in a village and then to begin rebuilding all the houses in an entire village. . . . While they are doing that, however, the plague has usually spread to the next town and by the time they have reached there it has gone still further.[110]

Home improvement, Heiser concluded, was "nothing more than a stern chase." It could not hope to catch up with the actual spread of plague, leading to loss of life that a more proactive strategy could prevent. The Dutch countered that they had a duty to protect local customs and daily village life until an outbreak forced their hand. Suggestions for improvement, Heiser noted, were met with "the invariable answer . . . that they have tried it but that it will not work."

Despite this critical assessment, Heiser was not entirely unappreciative. He labeled the home improvement scheme "stupendous" and its outcomes "impressive." Apparently, the Dutch could have done worse. The tour continued to the plague-stricken district of Kedoe, where Heiser visited multiple home improvement sites and wrote that the scenes he witnessed "again recall the stupendous task [the Dutch] are undertaking." On balance, his views on the matter were ambiguous. The slow and reactive nature of the scheme was certainly unsatisfactory. "The present plan is to rebuild 50,000 houses annually in towns already infected," but with an estimated five million houses in Java "this policy cannot hope to stamp out plague in anything like a reasonable number of years." It was an ambitious scheme nevertheless, he concluded: a challenge that "may well awe anyone except a determined Dutchman."[111]

The Eastern Bureau of the League of Nations

In February 1930, a visit by the Advisory Council of the Eastern Bureau of the League of Nations offered Dutch colonial health officials another opportunity to showcase home improvement to a select professional audience. Senior health officials from member states in Asia had descended on the thriving hill city Bandoeng for the fifth annual meeting of this regional health organization. As was customary, physicians and officials used this international and intercolonial meeting as an opportunity also "to visit diverse sanitary institutes" in the host country. Naturally, in Java, this included home improvement.[112] Sources documenting this visit are scarce, but the photograph discussed earlier (figure 3.4) of delegates inspecting a home improvement site in the district of Temanggoeng provides a unique glimpse into what such a visit looked like. We count about ten health officials in white and grey suits roughly in the center, who appear to be in conversation with each other, standing in the middle of a construction site. Laborers work in the foreground, residents stand in the background, materials and house frames occupy the remainder of the picture. The opinions of these delegates have largely gone unrecorded, but journalists were able to elicit a few comments that would be paraphrased across multiple newspapers. J. D. Graham of British India was reportedly "delighted with all they had seen and perceived." F. H. Guérin of French Indochina was much impressed with the "choses merveilleuses" regarding the provision of healthcare in Java in general and with home improvement in particular. The scheme was said to have entirely increased "his appreciation for the organizational skill of the Dutch in colonial matters." Should *his* colony suffer a new plague outbreak, he was quoted as saying, the methods employed in Java would certainly serve as an example.[113] If such was indeed their assessment, Dutch colonial officials must have been chuffed. Overall, the Advisory Council must indeed have looked favorably at the home improvement scheme, as Dutch health officials would presently be able to coax their international colleagues into a formal endorsement of their signature health intervention.

THE BANDOENG RURAL HYGIENE CONFERENCE

The FEATM, the League of Nations, and the Rockefeller Foundation certainly were the most prominent organizations to pursue international health collaboration in early twentieth-century Asia. Their professional support of home improvement—even Heiser's reluctant praise—could be construed by Dutch officials to reflect positively on their colonial project as a whole. But the strongest endorsement of the scheme was yet to come.

In August 1937, the Dutch East Indies hosted an Intergovernmental Conference of Far Eastern Countries on Rural Hygiene in Bandoeng under the auspices of the League of Nations. It became a landmark in the history of public health.[114] First, the meeting explicitly recognized that health was tied to broader social and economic processes. Second, it stressed the importance of local conditions and community participation to the success of health interventions. And third, it advocated an international health agenda focused less on the control and eradication of individual diseases but more on the provision of primary healthcare. To address the most pressing health questions facing South, East, and Southeast Asia, it sought to develop an intersectional approach. The Bandoeng Rural Hygiene Conference consequently connected physicians, agronomists, engineers, and other experts to articulate more complex responses to challenges in sanitary infrastructure, medical training, nutrition, education, the position of women, and indeed the high incidence of infectious disease. This focus was quickly lost again when—in the wake of World War II—new technologies such as DDT prompted a return to top-down disease eradication models. It was rekindled in 1978 with the Declaration of Alma-Ata on the importance of primary healthcare, which was explicitly framed as the "resurrection" of the health ambitions that had been articulated in Bandoeng.[115]

Shortly before the meeting, members of the Advisory Council paid another visit to Java. Home improvement was once more on the agenda. This time, delegates were offered a tour of villages undergoing improvement in the regency Tasikmalaja. It appears that delegates were equally interested in a new plague vaccine that had recently been developed by Otten and had achieved a dramatic reduction in plague deaths.[116] Indeed, at the time of the conference, the "considerable importance of vaccination emerged clearly both during the discussions and in the resolutions."[117] All countries in Asia, concluded the conference's committee on plague, sought to adopt a policy of vaccination when dealing with plague, citing Otten's "non-virulent live vaccine" as an example. But while vaccination certainly offered a more practical approach to plague control, the committee on plague gave discursive priority to "housing improvements" instead. In fact, the conference's final report went as far as to recommend home improvement to other countries and cited the Dutch East Indies as a model. In a list of formal resolutions, the committee on plague stated:

> 3. Apart from the destruction of rats . . . by trapping, poisoning, fumigation, etc., the Conference emphasises the necessity for improvement of existing dwellings and for the construction of new houses based upon rat proof designs. . . . The Netherlands Indies Government has set an excellent example with its approved bamboo dwellings, and similar principles may be applied in communities where timber, mud, straw, and the like are utilised.[118]

A stronger international and professional endorsement of the home improvement scheme was difficult to imagine. Member states, suggested panel members, could even submit their own designs for dwellings made of locally available construction materials to Dutch experts for evaluation.

There was no official tour of medical establishments or plague-affected districts this time. Instead, delegates and members of the public could familiarize themselves with examples of disease control in member states at a concurrent exhibition at the Bandoeng trade fair complex. Naturally, the section on health in the Indies did include materials on home improvement that could this time be compared to methods elsewhere. The section on British India, for instance, included examples of chemical plague control by means of fumigation: "a method," newspapers pointed out haughtily, "that the Dutch East Indies have abandoned."[119] Two model houses—one plague dangerous, the other rat-proof—were also present.[120] The Bandoeng Rural Hygiene Conference, in short, offered an opportunity for Dutch health officials to showcase the signature health intervention they had developed over the last three decades and to consolidate professional support into a formal declaration of approval. This endorsement came not a moment too soon. Now, a potentially fatal flaw in the home improvement scheme could finally be admitted to—as I discuss in chapter 5.

Conclusion

Between 1911 and 1942, Dutch scientists, physicians, and officials participated in a concerted effort to broadcast home improvement to lay and specialist audiences in the Netherlands and abroad. They took pride in their intervention. The home improvement scheme was documented in hundreds of photographs, in film, as well as in tables, graphs, charts, and maps to demonstrate its progress. Select audiences were even taken on tours to inspect home improvement at first hand. These materials captured the spectacular nature of the scheme: the dramatic improvement of houses, villages, and entire landscapes, and the contented (or at least productive) collaboration of Dutch and Javanese residents, laborers, inspectors, physicians, officials, and engineers in the face of plague. In other words, they conveyed an image of strong but benign colonial rule that was increasingly under pressure as anticolonial and nationalist voices gathered strength. This image, I reiterate, was grounded in a very material expansion of state power. While plague control in other contexts was often limited to urban areas, in Java it was methodically rolled out across the island and impacted the everyday life of millions. The episode with Heiser indicates that the Dutch brooked little criticism of their signature health policy. Indeed, the endorsement contained in the report of the Bandoeng Rural Hygiene Conference suggests that health officials were *intent* on receiving professional credit for the scheme. The home improvement scheme, it emerges, served a function beyond plague control: a function that hinged on its visual and performative character. It argued for the continued need of colonial rule in the Indies. It displayed Dutch medical and technological fitness to the task. And the scale at which it was implemented demonstrated Dutch commitment to its new ethical mission to Dutch, Indies, and international audiences alike. Indeed, the spectacle of home improvement may have been more important than its efficacy against plague from the start, as it quickly emerged that no measure of "improvement" would ever make a house ratproof.

CHAPTER 4

Plague Propaganda

> Alongside the *technical* comes the *domestic* improvement. To achieve this, an *obligatory house cleaning* has been introduced, the quintessence of the entire plague control scheme . . . and the nice thing is, that the Javanese begins to realize that he lives much more pleasantly within a neat environment than in a dirty one.
>
> —H. F. Lumentut, lecture at the *Indisch Genootschap*, 1921

Plague was perhaps the first and most prominent subject of a new and colorful health practice that flourished in late-colonial Indonesia: health messaging. Over the first half of the twentieth century, a suite of public health education initiatives was developed in the Indies by public and private actors that relied heavily on visual materials. Although the term "propaganda" already carried some of the more nefarious overtones it does today—to sway opinion through misleading information— these initiatives were commonly referred to as *medische propaganda*.[1] Its function was to overcome the severe shortage of medical personnel in the Indies and to improve population health. Effectively, medical propaganda placed responsibility for health with local populations themselves by instructing them how to prevent disease in the first place. True to its etymological origins of "propagating the faith," however, medical propaganda did not stop at the mere instruction of people on the nature, transmission, and prevention of disease. Rather, its long-term ambition was to exploit the success of health messaging to prevent some diseases—and of the highly visible results of mass treatment for a select few diseases such as hookworm and yaws—to convert local populations to European scientific medicine as a whole.[2]

Plague propaganda served two intermediate goals. First, it sought to instruct Javanese populations about the rat-flea-man transmission scheme. It explained the role of the traditional bamboo house in this chain, and fostered a new visual regime. Homeowners were to *see* and recognize the house as a space of multispecies encounters that facilitated plague transmission, thereby generating understanding of (and support for) the home improvement scheme. Second, it pursued a behavioral adjustment. Plague propaganda instructed populations in the hygienic inhabitation of the house: prompting them to regularly clean their dwelling and inspect it for the presence of rats and nests. In short, it sought to rat-proof the Javanese population along with their dwellings by making European standards of health, hygiene, and cleanliness *adat*.[3] Between 1911 and 1942, films, photographs, lantern slides, posters, maps, graphs, diagrams, pamphlets, stories, house models (life-sized and to scale), rat specimens, and microscopic preparations were paraded before the population of plague-stricken districts in village meetings, community demonstrations, house-to-house visits, public lectures, at schools, in youth health movements, film screenings, and in modest rural hygiene exhibitions, as well as at grand colonial fairs.

The home improvement scheme reduced nesting opportunities for rats inside the house and facilitated inspection. But the real key to breaking the chain of plague transmission between rat and man in Java rested less in the physical alteration of the house than in the behavioral modification of its inhabitants. After all, the emergency *dessa schoonmaak*, designed to bridge the divide between the first appearance of plague in a community and the implementation of home improvement, was often sufficient to stop an outbreak in its tracks—while improved villages could still host outbreaks. Consequently, if home improvement was the most visibly intrusive facet of Dutch plague control work, plague propaganda was its most insidious. This chapter cannot hope to do justice to the development of health messaging in late-colonial Indonesia as a whole. Instead, it concentrates on tracing the development of plague propaganda specifically and argues for its centrality to the Dutch plague control efforts in Java between 1911 and 1942.

Plague Intelligence

The origins of plague propaganda go back to the early days of the outbreak in Malang and had their basis in the organization of a plague intelligence service of sorts. After the disease was recognized in March 1911, state agents were faced with the question of how far the disease had already spread. An analysis of the available mortality statistics for East Java suggested that plague could have been present since November 1910 and had consequently had ample time to spread. Over the following weeks, Willem de Vogel of the BGD produced a series of maps that converted statistical and bacteriological information on the incidence of plague into a series of images that visualized the spread of the disease in the region.[4] For instance, the map for the week directly following the plague diagnosis (31 March–6 April) featured red dots indicating human plague cases in clusters to the northwest of the town of Malang, with a scattering of cases to the southeast. Over the following weeks, the maps traced its spread to *kampongs* north of the town, as well as the appearance of new foci to the south and east. Confronted with a severe shortage of medical personnel to cover the entire district, de Vogel's impromptu plague service was heavily dependent on intelligence on the spread of the disease being delivered by the population of these scattered communities.[5]

If a suspicious case of disease occurred in a village, residents were instructed to send a guide to the nearest road to await the passage of an itinerant physician who traversed his assigned area daily by car. A photograph highlights the sharp technological contrast of such an encounter, placing European modernity in the form of a Javanese physician wearing colonial dress beside his vehicle, approaching a traditionally clad Javanese man crouched by the side of the road with a pole and flag.[6] Furthermore, the scene—staged in so far as the photographer had to get in place—contains a strong power dimension. The crouching position in Java was, after all, not merely a common resting pose but also a deferential one (*jongkok*).[7] From here, the physician would travel onward on foot, horseback, or by cart to attend to the potential plague patient. If plague was indeed diagnosed the house of the victim would be evacuated and marked with red flags to caution others against entering. If a village was evacuated in its entirety, a warning sign likewise marked with flags would be placed at the entrance of the village to indicate the outbreak of infectious disease and to urge people not to take away any objects or to spend the night but to pass through quickly. In a way, such signs were the earliest forms of propaganda that sought to check the spread of plague by influencing behavior.[8] The results collected by this intelligence service were shared at the end of each day between local officials and physicians via telephone and ultimately communicated to de Vogel's headquarters to find their way into his weekly maps.

Intelligence on the spread of plague consequently required the instruction of local populations in recognizing a disease that had never before been seen in Java. As soon as possible, "Javanese and Dutch handbills were issued in which the symptoms of the disease were described."[9] These pamphlets were put up on police watch boxes as well as "portable restaurants" (*gerobak*) and contained similar information as the warning signs at affected villages. Given that most of the population was illiterate, however, the efficacy of handbills and warning signs was limited. It proved more helpful "to distribute these handbills among the school children" and treat their contents in class. "Eager to display their skills in reading at home, they will read the directions on plague to their relatives and neighbors."[10] This strategy—based on a rather optimistic estimation of the afternoon pursuits of school-age children—anticipated a much stronger focus on health education for children in years to come. Furthermore, physicians with the plague service were required to give instructions on the recognition of plague to "some intelligent natives" (i.e., those who could read and write). They also instructed rat catchers on how to safely handle specimens that were sick or dead.[11] The irony here was that Dutch plague physicians were mostly just as new to the disease as their audience.

Presently, at meetings "where the native officials were present," de Vogel demonstrated "by means of pictures and photographs" how plague control was organized elsewhere. "The work . . . in San Francisco with its many photographs has been of great service in this regard."[12] Stressing the educational uses to which such visual materials could be put, de Vogel provided a rationale for the extensive photographic documentation of plague in Java as well. These images, as I have argued before, helped to establish the role of the bamboo dwelling in plague transmission. They were later used in gatherings with "European planters . . . high native officials, and influential rich Chinese." By "plainly showing how plague in the house rat is communicated to man," Johannes van Loghem wrote, photographs were instrumental in persuading community leaders of the need to pursue an intervention in the built environment.[13] Before long, health officials gave public lectures accompanied by these and other images to audiences in Batavia and Buitenzorg.[14] Only afterward, it would seem, were lectures (accompanied by demonstrations or lantern slides that explained plague and plague control) extended to the broader population of affected districts.

Home Inspection

Almost immediately after home improvement was decided on as the principal plague control strategy—about August 1911—it became clear that this intervention alone could never build out the rat. On inspection, renovated houses were once more found to contain rats' nests. Villages from which plague had been eradicated fell prey to the disease once more. What was needed in conjunction with the *technical* intervention in the house, was a *behavioral* adjustment in the way in which it was inhabited. "Lumber, old boxes, and mats stowed away in dark corners, in lofts, or under balé-balés, must be cleared out from time to time to be examined or thrown away," admonished van Loghem, who had first recognized the vitality of such spaces to rodent populations.[15]

"Especially in the Chinese quarters, full of merchandise," he continued, but also in Javanese houses where the rice harvest was stored inside, frequent inspections were a laborious necessity.[16] A regular home inspection was imperative to prevent rat breeding inside, but this could in the long run never be managed by state agents alone. Instead, residents had to be persuaded to conduct a regular inspection and cleaning of the house themselves.

The importance of home inspection alongside home improvement was stressed repeatedly. In a pamphlet of 1912 that apparently sought to explain the home improvement scheme to government officials, the physician Otto de Raadt emphasized that "regularly exercised supervision of already improved houses will be absolutely necessary." After outlining different ways in which the scheme might be systematized, de Raadt pointed out that "for each system to succeed" the key remained the same:

> The instruction of the population. This is easy to achieve, by constructing in each dessa an expertly built rat-free house that may serve as a model, and furthermore to take care that different types of rat-free balé's serving likewise as models can be viewed with the dessa chief. . . . Propaganda in the widest sense of the word for this work of home improvement should thus primarily be designed for the Native official, so that they will realize what *woninghygiene* could mean for the future of the man in the dessa.[17]

Instruction on domestic hygiene was the key to plague control. Home improvement merely facilitated the process of inspection and importantly reduced the number of likely nesting sites. By placing model houses with village leaders in affected districts, residents were able to study the standards to which their own houses should adhere in order to make them ratproof. The features of these model dwellings have already been described, but physicians freely admitted that without a reformed understanding of cleanliness these technical improvements were bound to be ineffectual.

Photography, I argued in chapter 1, was instrumental in achieving a new understanding of the traditional bamboo house as a space of multispecies encounters. The house became recognized as a contact zone, facilitating a heretofore unsuspectedly close cohabitation of humans, rats, and other animals. Chapter 2 explored how these insights resulted in targeted interventions to guard part of the construction against infiltration by the rat—which were likewise documented by the camera. Most striking, however, were those images that combined a potential rat shelter, a technical improvement, and a demonstration of a new gaze and habit that Dutch health officials hoped to instill in Javanese populations. A set of two such images in de Vogel's report in the

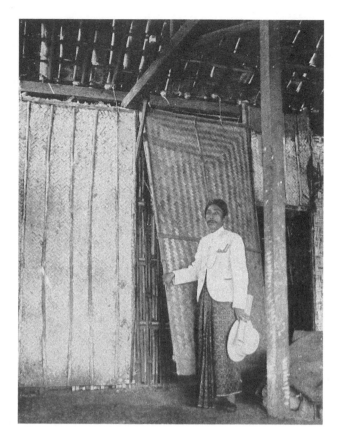

FIGURE 4.1.   Photograph of a *mantri* inspecting the inside of an improved dwelling, 1911.
Willem Thomas de Vogel, "Uittreksel uit het verslag aan de Regeering over de Pest-Epidemie in
de Afdeeling Malang, November 1910–Augustus 1911," *Mededeelingen van den Burgerlijken
Geneeskundigen Dienst in Nederlandsch-Indië* 1a (1912): 30–111, inset between 84–85 (fig. 29).
Courtesy of the University of Leiden Library.

Mededeelingen, for instance, focused on the "dead space" inside the house that
was inhabited by the rat. Figure 4.1 reproduces one of the images. It shows a
Javanese *mantri* standing inside an improved dwelling looking directly at the
camera and gingerly lifting an inner wall that has been mounted on hooks.[18]
Our attention is drawn to the previously obscured space between the inner
and outer walls made of woven bamboo mats, which has been made amenable to inspection. The photograph familiarizes the viewer with the inner
anatomy of the house (to return to this argument) and urges them to inspect
such spaces for the presence of rats and nests themselves. A second photograph in the report shows another *mantri* again looking directly at the camera as he holds down a newly installed hatch in the *pyan* while another man
holds open a door (presumably for better lighting).[19] Again, the photograph

alerted residents to the hidden spaces inside their homes: spaces with a life of their own, that required inspection in order to safeguard human health. Both photographs sought to direct the viewer's gaze toward spaces that were potentially plague dangerous and thereby to reform their understanding of the house. Both photographs also demonstrated behavior to be emulated to render such spaces safe or healthy. And both photographs were the product of an apparently firm conviction among physicians that sight led to understanding and to corresponding action.

Early plague propaganda consequently sought to familiarize people with the symptoms of plague, its transmission (including the role of the house), and methods of control. The efficacy of early health messaging attempts to achieve these objectives is difficult to determine, especially since vernacular sources are hard to come by. Government sources are notoriously silent about any forms of resistance to colonial interventions. Instead, they tend to emphasize how residents understood "the wisdom of our advice to leave the houses, where evidently the evil spirit had taken up its abode, and offered no resistance."[20] Newspapers, however, deviated from this narrative left and right. They offered generic complaints of residents willfully skirting European health instructions or recounted specific incidents where locals displayed a "characteristic" fatalist attitude toward plague and the *soesa* stirred up by health officials.[21] Overall, sources suggest that responses varied: ranging from uncomfortable acquiescence to active disobedience. Either way, it is helpful to call to mind an observation by the anthropologist Joshua Barker. In his study on state regulation and surveillance in Bandoeng he notes that the appearance of something "visible" and "new" in a community—home improvement, as happens to be the case for his interlocutor—is normally a memorable event.[22] By extension, the novelty of plague and plague control was bound to have an impact on local populations and to elicit a response.

The Plague Service

The independent DP that was active between 1915 and 1924 was a technical rather than a medical organization. Although it was led by thirty-three physicians, the DP employed nearly 900 staff in 1916 that were primarily engaged with tracking the spread of plague (forty-eight), disinfection and emergency interventions in the houses of affected districts (100), and—overwhelmingly— in home inspection (542 *mantris* and 126 supervisors).[23] The reports published over its years of operation are silent on efforts on the part of the DP to instruct the Javanese on plague, home improvement, or domestic hygiene. These facets of plague control remained under the control of the BGD. Nevertheless, the leaders of the DP were acutely aware of the fact that ratproofing the house was ultimately secondary to ratproofing its occupants. And over the years, the organization was instrumental in disseminating knowledge on the technical as well as the behavioral adjustments necessary to eliminate rats from the dwelling—concentrating on its Javanese employees.

Starting in 1915, the DP set out to standardize the home improvement scheme. As de Vogel had already observed during a tour of East Java in 1912, the execution and efficacy of home improvement differed considerably between districts.[24] To overcome this, an education program was established to train both European and Javanese staff. Heavily reliant on visual and practical methods of instruction, the scheme was set to deliver three to four hundred graduates a year.[25] In its first year, the DP trained 184 European and 636 Javanese house inspectors who were subsequently employed by the plague service.[26] A *modelkampong* in Malang allowed for hands-on instruction. It featured various building designs common in East Java, both in their original and improved forms. The former type was used to demonstrate the range of nesting spaces available to the rat, the latter to explain the interventions that neutralized them.[27] As previously discussed, the use of native building materials such as bamboo and *atap* was increasingly restricted under the reign of the DP on account of their plague dangerous nature. Crucially, however, the first director of the organization, Wilhelm van Gorkom, confessed: "I have repeatedly been convinced that the benefit of home improvement is illusory, when the *inhabitation* of houses does not conform to a way that does justice to the technical improvements."[28]

The irritability of Dutch plague officials over the return of rats to renovated houses—and of plague to villages from which it had been cleared—reached such heights that some suggested criminalizing and fining the discovery of rats in "technically perfect dwellings." Through such measures the Javanese *kampong* dweller was to develop a sense of civic responsibility. "He must be educated" in the art of keeping the house rat-free, conceded van Gorkom, "but educated strictly" until home inspection and the weekly *dessa* cleaning had become *adat*: part of the local assemblages of Islamic and pre-Islamic (animist) values, practices, and beliefs.[29] But what did an antiplague *woningschoonmaak* entail? In order to clarify this, the physician L. Krol prepared a short set of instructions for his colleagues. The pamphlet reflected Krol's belief that the success of home improvement depended on the subsequent cleaning and inspection of the house: by residents ideally, but under professional supervision. All furniture (shelves, *balé-balé*, and other objects) as well as "the harvest" (*padi* stored inside) would have to be carried outside once a week. The dwelling then had to be swept (floor, *blandar*, etc.), followed by a search for hiding spaces of the rat. Finally, this process was to be checked once a month by an inspector of the DP, though personnel shortages likely reduced this frequency to once every three months.[30]

The high-handed nature of this attempt to instill a new hygienic conscious-ness in Javanese homeowners was made clear in the first annual report of the DP. It stressed that home inspection ought to have a *politioneel-huishoudelijk* (domestic policing) character as it was vital to the success of the entire plague control scheme.[31] Indeed, the DP repeatedly discussed the desirability of amending the government's plague ordinance (that legally underpinned home improvement) to encompass regulations and fines for the improper "inhabi-tation" and "use" of renovated dwellings.[32] Such an amendment was, to the best of my knowledge, never enacted but perhaps local or regional fining sys-tems were. For instance, H. F. Lumentut, who oversaw plague control in the residency of Madioen after 1915, recounted how he sought to force the coop-eration of local populations by targeting the perceived laziness of the inhabit-ants of improved houses. If they failed to clean their dwellings regularly, and if rats' nests were discovered, he said, they would be punished. The nature of these punishments was not stated, though elsewhere Lumentut spoke of fines and forced evictions. Just one or two such punishments, he stressed, had served as an example for the remainder of the population. Afterward, "the entire plague *dessa* is reshaped in a perfectly neat Eastern village with *snoezige* little flowerbeds surrounding the whitewashed bamboo houses with their red-brown tiled roofs."[33]

In 1916, K. van Roon, the interim director of the DP, reiterated the views of his predecessor that the utility of regularly inspecting and cleaning the im-proved house was imperative throughout the plague-affected area. If the *actual* cleaning and inspection of houses in plague-affected regions was not yet up to scratch, he continued, "it is pleasing to see that here too we gradually see improvement."[34] At the end of the year, van Roon reflected that the in-spection of over 1.6 million improved and unimproved houses in the districts of Malang, Bangil, and Pasoeroean had once more demonstrated that rats' nests could be found "in the most diverse parts of the house." Consequently, when it came to the *woningschoonmaak*, "not a single corner of the floor, wall, or roof can be allowed to remain unobserved." No matter how simple the in-spection and cleaning of the house appeared as a plague control measure, he continued, it had to remain under the supervision of "specially trained and experienced personnel" for the foreseeable future.[35] At the same time, he stressed, the combination of home improvement and domestic reform was beginning to generate results. The yield of rats per house inspected was dramatically lower in districts such as Malang (where these measures had been implemented longest) compared to districts such as Soerakarta (where populations "have only been made aware of the great importance of the good and hygienic inhabitation of the house more recently").[36]

In 1921, the last annual report of the plague service by Louis Otten declared that the organization could no longer hope to control plague "by repressive means." In other words, he acknowledged that home improvement was insufficient. It could not hope to build out the rat in order to control plague. Instead, home improvement had to be understood as "a means to an end." It facilitated the discovery of rats and nests by the inhabitants, who could then take action to remove the animal and the plague "virus" from their abodes.[37] Home improvement, said Otten, consequently required a simultaneous improvement in how people saw and inhabited their dwellings. Since his service was only responsible for the former, however, he did not consider the latter. Surprisingly, Otten *did* make brief note of the unpopularity of the home improvement scheme. "The complete revolution in life and domestic habits that [home improvement] entails, means that it will never be able to bask in the popularity of the population," he admitted, and the interventions of the plague service were consequently not received with any enthusiasm. The unwillingness among the "lower societal classes" stemmed in part from their failure to understand the need for these interventions, he concluded, tacitly reiterating the need for further public health education.[38]

The Department of Medical Propaganda

Concurrent to the development of the plague service, the BGD began to experiment with public health education. Specifically, it developed visual materials to instruct lay populations about the nature and prevention of different health threats—including plague. These materials remained remarkably on message over the years. They instructed populations about the nature of plague and continuously emphasized how rats and dwellings were implicated in its transmission. This plague propaganda sought to justify home improvement, cleaning, and inspection by state agents, as well as the need to reform individual behavior. Many of the materials that educated the Javanese in the basic principles of European scientific medicine also found their way into the lectures and exhibitions discussed in chapter 3, thus serving a secondary goal of broadcasting the ethical, emancipating nature of Dutch colonial governance to metropolitan and foreign audiences. Sometimes these goals overlapped. At the Colonial Exhibition in Semarang in 1914, for instance, the BGD contributed several displays on the control of plague, cholera, and rabies to the govern-ment pavilion. Ostensibly targeting an international mercantile audience, the plague display was situated in the "native" section of the fair and certainly addressed more local audiences as well. It included maps of the spread of plague through East Java, a complete model of a rat-free bamboo house, and photographs of the plague bacillus and plague symptoms. These explicit med-ical images were then juxtaposed with others showing the full array of in-struments deployed to control and study the disease, including the laboratory materials required for the examination of the spleen in plague-suspicious corpses. A memorial booklet of the event pointed out, "With regard to the control and prevention of the disease there were models of a disinfection car (scale 1:10) and of a de-fleaing station with fumigation chest (scale 1:5)," even though these techniques had been largely abandoned since 1911. "Alongside these were demonstrated the measures such as they are employed today," in-cluding "models of evacuation and pneumonic plague barracks and examples of home improvement." Proceeding to describe several houses renovated in both wood and bamboo, the pamphlet concluded:

> Furthermore, there were displayed a range of instruments deployed in the fumigation of rat-attracting materials and houses. Otherwise photo-graphs (enlargements) of rat fleas, rats, and rat nests, and, pertaining to the laboratory research, there was a photograph (enlarged) of a plague marmot, after death entirely opened up for a post-mortem.[39]

It certainly was a timely display. Semarang was confronted with its first plague cases only a year later.

Plague may have been the first disease for which such a range of educa-tional materials was produced. But after de Vogel became the head of the BGD in December 1912, disease prevention quickly became a top priority. "Diligent propaganda" targeting specific diseases, he argued, would result in fewer cases and generate a broader appreciation of European medicine among the popu-lations. Health messaging consequently served a higher purpose: to spread the gospel of scientific medicine as a whole. Reflecting on the task of the colonial health service at the Koloniaal Instituut in September 1915, de Vogel stressed that the "education of the native population in Western medicine" was im-perative to encourage this appreciation further still.[40] A few years later, in a summary of the BGD activities between 1911 and 1918, de Vogel outlined the reforms he made to focus on the control of endemic infectious diseases. He also announced a new foundational principle.[41] Driven by idealism as well as pragmatism in the face of an overburdened and underfunded health organ-ization, he declared that "the chief task of the BGD henceforth shall be in the realm of hygiene . . . and thus consists in the *prevention of disease*."[42] Health messaging was central to this endeavor. "It is the intention of Headquarters," de Vogel announced, "to create a separate division for medical propaganda" to instruct people in the nature, transmission, and prevention of infectious disease. This medical propaganda was to take oral, written, and visual forms. In fact, the BGD had already started the publication of a periodical—the *Korte Berichten*—that discussed health-related topics, and which were translated into Malay by the semigovernmental Commission for Popular Reading (Commissie voor de Volkslectuur).[43] "Furthermore," concluded de Vogel, "propaganda will be conducted by the screening of suitable cinematic films."[44] In fact, following promising experiments with this method, the BGD was awarded a *f.* 10,000 government grant to trial the development of propagandistic health films in the archipelago itself.[45]

In 1920, the BGD formally created a dedicated Department for Medical Propaganda (Departement voor Medische Propaganda, DMP) under the leadership of Lucien von Römer.[46] Over the next three years, the department published several pamphlets, a series of wall plates on yaws, three general hygiene posters, and a colorful series of posters on poisonous snakes. The emphasis of the DMP was not on plague, but its work contributed to developing a culture of health messaging in the Indies that would flourish through the 1920s. Meanwhile, on a tour of neighboring Asian states, de Vogel further demonstrated his commitment to public health education by noting that he made local enquiries into the organization of both professional medical education and medical propaganda for local publics.[47] He failed to elaborate on the subject in his presidential speech at the FEATM meeting in Batavia of 1921, but a concurrent hygiene exhibition at the School for the Education of Native Doctors (School tot Opleiding van Inlandsche Artsen, STOVIA) curated by von Römer reveals their continued interest in this approach. Importantly, this exhibit *did* feature plague materials. For instance, there were "several models of Native houses fitted as required for combating plague," as well as a "new bamboo-house" designed by the architect Henri Maclaine Pont (see chapter 2).[48]

Over the first decade of plague control and up to the liquidation of the DMP due to budget cuts in 1923, several more educational materials on plague were produced under the supervision of the BGD.[49] In 1915, for instance, the Commission for Popular Reading published a booklet by de Raadt called *Penjakit pest Ditanah Djawa* (Plague disease in Java). The fifteen-page pamphlet appears to have targeted a Malay-speaking literate middle class. It contains no images, but describes plague disease, its method of transmission, and the steps necessary for its control. It prompted readers to keep houses clean and free of rats, and explained why home improvement was implemented in affected districts.[50]

A similar leaflet was published in Sundanese, the principal language in West Java.[51] A second Malay-language pamphlet on plague, *Dari hal penjakit pest (Sampar) dan pendjaganja* (The plague disease and the means to prevent it) was published in 1919. It provided detailed descriptions of the rat's ability to live inside the bamboo frame and the *atap* cover of the house, and the interventions necessary to prevent the rat from nesting there.[52] The pamphlet appears to have been published in Sundanese as well.[53] And in 1920, a similar publication by the interim leader of the DP appeared in Buginese—possibly in response to a case of rat plague in Celebes (Sulawesi).[54] A fourth leaflet on plague was written by Otten in Dutch and summarized the state of plague control in 1921. Its audience is not readily clear. It provided detailed technical instructions on the implementation of home improvement. It also included a copy of the plague ordinance of July 1914 that underpinned the scheme. Furthermore, there was a detailed list of instructions that the inhabitants of improved dwellings were required to adhere to—detailed enough, in fact, to explain why some form of instruction or supervision would have been required (see appendix 2). The emphasis this document placed on lighting of the dwelling is noteworthy. While light was naturally regarded as necessary for visual inspection, light—sunlight—also continued to be regarded as an excellent disinfectant against plague bacilli.[55]

Were any visual materials used over this period to instruct local populations about plague? The archival record is unclear. The historian Dafna Ruppin writes that an unknown "instructive, scientific" plague film with "pedagogical qualities" was ordered from Europe in June 1911 and was shown in a theater in the Semarang city gardens. Its first screening was attended by local notables as well as Dutch and Indies physicians, followed by screenings to the general public (at a possibly prohibitive fee).[56] There also is a short newspaper report of a film on plague and plague control being shown at the historic Pasar Baroe in Batavia in June 1911.[57] The BGD may have provided materials to the exhibition in Semarang in 1914 that were used more widely. In 1915, a Chinese individual who had recently traveled from Hong Kong was the first to be diagnosed with plague in Batavia. Several cases of rat plague were also identified in the inner city and in the government suburb of Weltevreden.[58] In response, several emergency interventions were implemented that reportedly included visual health messaging. According to an anonymous witness, writing in the *Sumatra Post* two years later:

> The people [in Batavia] worked with brightly colored posters, in which the principal instructions were printed as concisely as possible, in Malay and in Chinese. These posters were put up at the entrance of every

kampong and furthermore everywhere where natives congregate in large numbers: at the *passar*, at stations, cinemas, and schools.

At Batavia these instructions were complemented by simple drawings, and these posters became the principal topic of conversation in the *kampong*, which thus worked excellently.[59]

Given that the Sumatran port city Medan was presently facing an outbreak of its own, the author suggested this method could be adopted to provide instructions to the local population. I have found no further evidence of the existence of such brightly colored posters at this time. But if nothing else, the article intimates the value some members of the public attached to visual methods of instruction. In Medan, meanwhile, the local physician H. Vervoort pursued the instruction of local populations on plague and plague control via a series of lectures accompanied by lantern slides. In the battle against plague, he stressed, the *echt-oud-Hollandsche schoonmaak* (typical old-fashioned Dutch cleaning) assumed an important role. The historical frenzy with which Dutch housewives and maids were said to clean their homes had in fact been proverbial since the seventeenth century and was—as historians have recently argued—an important driver of Dutch economic success.[60] According to Vervoort, a similar passion for domestic hygiene now had to be inculcated in Indies populations in order to bring plague to heel. After a first lecture that counted European colonials including the governor and his wife among the audience, Vervoort specifically addressed local leaders and plague control workers at later events.[61]

Private Plague Propaganda

Medical propaganda in the Indies was not produced by state agents only. While the DMP's existence was short-lived, its activities were generally viewed positively and shored up broad support for the undoubted, if unquantifiable, benefits of public health education with visual materials. Over time, diverse private individuals and organizations with or without government ties also began to produce health messaging materials in order to address a range of health challenges.

The Rockefeller Foundation was a key player in this domain. Since 1913, this American philanthropic organization had pursued "the well-being of humanity throughout the world" with a strong emphasis on improving population health.[62] Its initial focus was on hookworm, since its directors believed that the control of this prevalent and debilitating intestinal disease would not just benefit health but have a broader societal impact by increasing economic productivity.

In 1924, after repeated offers, the new head of the Dutch colonial health service, van Lonkhuyzen, finally allowed Rockefeller agents to arrange a demonstration of its hookworm control methods.[63] Broadly speaking, such demonstrations were similar to plague control. After a survey to estimate the incidence of hookworm in a community, the Foundation financed the construction of latrines in rural *kampongs* and initiated an education campaign that instructed local populations in the art and health benefits of proper defecation. Next followed the communitywide administration of medications to kill and flush out the worms. Following such a demonstration, the increase in health and productivity of a population had to inspire governments and corporations to continue these activities elsewhere. The relationship between the Rockefeller representative John Lee Hydrick and Dutch health officials had been strained at first, as the Dutch were skeptical of the hookworm program and its benefits.[64] In due course, their collaboration improved and Hydrick was able to expand his rural hygiene demonstrations to other districts and, as I discuss below, to focus on other diseases.

Another prominent figure here was H. F. Tillema. The pharmacist, entrepreneur, and former city councilor of Semarang was disturbed by the poor housing conditions that prevailed across the Indies and correlated them with both poor health and immorality. In a series of heavily illustrated books, Tillema pointed to the ethical mission of the Dutch colonial state to argue for sanitary reform and proper house construction in an attempt to improve health conditions across the archipelago. As it happened, Tillema was critical of the disproportionate focus of the colonial health service on plague and its express refusal to improve dwellings to guard against other diseases such as cholera and malaria. But while his own publications effectively produced propaganda *against* plague, as it were, they also elaborated at length on the tactics deployed by state agents to counter this disease. For instance, in the first issue of his six-volume series *Kromoblanda*, published in 1915, Tillema recounted two fables. The stories had been relayed to him by the regent of Temanggoeng, who said they were used by a *doctor djawa* in Djokjakarta to instruct populations how to prevent cholera and plague. In the first story, a princess had been banned from the court of Solo (Soerakarta). She now roamed the land, defecating in every well she passed, and all who drank from such a well became sick and died of diarrhea. The second fable went as follows:

A native once owned a pigeon, which overheard a conversation between two evil spirits.

The first ghost said: "I spread disease and death around me by mixing my poison into water. Everyone, who drinks this water, will die of vomiting and diarrhea."

The second ghost said: "I spread disease and death by spreading my poison among rats, who transfer it to man."

The pigeon recounted this story to her owner, who informed a meeting of the old and wise of the dessa.

Long they discussed the ways in which this evil could be met, but none knew what to do.

Finally, the oldest man of the dessa joined the meeting, and he was asked for his advice. And his advice was:

"Avoid water and rats at all cost, and if you meet them anyway only fire can save you. Never drink other than boiled water, and burn every rat that you may find."[65]

Rather than trying to familiarize local populations with biomedical concepts such as pathogens or vectors, or explaining the finer points of plague transmission via the flea, this *doctor djawa* reportedly sought to translate European medical knowledge back into a more practical superstition. In a later issue of *Kromoblanda*, Tillema provided a "nice" and perhaps more regular "example of instruction and propaganda against plague", copied from a newspaper article of October 30, 1915. It noted that the *assistent-wedono* of Semarang-Wetan had invited the village headmen in his district to attend a demonstration at the local medical laboratory to witness a demonstration of "what happens to rats" during an outbreak of plague.[66] The idea behind such demonstrations (as with de Vogel's lectures to community leaders in Malang in 1911) was that the knowledge distributed would trickle down into the community from local authorities and thereby generate wider support for the plague control efforts.

Tillema's propaganda appears to have mainly targeted Dutch officials and physicians rather than a broad segment of the Indies population. Still, his activism inspired other initiatives—and his publications and photographs were often cited and widely used. Other public health education initiatives developed that directly catered to local populations. The Vereeniging tot Bevordering der Hygiëne in Nederlandsch-Indië (Hygienic Society), for one, published short pamphlets in the mid-1920s on a number of health matters such as dental care and the adulteration of food. A booklet with "gentle reminders" to maintain health in the tropics written by the retired army physician Henricus Neeb contained several instructions on plague. It supported the government policy of home improvement, home cleaning, and home inspection and urged people to eradicate vermin such as fleas. Neeb further argued that "hygienic city and kampong construction" combined with a well-organized "hygiene inspection and intelligence service" were instrumental to improving population health in the colony.[67]

A different pamphlet by Leopold Kirschner (a government physician), M. L. A. Cordesius (the director of a girls' school in Bandoeng), and W. Hoogerbeets was entitled *The Ten Commandments of Hygiene in the Tropics*—nicely accentuating the proselytizing mission of medical propaganda. It contained ten health instructions that were delivered in rhyme in Dutch, Malay, and Sundanese, and accompanied by instructive illustrations. The tenth commandment was again dedicated to the control of vermin. It went:

> *Keep not just your dwellings, but also commons clean.*
> *Since puddles offer mosquitoes good breeding sites.*
> *The rats and insects feast on garbage.*
> *Which for humans increases chances of contagion.*[68]

The accompanying sketch features a bamboo-*atap* house with an unkempt garden containing several puddles (figure 4.2). Rats frolic in the foreground, mosquitoes (a mass of small black dots) flutter overhead. To anyone familiar with recent advances in scientific medicine, the message was clear: dirt and disorder around the house breed malaria and plague.

The Hygiene Exhibitions

Public health education by means of visual materials took flight after the mid-1920s. It covered plague and a steadily increasing number of other infectious diseases, and ultimately expanded to topics such as food, midwifery, and infant care. Already in 1926, the DVG considered restarting a propaganda department. The undoubted highpoint of public/private health education, however, was the EHTINI—the First Hygiene Exhibition of the Dutch East Indies—held in Bandoeng in 1927. The organizing committee met under Neeb, and though it involved a score of government scientists and physicians the event was organized privately by the Hygienic Society. The EHTINI was an *interlocaal* event with international aspirations, explicitly modeled on the Dresden Hygiene Fair of 1911. In two months, it drew an estimated 200,000 visitors.[69] The fair's end date was postponed twice, the governor-general visited multiple times, and a special train service was operated from Batavia on its final day to accommodate the visitors.[70] In the run-up to the event, Neeb had enthusiastically promoted the event in neighboring colonial states and secured foreign contributions to various displays.[71]

Through posters, photographs, and film, visitors were invited to study the myriad facets of healthcare in the Dutch colony—public, private, and corporate—and learn more about the ways in which different diseases were spread and

Tiende Gebod

~

Larangan kasepoeloeh — Tjegahan kasapoeloeh

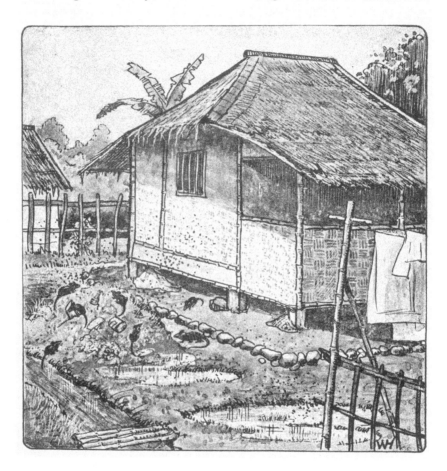

FIGURE 4.2. Drawing accompanying "The tenth commandment of hygiene in the tropics," 1927. L. Kirschner, M. L. A. Cordesius, and W. Hoogerbeets, *De Tien Geboden voor Hygiëne in de Tropen* (Bandoeng: N. V. Drukkerij, 1927). Courtesy of the University of Groningen Library. Photograph by Dirk Fennema.

could be countered. Maps, charts, and graphs documented diseases' geographical range or broadcasted the gains that had been made in controlling them. In short, the EHTINI was a treasure trove of demonstration materials used to instruct the Indies public in hygiene and disease control. The value of these materials, lectured a memorial book of the event, rested in a simple axiom: *"seeing* leads to better *understanding*." Once in possession of this understanding and armed with a European medical gaze, the public surely could not fail to act in the interest of its own health.[72] The purpose of the EHTINI (or rather, the purpose of the materials on display) was thus explicitly stated to foster people's own sense of responsibility in safeguarding both personal and public health.[73] At the same time, as I have argued above, the event was another spectacle of "ethical" colonial governance.

The EHTINI featured two large displays on plague, photographs of which were included in this memorial book. In one, we see how maps were mounted on a divider that documented the spread of plague in Java alongside several photographs that focus on plague's connection to the house (figure 4.3). We can make out photographs of split pieces of bamboo undoubtedly containing rats or nests, and of other building components prone to infestation by the rat. Some of these photographs appear to show houses that have been improved, while a small set at the back of the display has captured four patients presumably with buboes. On a table underneath, there is an encased microscope, several mock preparations of plague rats, and five models of Javanese houses featuring local roof designs. As discussed in chapter 2, Dutch health officials believed that Javanese roof shapes such as the *limasan* and the *joglo* facilitated plague transmission. These models presumably sought to explain this assumption.

The display continued on the other side of the divider, where it combined scientific imagery of plague with more artistic representations. More graphs, charts, and maps document the spread of plague between 1911 and 1926. To the far left are two diagrams of the rat flea and its proventriculus. The lower middle row features what appear to be five watercolors that are described in a catalog of the event. On the left are two paintings of the exterior of two Javanese houses with one featuring what appears to be a very large rat. The other three are more difficult to identify. According to the catalog, one depicted:

> (in the background) a man, sleeping on a baleh-baleh. In the foreground (to heighten the contrast) a dead rat: from here the fleas relocate to the man and a rat. Enlarged on this image: plague microscope slide with rat blood, flea, proventriculus flea with plague bacilli, beak flea filled with plague bacilli.[74]

This rather complex image effectively bridged facets of human behavior around the house with the nature and transmission of plague. Another image represented a plague victim and included an enlargement of "bubo liquid with plague bacilli" and a dead rat whose fleas were "biting the child." At the top of this display there was an enlarged representation of plague bacilli as seen through the microscope.

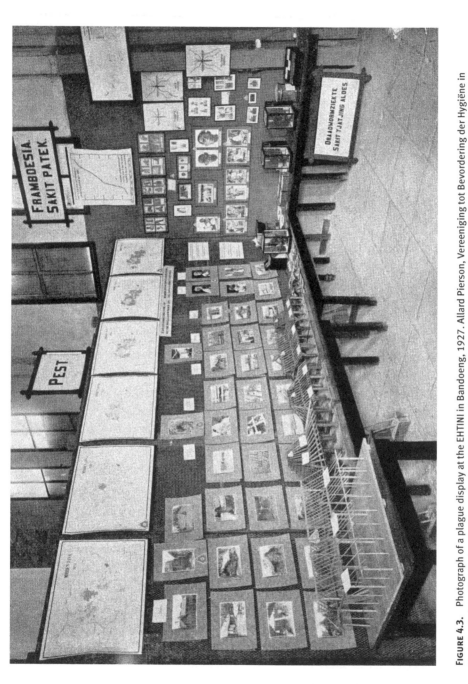

FIGURE 4.3. Photograph of a plague display at the EHTINI in Bandoeng, 1927. Allard Pierson, Vereeniging tot Bevordering der Hygiëne in Nederlandsch-Indië, *Verslag der Eerste Hygiëne-Tentoonstelling in Nederlandsch-Indië* (Bandoeng: 1928), 22, HL 86–64. Courtesy of the University of Amsterdam.

The EHTINI combined such displays with lectures and the screening of health films, including the plague film introduced in chapter 3. But "one of the most important contrasts" of the entire event, wrote one commentator, was "shown separately on the fairgrounds: a complete plague-dangerous Native dwelling of Central Java, with its countless sites for the nesting of rats."

Here, the various bamboos of the house and its furniture have been opened up in places to reveal the rat nests and dead rats within. In a corner there is a pile of rice, from which a rat rears its head, etc. etc. Everything corresponds closely to the original, including the neighboring rat-free construction: neat and practical. If only one could show these two houses to the entire population of Java.[75]

Sadly, no images of these house models survive. We may remember that a similar contrast had previously been presented at the Colonial Exhibition in Semarang in 1914, when the ratproof structure was still made primarily of bamboo. It would have been interesting to see how these models compared.

We do get a sense of how such models were used to instruct the public about plague and plague control from hygiene fairs elsewhere. The organizers of the EHTINI had expressed the hope that their exhibition could be transformed into a permanent museum. While this would not be the case, it appears that parts of it went on tour through Java. At a hygiene exhibition at the Pasar Malam in Klaten, for instance, two photographs captured a large display on plague and plague control that contained largely the same materials. In addition to the maps, charts, and photographs shown in Bandoeng, there was a collection of bamboo beams supposedly retrieved from plague houses with arrows bearing the word *tikoes* (rat) that pointed out potential nesting spaces of the house rat. This event also featured a model ratproof house for which photographs *do* exist. In one, we see Governor-General Andries de Graeff with several other officials inspecting this dwelling made of wood, *gedek*, and roof tiles.[76] In two photographs of the structure's interior, we see signs explaining the interventions that had been made as well as articles of furniture that had also been made ratproof.[77] The gable consisted of slotted laths and in one corner was a cooking compartment with a smoke vent: making it light, airy, and (as we will see in chapter 5) dangerously hospitable to mosquitoes.

Similar exhibitions were organized at other events through the 1930s. Most prominently, the BGD and DVG contributed displays to the annual Pasar Gambir at Weltevreden to showcase its achievements or highlight a particular topic.[78] In 1929, its focus was explicitly on plague and plague control. One Indies newspaper praised the government pavilion for its clear graphic representation of the historic spread and current status of plague and plague control in Java. "We could also see the home improvement as the only means by which plague could be controlled in the form of miniature dessa houses before and after improvement."[79] Even a complete layman, it reported, would emerge from the exhibit with a clear understanding of the disease and its method of control. A week later, the same newspaper took readers on a tour along the various activities at the Pasar Gambir and once more lavished praise on the health display:

> One of the most interesting exhibits must be the one of the Public Health Service. . . . Whoever visits this exhibit must not forget to tour the display of the Hygienic Propaganda service. Here the native, and indeed the European, is shown the severe risk of plague infection. . . . The drawings, that have been put up in the pavilion, stem from the film viewing about plague control. After viewing the film, the school children are invited to draw what they have understood. . . . Here we can see the real results of the hygienic propaganda, and we must say that the fact that the core principles have been deeply instilled into the children must not be underestimated.

This author was certainly convinced of the effect that health messaging had on the minds of Javanese and European audiences alike. The impact of the plague film on children in particular has a somewhat eerie ring to it, and plague was only one of several topics of health messaging that directly targeted children. Meanwhile, leaflets on plague transmission were also distributed to visitors of the Pasar Gambir (figure 4.4). Their message was simple: "The plague is transmitted from rat to rat and from rat to man by a flea," it read at the top in Dutch and Malay. Below this caption was a collection of small dots ("rat fleas to scale") and beside it a diagram of the rat flea ("as seen through a magnifying glass"). The pamphlet is dominated by an image of a rat sheltering its young, however, accompanied by a core message: "no rats in your house or commons, no fleas. No fleas, no PLAGUE," and a simple instruction: "keep your house and commons free of rats."[80] Over the last decade of Dutch colonial rule, the health exhibit at the Pasar Gambir was dedicated to plague control at least once more, in 1937. Despite the recent, dramatic impact of a new vaccine, its emphasis remained "on house construction and its use in the control of rats."[81]

The Department of Medical-Hygienic Propaganda

The above-mentioned initiatives appear to have given health messaging a boost. From letters exchanged between Hydrick and his superiors at the Rockefeller Foundation we learn of a growing enthusiasm with the DVG for its hookworm program specifically and its method more generally. Indeed, they

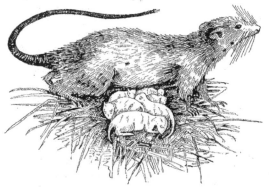

PEST.   3

De Pestziekte wordt van rat op rat en van rat op mensch overgebracht door een vloo.

Koetoe inilah jang membawa penjakit PEST dari tikoes jang satoe ke tikoes jang lain, dan dari tikoes menoelar ke orang-orang.

Rattenvlooien ware grootte

Rattenvloo, gezien door vergrootglas.

Koetoe tikoes, besar jang sebetoelnja.

Koetoe tikoes dilihat pakai katja, jang akan mendjadi besar.

Geen ratten in Uw huis of op Uw erf, geen vlooien.
Geen vlooien, geen PEST!

Kalau didalam roemah atau dipekarangan tiada ada tikoes, disitoe akan tiada ada djoega koetoenja.
Kalau tiada ada koetoe, tentoe tiada ada sakit PEST itoe.

Houdt dus erf en huis vrij van ratten. Maakt het de rat onmogelijk zich daar te nestelen en vangt alle ratten weg.

Djadi djagalah roemah dan pekarangan kamoe soepaja djangan sampai ada tikoesnja. Djagalah soepaja tikoes djangan bisa bersarang disitoe, dan tangkaplah segala tikoes-tikoes itoe.

FIGURE 4.4. Pamphlet describing plague transmission and prevention in Dutch and Malay, 1929. "Pamphlet," ca. 1929, RG 5, series 5, subseries 655, box 228, folder 2830. Courtesy of the Rockefeller Archive Center.

suggest something of a charm offensive to convert a reticent van Lonkhuyzen to the utility of such initiatives.[82] Already in July 1925, Hydrick reported that van Lonkhuyzen was "not so pessimistic" about the Rockefeller method "as he was at first."[83] Toward the end of 1926, Hydrick reported that, as per the original agreement, the DVG was increasingly taking over responsibility of the

Foundation's demonstration units. In fact, it was steadily expanding its investment in hygiene education across the board. The DVG was so impressed with a "Healthmobile" that enabled lectures accompanied by lantern slides and film screenings even in remote villages, for instance, that they offered funding for a second.[84] By September 1926, the Dutch colonial government allocated ƒ 70,000 with which to restart a new Department for Medical-Hygenic Propaganda (Departement voor Medisch-Hygiënische Propaganda, DMHP) that came into being in early 1927. The department was led by Hydrick, who was incorporated into the DVG as an adviser.[85] By July 1928, the DMHP had expanded its activities to cover multiple health challenges and a fully converted van Lonkhuyzen himself proudly demonstrated its materials and achievements at an exhibition for a select audience of colonial officials, including the Governor-General.[86]

The Plague Film

The growing appreciation for health education prompted the DVG about the same time to commission the Dutch film producer Willy Muellens to produce a feature-length film on plague in Java. On September 11, 1926, the *Bataviaasch Nieuwsblad* reported that following negotiations Muellens had agreed to produce a *propagandistische* hygiene film to be paid for by the state.[87] The finished product was a seventy-minute long, three-part assemblage (briefly described in chapter 3). The film combined animated sequences that illustrated how fleas moved between rats or how bacteria circulated within the body with live-action shots of scientists, villagers, and rats, as well as static and stop-motion maps and diagrams.[88] Special effects clarify how plague moves across Java or how it spreads from house to house within a village. Magnification is used to show fleas and plague bacilli. The film is a curious blend of the ethnographic and the educational. Its primary focus was on instructing the viewer in the method of transmission of plague from rats to man and on the role of home improvement in containing the disease. But at the same time, long shots of Javanese village life and European laboratory life gave viewers a glimpse into different lifeworlds. After its screening at the EHTINI, the plague film would be shown across Java.

The first part of the plague film considers "the nature of plague infection." It starts with laboratory scenes and moves to plague-affected villages where "happiness returned" as a result of home improvement. Part two focuses more specifically on "the control of plague." Viewers are introduced to the hiding spaces of the rat and the way in which rats and plague spread across Java. Here, there was a clear attempt to reform the behavior of Javanese audiences by means of practical demonstration. In one section, for instance, subtitles announce that regular inspection of the house leads to the timely detection of rat nests and live rats. We are then shown four Javanese men who follow the instructions of the DP laid down a decade earlier: they carry the furniture outside, search the house, sweep the floors and the rafters, and clean all items. A *mantri* walks by and inspects whether the bamboo poles of the roof have been properly sealed against the entrance of the rat. These men all display desirable, plague-resistant behavior.

Elsewhere, a scene explains the erratic spread of plague between villages. We are introduced to the narrative character Pa Wongso, a generic agricul-turalist off to buy *padi* at the market. Subtitles ask, "Where did this *padi* come from?" Why, surprise, it came from a plague-infected district. In a flashback, we see the original owner of the rice grabbing several bushels of rice. Under-neath, he finds a dead rat and carelessly tosses it away. Subtitles inform us that infected fleas have taken shelter inside the *padi*, which is next demonstrated in a cartoon-like sequence. The viewer is now given a closer look at fleas "as seen through the magnifying glass" busily moving across the screen. Hiding in small amounts of food, these fleas transmit plague from *dessa* to *dessa*. We return to Pa Wongso, walking home and placing the *padi* in his storeroom. Rats appear. Fleas relocate. Plague begins among the rats. Pa Wongso finds dead rats in his *padi* and after a long searching look, he too tosses them aside—though his expression of wonderment suggests surprise and ignorance rather than malevolent intent. Soon after, a family member falls ill. In brief, the scene demonstrates the dangers of being unaware about the transmission of plague, as well as the risk of certain domestic practices thought to aid it: in this case, storing rice in easily accessible storerooms.

Muellens's plague film was shown both in the Indies and back in the Neth-erlands, where a copy was held by the Koloniaal Instituut. In October 1927, the film was shown at a cinema in The Hague before diverse health authori-ties, as well as the minister of colonies. Van Lonkhuyzen introduced the film and observed that the Rockefeller Foundation had donated a third car to the DVG that allowed the film to be shown in *kampongs* across Java: undoubtedly generating wider support for plague control as a result, he claimed.[89] The film was a modest hit in the Indies. For a period of time, it was shown at a new outdoor cinema in the central Koningsplein (the present Merdeka Square) in Weltevreden.[90] In 1929, records of the DMHP inform us that two films on plague control and home improvement had been shown forty-five times in the projection hall of this department over a period of three months. The num-ber of lectures and demonstrations on plague and housing by the Department numbered 819 over the months of April, May, and June of that same year. Fur-thermore, the DMHP employed a school bus to bring students from around Batavia to visit its studios. *Mantris* went around the city with handcars packed with health education materials that certainly covered plague. And, as mentioned, automobiles carrying propaganda materials and equipped with a film projector toured Java to reach remote districts.

The Health Brigades

One facet of the DMHP's work was especially blatant in its attempts to convert local populations to the complex of European scientific medicine as a whole. Already in 1911, there had been a focus on the instruction of school-age children to explain the plague threat and gather support for government control measures. This focus was institutionalized, as it were, with the formation of the Health Brigade (Gezondheids Brigade) in 1928: an organization modeled on youth movements elsewhere about 1930, complete with shield, flag, and anthem. At one point, the organization counted 700 groups across the archipelago that were classified as "Dutch," "Javanese," or "Mixed"— apparently referring to their operating language rather than the ethnicity of their members. Hydrick described the organization to his superiors in 1929:

> Children's health clubs: (Gezondheids Brigade). Organized along lines of the Health Crusaders; developing satisfactorily; 1,824 members now enrolled in 54 brigades.[91]

In a short note of 1932, one Rockefeller official reflected on the medical propaganda work in Java. When it came to public health education, he stressed, the importance of visual materials and a focus on children could not be overstated:

> The work is now beginning to reach the outlying islands and is constantly gaining in support. Public health lectures with moving pictures are given twice weekly in the public garden of Batavia. These are attended by thousands and have become a part of the life of the people. Much study has been given during the past year as to whether hygiene can best be conveyed through stories or by statements of fact in pictures and illustrations. Experience emphasizes the fact that the best hope lies in the teaching of school children.[92]

What is perhaps most noteworthy here is the assertion that public health lectures and films had "become a part of the life of the people." In parts of the archipelago, medical propaganda was ubiquitous.

In 1934, director P. Peverelli, claimed that some 30,000 children were enrolled in the Health Brigade. For reasons that are unclear, responsibility for the organization was transferred from the DMHP to the Indies' Youth Red Cross Society in 1935. Afterward, a pamphlet published by the Health Brigade a few times a year no longer focused on health issues alone. It also began to feature explicitly pacifist stories and announcements.[93] It is tempting to frame this shift as a response to the growing war threat around the world, but the local political context seems just as important. As nationalist movements were becoming increasingly assertive and calls for decolonization grew louder, the intent of these pamphlets may have been to urge young Indies populations not to resort to violence against the colonial state. The popularity of the brigades waned over the 1930s, but the organization appears to have existed up until the Japanese invasion in 1942.

The main focus of the Brigade, of course, remained on health. Its periodical addressed myriad health concerns that schoolteachers were urged to treat in class. Plague was a frequent topic. Through the 1930s, articles and stories focused on explaining plague transmission and the need for home improvement, inspection, and cleaning. One example was the fable *Sidin and Tikoes*, published in 1935. Sidin, a native boy, returns home from school one day reminiscing about the beautifully colored posters on plague transmission that his teacher had put in the classroom. As he is sitting on his *balé-balé*, a rat emerges from the bamboo frame and introduces herself as Tikoes. They befriend each other, and Tikoes tells Sidin how she lives with her children inside the bedstead, while her sisters have settled up in the rafters of the house. They feed on the *padi* stored in a separate shed next door. Tikoes recounts her fortunate escape from plague in another village by hitching a ride in a basket of *padi*, but plague caught up with her. She "heard it mentioned that in the houses next door many rats have also died." That evening, Sidin's father is called to a meeting with the village headman. Later, the family is visited by a *mantri* who offers a biomedical explanation of plague transmission using more demonstration charts. The *mantri* tells them that their house must be kept clean, that it will be renovated in the near future, and that they must kill any rat they find. Sidin's family diligently follows the instructions of the *mantri*. Tikoes is never heard of again. The family survives the outbreak in their village unscathed. Presently, workmen arrive who "break down almost the entire house and clean it and now they have received a beautiful house covered in tiles instead of with atap, with sheet metal covering the ends of the bamboos, and a baleh-baleh constructed all of wood." And the family lived happily ever after under vigilant and benign Dutch colonial rule.[94]

Other publications that considered plague sought to convey a similar message but tended to be brief and straightforward. For instance, in a short and rather graphic snippet, Peverelli recounted how one day he noticed a mass of people that had gathered round a rat in the street. Its hindlegs had been nailed to a wooden plank and the frightened animal had nowhere to run.

> Personally, I wish to kill all the rats, though to torture them not one. I duly picked up a stone and crushed the beast.

The audience was less than pleased with his interference and Peverelli fled the scene in a taxi. The thing was, he continued, that the ability to catch a rat suggested its suboptimal physical state. In other words, it might be sick, possibly with plague. A Javanese man renowned locally for his ability to catch rats with his bare hands had soon after succumbed to plague, he wrote, indicating that the rats he was able to catch had been sick and carried infected fleas.[95] Later, in 1939, another pamphlet reproduced a school poster that had been published in 1933.[96] The image showed four "enemies of the body" that included both rats and fleas. An accompanying description repeated familiar information: that these species inhabited hollow pieces of bamboo—even the *balé-balé*—and that their cohabitation with humans was the key link that connected rat plague to human plague. Home improvement was the key to its control, and though it cost "quite a bit of money . . . it is necessary." "About plague, home improvement, and vaccination," Peverelli concluded with vaccination as a late addition, "I will tell you more later."[97]

Conclusion

Between 1911 and 1942, public health education that relied heavily on visual materials—medical propaganda—developed into a key public health practice in the Dutch East Indies. Plague was a catalyst for its development, as well as a sustained target. These health messaging materials and activities aimed to instruct the Javanese in a new understanding of this disease as a bacterial, vector-borne disease hosted by rats, conveyed by fleas, and contracted within (or indeed *through*) the house. On the one hand, plague propaganda aspired to generate broader awareness of biomedical explanations of plague and to thereby facilitate interventions designed to counter the disease—home improvement. On the other hand, it sought to instill new ways of seeing and inhabiting the house to keep "improved" structures free of rats. From the inception of the home improvement scheme, plague physicians admitted that technical interventions in the house were moot if its occupants could not be brought to properly clean and inspect the renovated structure. The persistence of this two-pronged approach—home improvement and plague propaganda—through the 1930s indicates how this far more laborious and costly intervention was favored over vaccination (which became available in 1935): possibly because of its "permanent" character, but certainly also for the unprecedented degree of surveillance and cultural influence this method of plague control offered over local populations, and—not least—because of its powerful appeal to metropolitan and foreign audiences.

CHAPTER 5

Plague, Malaria, and Vaccination

> With the present state of medical science and under the given circumstances of the land and the people, a more efficient means of plague control is impossible. The results of the current system, which has been built over the course of twenty years of struggle and experience, can be called satisfactory.
>
> —H. J. Rosier, memorandum to the Volksraad, 1935

In 1934, over 23,000 deaths were attributed to plague. It was the highest annual mortality figure in the three decades that this disease was endemic in Java (see introduction, table 1). The global economic downturn that began in 1929 had prompted severe budget cuts in all branches of the colonial government, including plague control. As the budget shrank, cases went up. Yet by the time of the Japanese invasion and the effective end of Dutch colonial rule in March 1942, the number of plague cases had dwindled to just a few hundred a year. What caused this dramatic improvement? The development of a new "live vaccine" by Louis Otten in 1935 had proven a game changer. Although its efficacy was limited to around six months, widespread vaccination and revaccination bought much-needed time for the reduced plague service to implement permanent control measures in the form of home improvement and plague propaganda. Rat plague might persist, but by the outbreak of World War II human plague had nearly been eliminated.

But this is only half the story of plague's final years in Java. Soon after an efficacious vaccine became available, physicians with the plague service began to publish studies that suggested how home improvement—the signature health intervention of the Dutch late-colonial period—was implicated in the spread of an arguably worse disease: malaria. This mosquito-borne parasitic disease was consistently described by colonial officials as "undoubtedly the worst scourge of the population of the Dutch East Indies archipelago."[1] Anecdotal and epidemiological evidence that correlated home improvement to fresh out-breaks of this disease dated back as far as the mid-1920s. The belated acknowl-edgment of this phenomenon *after* an alternative plague control strategy became available may consequently strike us as a bit Machiavellian. The so-called Otten-vaccine offered a new medical breakthrough that demonstrated Dutch scientific prowess that helped to obscure the deadly fallacies of an earlier innovation—one that physicians and officials had staked their national and in-ternational professional and political reputations on. Then again, between "plague rat and malaria mosquito," which was the greater health threat?[2]

In this final chapter, I examine the last years of plague and plague control in Java. Originally, it was envisioned as demonstrating the continued domi-nance of home improvement and domestic reform through the remainder of the Dutch colonial period. But as I discovered more sources, this picture be-came more complex. Yes, officials and physicians emphatically defended the role that housing reform could play in bringing plague under control, even if vaccination was vital to its ultimate demise. Together with the challenge posed by *woningverbeteringsmalaria*, however, several questions presented themselves. Why had vaccination not been deployed in the Indies much earlier, as it had elsewhere? What prompted new vaccine research this late in the game, so to speak, when home improvement had already been "perfected" over the course of twenty years? How did health officials navigate the ethical challenges posed by the correlation between plague control and malaria? And, returning to themes discussed before, what were the real ambitions of the home improve-ment scheme? How were ideas about health and disease as a product of human-animal relations within their shared environment reformed in response to this development?

Plague and Vaccination

Immediately after the identification of the plague bacillus in 1894, scientists sought to use this breakthrough to develop new treatments and prophylactics. Alexandre Yersin himself returned to Paris with plague bacilli from Hong Kong to work on a vaccine with colleagues at the Pasteur Institute. They grew cul-tures of plague bacilli on *gélose* (agar plates), diluted them "in a very little bit of *bouillon*," and then killed the bacilli by heating them to 58°C for one hour. This "killed whole-cell" vaccine protected small animals from bubonic plague for a short period of time (but offered no protection against pneumonic plague).[3] Furthermore, the team sought to produce a treatment by copying a method that had recently been developed to treat diphtheria. Yersin injected plague bacilli into a horse, hoping that the animal's immune system would produce an "anti-toxin." After drawing blood from the horse, a serum containing any such anti-toxin could be distilled and injected into humans as either a prophylactic or a cure.[4] The serum produced a strong response (fever, hives) and yielded mixed results. A trial on human plague patients back in Hong Kong in 1896 was promising: only two out of twenty-three patients died.[5] But when Yersin traveled on to Bombay, where plague broke out in September of that year, his serum was less successful. Nineteen patients out of fifty-seven treated died.[6]

Simultaneously, the British colonial government had sent for the Jewish-Russian, French-trained bacteriologist Waldemar Haffkine. A former colleague of Yersin, Haffkine had studied cholera in India and successfully trialed a vaccine against this disease in Calcutta. When plague broke out in Bombay, officials asked him to bacteriologically confirm the outbreak and, if possible, to develop another vaccine.[7] Over the following months, Haffkine devised a new method to cultivate plague bacilli in large quantities in a nourishing broth contained in large glass jars. This suspension was heated to 65°C to kill the bacilli and then injected into various test animals. Two rabbits treated this way survived a subsequent encounter with live plague bacilli, prompting Haffkine to trial it on himself in January 1897. There were no side effects beyond a slight fever. Following a successful trial with protecting the inmates of a local prison where plague had broken out, Haffkine's formula was mass produced at a dedicated laboratory. The vaccine would play an important role in plague control in India. Over one million doses were produced in 1899 alone. Its efficacy was of short duration, however, while the practice of vaccination was widely unpopular in India, whether for smallpox, cholera, or plague.[8] The Haffkine vaccine consequently failed to contain the disease—whose mechanism of transmission also remained unclear—while a series of fatal mishaps with the vaccine further eroded public trust. It took a decade before Haffkine's name was cleared and his vaccine was widely deemed safe again. The degree of protection it afforded remained a matter of international debate.[9]

Over the following years, scientists around the world experimented with other formulas. In 1899, members of the German Plague Commission sent to investigate the outbreak in India tried to grow cultures of live plague bacilli on agar plates. They killed them with heat using as low a temperature as possible and added carbolic acid (a stabilizing agent still used in vaccines today).[10] The product succeeded (experimentally) in immunizing monkeys and rats against plague.[11] About the same time, researchers in Brazil sought to modify Haffkine's recipe.[12] And somewhat later, in the US-occupied Philippines, Richard Strong sought to develop a "true" vaccine. He inoculated guinea pigs, monkeys, and ultimately human prisoners with attenuated nonvirulent plague bacilli that had been long-cultivated on agar plates. In the process, Strong caused the deaths of thirteen Filipino prisoners who were involuntarily injected with a cholera vaccine contaminated with live plague bacilli. The incident prompted ethical questions about the testing of medical products on colonial subjects though it sparked little immediate change.[13] According to a review of these and other formulas published in 1912, Strong's "live" vaccine had a significantly higher efficacy rate than its "killed" competitors and conferred a longer-lasting immunity. Nonetheless, a live vaccine would not come into general use at this time as researchers feared that cultures might be insufficiently attenuated or could regain their virulence in people who were "peculiarly susceptible to the infection."[14]

Plague Vaccination in the Indies

When plague was recognized in Malang in March 1911, there consequently were several treatments and prophylactics for Dutch health officials to choose from. Both vaccination and serum treatment were included in the initial response organized by Willem de Vogel. Small quantities of plague serum had regularly been imported and distributed to key port cities in case of an outbreak.[15] Since it could not be stored for very long, early attempts at serotherapy relied on dried serum instead. "The results," wrote Augustinus Deutmann after trials on fourteen patients, "were nil."[16] Meanwhile, the government bacteriologist J. de Haan had immediately started to grow bacterial cultures of plague bacilli retrieved from human and rodent cases in the hope that immunizing material could be developed in Java itself. This endeavor could not take place in his makeshift laboratory in Malang, he stressed, nor even in the halls of a royal palace. Only a modern, well-equipped laboratory would do. A chest containing several cultures was accordingly sent to the Landskoepokinrichting and Pasteur Institute in Weltevreden on April 14 via a special express train and under police escort. Two weeks later, the first batches of vaccine were returned to Malang and distributed in the *dessa* Kapong Pajaman.[17]

Two photographs of this event have survived. In the first, four men dressed in white colonial uniforms are standing in the village square to give a demonstration (figure 5.1). The male population is seated on the ground behind them. Two local officials stand on the edge of the frame toward the right. The man at the center, a Javanese *mantri* or *doctor djawa*, has exposed his back to allow one of his colleagues to inject him with vaccine. The vaccinator—Deutmann—is holding a bottle and a syringe. An assistant holds a bottle of iodine, an antiseptic used to disinfect the skin before vaccination. The man being vaccinated

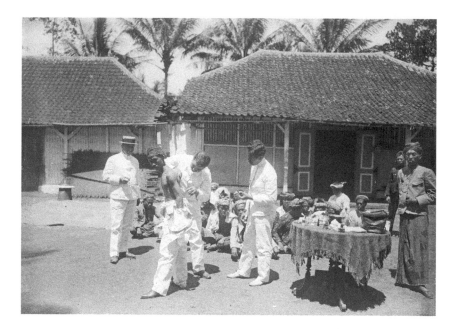

FIGURE 5.1. Glass plate positive of plague vaccination in *dessa* Kapong Pajaman, 1911. Unknown, *Vaccination against Plague in Java*, 1911, TM-10024179. Courtesy of the Nationaal Museum van Wereldculturen.

looks directly into the camera: inviting us to witness his experience in a manner that reminds us of the contemporary photographs of *mantris* demonstrating desirable hygienic behavior inside an improved house (chapter 4, figure 4.1). The European official left of center observes the scene with a contented smile. On the right, we see a table with an assortment of papers and utensils.[18] A second photograph more or less repeats the scene. This time, the man that was vaccinated has taken up position behind the table and continues to look directly at the photographer while one of the villagers has taken his place as the person being vaccinated.[19] In the background, the male residents of Kapong Pajaman look on. These photographs were not included in Deutmann's plague report in the *Mededeelingen* and their origin is unclear. The first is a glass positive held by Nationaal Museum van Wereldculturen. The second was reproduced in a paper that argued for additional vaccine research that was published in the journal of a catholic missionary society in 1915. According to this paper, these photographs were taken by the amateur photographer F. Stucky who worked on a local sugar estate.[20] Their purpose appears to have been both evidentiary (to demonstrate that vaccination took place) and educational (to inform physicians how to gain the trust of local populations, or to show local populations how their peers in other villages had submitted to this practice).

As for the vaccine itself, this had been produced by the director of the laboratory at Weltevreden. A. H. Nijland had chosen to follow the method proposed by the German Plague Commission. Additional vaccine was ordered from Bombay that had been prepared according to Haffkine's method. Both formulas were used as soon as they became available in the hardest hit dessas, making a comparative trial impossible. In the subdistrict Karanglo, Deutmann and *doctor djawa* Soedirman vaccinated 11,919 and 3,764 people, respectively, with the Nijland and Haffkine vaccines.[21] The vaccine was administered via subcutaneous injection "in between the left shoulder blade and the spine" after disinfecting the skin with iodine tincture.[22] The pair worked with one needle each, disinfecting it in between subjects in a metal container filled with boiling glycerin. A photograph of this process taken some time after the previous set features Soedirman and Deutmann seated in the village commons. A table of equipment is set between them. The glycerol sterilizers stand at their feet. Javanese men and women receiving the vaccine crouch or kneel in front of them and the whole set is surrounded by local residents and officials.[23] The population, stressed Deutmann, was quite willing to be vaccinated and was presumably quite familiar with this process due to regular smallpox vaccination. Since all three photographs appear to corroborate this claim and present a rather positive image of colonial relations, it is surprising they were not published at the time. Perhaps it had something to do with the success—or lack thereof—of vaccination. Neither the Nijland nor the Haffkine formula offered any protection. "Plague," wrote Deutmann, "spread as if nothing had happened."[24] Similarly disappointing results were obtained elsewhere. In October 1911, vaccination was halted to concentrate on evacuation and home improvement instead.

Three years later, when the number of plague cases soared and the disease expanded into Central Java, the early abandonment of vaccination began to draw criticism. In parliament, the leading colonial "ethicist" Conrad van Deventer asked whether the government had not abandoned "established tools" of plague control too early. Other questions also emerged. Had the Nijland vaccine perhaps been defective? Why should the Haffkine vaccine have no effect in Java? Why had further trials with a curative serum not taken place? And on that note, why was such meager care available for those infected?[25] Indeed, treatment and nursing of plague patients was left almost entirely to the local population itself. In a series of publications, J. G. Sleeswijk, a professor of technical hygiene at the University of Delft, contested the narrow focus on home improvement that was advocated by Johannes van Loghem. Rather than "hollow resignation" at the outcomes of vaccination, health workers had a duty to investigate further. Drawing on the language of the *ethische politiek*, Sleeswijk voiced a broader societal concern with the perceived neglect of the Javanese plague patient (see below).[26] In response, van Loghem published a vigorous defense of the choices that had been made. He reiterated the arguments in favor of home improvement and stressed the lingering uncertainty regarding the efficacy of serums and vaccines presently available.[27]

The escalating situation in Java demanded a reevaluation of the plague control measures. I previously described how new experiments with fumigation were quickly abandoned, while a solution for the slow pace of home improvement was found in the *dessa schoonmaak*—an emergency renovation followed by weekly cleanings and inspections. At the same time, W. A. Borger at the Landskoepokinrichting and Pasteur Institute began developing plague vaccines with bacterial cultures sourced from Java. But just as he completed his first publication, Borger contracted a laboratory infection and developed a fatal case of pneumonic plague. His colleagues praised his contributions, but of the eleven formulas tested on 676 rats none proved suitable for continued experimentation.[28] The vaccine research was only picked up again four years later by Paul Christiaan Flu, the new director of the Geneeskundig Laboratorium. He began with an exceptionally broad-ranging survey of the existing literature on the subject, followed by experiments with a number of different formulas that he tested on rats, guinea pigs, rabbits, and monkeys. The most promising results with vaccinating animals were yielded by a vaccine made with what he referred to as "watery aggresines." These were "extracts" from plague bacilli that were blended with either distilled water, glycerin, or carbolic acid. The different formulas were all cultivated and stored in empty gin bottles, before the bacteria were killed by being heating to 44°C for three hours.[29] For unclear reasons, these experiments were not carried forward and no human trials appear to have taken place.

It was not until 1920 that Louis Otten—the last director of the independent plague service—initiated a new field trial with vaccination in the residency Temanggoeng.[30] This district presented considerable challenges for the DP. It was mountainous, inaccessible, and the houses were built of loam and did not lend themselves well to the usual renovations.[31] Vaccination offered a practical alternative. Otten devised a proper trial and opted to use the Haffkine vaccine instead of the formulas developed by Nijland, Borger, or Flu. He began with "original" vaccine imported from Bombay. Two years later, he introduced a vaccine produced at the Landskoepokinrichting and Pasteur Institute according to Haffkine's method. In the wake of these trials, Otten concluded:

> As for the outcomes of vaccination, it appears . . . that these are far from satisfactory: although in 1921 plague mortality was reduced to below 30%, the mortality in 1922, when most vaccinations took place, rose to

more than double that, so that the end result was a reduction in mortality of up to 48.2% or just a little bit less than half of all cases.[32]

Considerably better results had been obtained with the imported vaccine, wrote Otten, but results were inexplicably skewed between batches. Both the imported and the home-grown vaccines could still achieve a significant reduction in plague mortality. Nonetheless, the practice was abandoned. According to Otten, the Javanese population could in principle be won over to regular vaccinations if the results were "obvious," but the Haffkine vaccine offered "a too limited efficacy" to achieve this. Plague control in Temanggoeng reverted to home improvement and hygiene education after all.[33]

Plague Nursing

In response to growing criticism over the dominant focus on home improvement, the failures of vaccination, and the neglect of the Javanese plague patient, the Dutch government felt compelled to strengthen its medical presence in the affected districts. It was faced, however, with a severe shortage of medical personnel. In February 1914, it consequently issued a call for "twenty young physicians" to travel to the Indies and join the plague service for a period of one year.[34] "What a wonderful opportunity to broaden their horizon and increase their knowledge," gushed the Dutch press.[35] But the minister of colonies faced considerable difficulty in filling these vacancies, as graduates considered the pay low and the work dangerous. After several weeks, newspapers up and down the country reported that while a handful of female physicians had submitted themselves for consideration, no male physicians had come forward. Commentators offered "a word of praise for these women" but otherwise expressed their "bitter disappointment" in the Dutch educated elite.[36] Two Indies physicians studying in the Netherlands would also volunteer. The government had to reissue its call several more times, now stating explicitly that female physicians were also eligible.[37] This provision was quite revolutionary. Since 1913, de Vogel had debated with the governor-general over the desirability of hiring women as *gouvernementsarts* with the civil medical service. After a first experiment, de Vogel insisted that the services of female physicians were certainly welcome but to prevent any "disruption" they should form only "a relatively small part" of the health service. Consequently, he offered "no objection" to hiring more women—as long as their number was limited to two.[38] With regard to the plague vacancies, however, he had little choice. In June 1914, the required number had finally been reached and five female and fifteen male physicians departed for the Indies.[39]

Concurrently, several individuals and organizations in the Netherlands sought to offer additional support. The Dutch Red Cross had offered its services, and at the end of March 1914 colonial civil servants proposed "to set up a popular movement to provide financial and medical assistance in the plague districts of Java." To structure such initiatives, the governor-general formally requested aid from the motherland in the form of nursing staff and field hospitals.[40] The response was quite significant. Before the end of April, the Red Cross had formed a committee under the chairmanship of the prince-consort to gather funds and attract volunteers in order to send over a "plague ambulance." The Indies Missionary Society also prepared a mission consisting of "physicians, nurses, spiritual brothers and sisters, and laymen," but ultimately supported the Red Cross initiative instead. In July, just before the onset of World War I, the committee had collected over ƒ 177,000 and had sent no fewer than four separate ambulances to the Indies.[41]

The plague ambulances each consisted of three female nurses who carried along equipment to set up a proper field hospital. They were placed under the supervision of a physician assigned by the BGD and could each care for ten patients at once, with spare capacity for another ten. Furthermore, they were equipped for bacteriological and chemical research, surgery, and disinfection. The ambulances also boasted a policlinic tent where patients suffering from other diseases could be treated "with the objective of gaining the confidence of the population."[42] Through 1915, three of the ambulances operated in the district of Malang and the fourth was set up in Kediri. Medical treatment of bubonic plague patients consisted primarily of incisions of the buboes, bloodletting, regular nursing, and the provision of proper food.[43] The nursing of pneumonic plague patients, admitted one physician, "was out of the question." They were placed in isolation barracks where they succumbed within a few days. The plague ambulances received a fair amount of attention in the Dutch and Indies press, but wartime developments in Europe likely overshadowed the mission and other sources are scarce. Several nurses and physicians wrote to newspapers to tell of their experiences, and the physician Henri van Dijk reportedly produced a photographic album of the mission. According to a description, his photographs contained both familiar subjects (e.g., rat cadavers inside hollow bamboo beams) as well as less familiar sights (e.g., a plague house being burned).[44] Another set of fifty photographs is held by the Nationaal Museum van Wereldculturen. They contain scenes from daily life in and around the plague ambulances, such as the setting up of tents, the treatment of patients (for plague and other diseases), childcare, tea breaks, a visit by the governor-general, and even outings into the country. Surprisingly few of them appear to relate to plague directly.[45]

The afterlife of this temporary expansion in medical care is difficult to determine but appears to have been slight. Both the plague physicians and the Red Cross plague ambulances had been intended to support the regular health service in Java for just one year. In August 1915, seven of the original nurses had chosen to remain in the Indies for the time being.[46] One later contracted plague and died. In the meantime, several Javanese women had been taken in to receive hands-on training in European "nursing virtues."[47] The plague physicians likewise were incorporated into the regular colonial health service or returned to the Netherlands. Over the 1920s, sources specifying medical care for plague patients are virtually absent. After 1930, the "statistical abstract" attached to the *Indisch Verslag* (formerly *Koloniaal Verslag*) provided detailed numerical information on different facets of medical care and public health. It offered an overview of the number of plague cases and deaths, the number of houses improved, and later the number of vaccinations given. When it comes to the number of patients treated for specific diseases in government hospitals, however, we notice that plague is almost completely absent.[48]

Plague in Priangan

In 1928, plague entered the residency East Priangan in West Java. This large, mountainous region was the heartland of Sundanese culture and featured prominently in Dutch imaginations and representations of the Indies. When home improvement in Central Java was "not even half completed," plague now threated to gain a wide diffusion in the cherished and profitable Preanger regencies.[49] Consequently, "the question of vaccination became acute once more."[50] This sense of urgency increased after the Great Depression of 1929 began to impact on government finances. Following an initial round of budget cuts across the colonial civil service in 1931, a second reduction was announced in 1933. In response, the head of the DVG appealed to the governor-general to spare his department. Pointing to the importance of public health in a tropical country with "primitive hygienic conditions" and the terrible sacrifice in human lives that had been brought to tropical diseases over the centuries, J. Offringa concluded:

> We may remind you that the DVG has been serious about these reductions, and that when in 1931 the Government asked for f. 1.6 million in budget cuts, the Head of this Service could offer f. 3.2 million. This freely given sacrifice . . . might now become fatal to us.[51]

But further cuts were demanded still. According to the health department's annual report for 1933, the budget for plague control was slashed in half. The number of epidemiological informers, home improvement supervisors, and home cleaning inspectors was reduced by nearly 300. The most significant reduction was achieved by lowering the budget for monetary advances provided to homeowners with which to finance the renovations by more than *f.* 900,000.[52] From 1933 to 1934, ordinary funds for the department dropped by another *f.* 50,000 and extraordinary "material expenses for home improvement" were reduced by *f.* 160,000. The budget now covered the cost of renovations in about three districts in Priangan a year, while sixty were slated for improvement.[53]

In the meantime, plague incidence rose sharply. From a low of 3,980 deaths in 1930, plague mortality increased to 4,539 and 6,442 in 1931 and 1932. It next reached an unprecedented 16,880 deaths in 1933 and a final peak of 23,239 in 1934. As the demographic historian Terence Hull observes, plague deaths in Priangan over these years far exceeded those in East Java since the start of the outbreak in 1911.[54] In August 1934, Offringa wrote to the governor-general to express his concern over this development. Diplomatically, he concluded:

> While I am convinced that for the moment there is no direct cause to correlate the financial reductions to the increase in plague cases, I cannot pretend that financial matters in specific circumstances do not have an impact . . . : *one ends up in a "dangerous zone" in which further reductions can create or influence conditions that can have a significant influence on the conduct of the epidemic.*[55]

Unsurprisingly, a causal link *was* evident to most observers. If nothing else, the evisceration of both budget and staff was hardly constructive at a time when plague was expanding its range.

In the annual report of the DVG for 1934, Offringa admitted that plague was indeed resurging. "If 1933 was already a peak year, the number of recorded plague cases in 1934 was significantly higher." Indeed, they were "the highest since the epidemic in Java commenced." But on the upside, it was gratifying to see that where home improvement and home inspection *had* been implemented, they had made a lasting impact (see chapter 3, table 4). Only two plague deaths were recorded in East Java (where home improvement in plague-stricken districts was complete) and another 2,668 in Central Java (where home improvement was ongoing). Even in West Java, the "success of home improvement" was apparent. Few villages had been renovated, but those that had saw the incidence of plague fall, "as is the rule."[56]

Upside or not, back in the Netherlands the minister of colonies was confronted with significant criticism over the advance of plague. His defense was the same as Offringa's, that while the health budget had been reduced from nearly *f.* 21 million in 1930 to less than *f.* 12 million in 1935, "vital parts" of the system had remained intact. But both in the Indies and in The Hague politicians protested. In the Volksraad, the prominent representative *Raden* Oto Iskandar di Nata asked why "special interventions" that were promised in 1934 had not been implemented in Priangan—and if they would have been if the victims were European.[57] In parliament, Agnes de Vries-Bruins, a member of the opposition Labor Party and a physician, cited back official documents to the minister to the effect that the DVG could not function with any further reductions. She stressed that the DVG had not only lost staff, it had lost oversight. Outbreaks of malaria and other diseases had gone unnoticed. Meanwhile, economic hardship among the population had exacerbated existing health challenges. Offringa had argued that the efficacy of home improvement was not in doubt as there had been no resurgence of plague in previously improved terrain. Since it was a purely reactive strategy, budget cuts could not be blamed for plague's more recent rampage through Priangan. If so, what was being done in this district instead? What of the impact of the reductions on the *dessa schoonmaak* and other temporary interventions? And what of the scheme's future? Indeed, commented another parliamentarian, if home improvement continued at its current pace the program would not be completed for another thirty years.[58]

The upward trend in plague mortality had also caught the eye of Queen Wilhelmina. In April 1934, a rather assertive note by the queen's secretary found its way to Hendrikus Colijn, the prime minister and minister of colonies. It read:

> In response to Her Majesty the Queen's command I have the honor to inform Your Excellency that it came to Her attention that the number of deaths for plague over 1933 . . . is so much higher than that for 1932. Her Majesty asks Herself whether reductions in healthcare have contributed to the undesirable factors behind this. Her Majesty would very much like to be informed of the chief cause to which this increase in the number of plague cases can be attributed and will very gladly receive further details in due course.[59]

If this "royal commandment" conveyed Wilhelmina's concern for her colonial subjects (as newspapers gushed afterward), it is poignant that demographically more relevant diseases did not attract her attention to the same degree.[60] On the other hand, given its high profile, plague incidence may have served as a barometer for the success of colonial health policies more generally. In any case, her note appears to have been a slap on the wrist. Colijn relayed the message to the governor-general at Batavia. Meekly, the notorious austerity politician added that the budget cuts in public health "had gone a bit too far."[61] "The great mortality for plague draws widespread attention," he continued, and added that the foreign secretary had received enquiries into the cause behind the increase as well. In another demonstration that plague control was tied to Dutch scientific and imperial prestige, Colijn noted that the increase "might very well tarnish the reputation of the Netherlands as a colonial power." "The purely humanitarian side" of this affair, he concluded, was "of course of even greater importance."[62]

Over the 1930s, in sum, plague posed a growing challenge. Its geographical expansion and the rapid increase in the number of cases were both troubling. The disease edged closer to Dutch centers of colonial control in Batavia and Bandoeng. Efforts at controlling it were hampered by financial constraints. The home improvement scheme progressed at a snail's pace, and foreign powers were perceived to look for weaknesses. An alternative was urgently required.

The Man with the Syringe

In September 1929, plague broke out in the *kampong* Tjiwidej in the residency of Central Priangan.[63] Otten, now the director of the Landskoepokinrichting and Pasteur Institute, led an investigation. His team collected various materials for investigation, including a dead plague rat. On returning to his palatial new laboratory in the nearby hill city Bandoeng, Otten isolated the plague bacillus from this cadaver. He passaged it through a guinea pig, isolated the bacterium again, and set it aside as a deep culture on an agar plate. About the same time, Otten started another survey of existing plague vaccines and began to experiment with his own formulas.[64] In March 1930, according to his own account, he required a "virulent" plague strain with which to infect his laboratory animals and happened to select the sample from Tjiwidej. He grafted the culture onto a broth and injected some of it into a fresh guinea pig. The guinea pig "did not care for this at all" and remained perfectly healthy. Such things happened. But upon being inoculated with the preparation once more:

> the infection did not catch again, and when this phenomenon recurred with a large dose, up to a whole culture, and was repeated with numerous rats and guinea pigs, I understood to be dealing with a plague strain that had spontaneously and in a short period of time become avirulent.

Given the disappointing outcomes of killed vaccines, Otten explained at a medical conference in Amsterdam in 1934, "I could not resist the temptation to see whether a live vaccine of the 'Tjiwidej' strain could generate more encouraging results." A first series of tests with a reworked formula were encouraging indeed. Nine out of ten rats survived after being injected with Otten's vaccine first and ordinary plague bacilli after. Fifteen guinea pigs all survived this procedure, as did fifteen white mice. Of fifteen monkeys, only one succumbed. Over time, Otten developed a vaccine whose protective powers lasted about six months. His fear, however, was that an avirulent strain could somehow regain its virulence and induce the disease it was supposed to contain. Only after four years of research did Otten feel confident that his live attenuated vaccine was ready to be tested on human subjects. And, he told his colleagues, "I shan't commence by trialing it on a prisoner, as Strong did, but on myself."[65]

In October, "the highly anticipated moment" arrived.[66] In the presence of witnesses, Otten had his plague vaccine injected into himself, followed by a second dose when no negative consequences manifested. Next, twenty volunteers working at the Pasteur Institute allowed themselves to be vaccinated. Again, there were no adverse side effects.[67] Otten duly informed Offringa that the vaccine was safe to use. A meeting was arranged between themselves and the head of the department of plague control, H. J. Rosier, to devise a field trial. Their plan was submitted to the governor-general, who gave it his blessing and urged them to start at once. Funds were made available, and as soon as November 2 a test began in the plague-stricken districts Bendjaran and Batoedjadjar near Bandoeng.[68] That morning, a team of six Dutch and Indies physicians had arranged a vaccination station at the *pendopo* of a local headman. According to detailed press coverage, the local community had gathered and awaited the arrival the regent of Bandoeng, who was also vaccinated to shore up confidence.[69] "In a tightly packed crowd, the population of Bendjaran and the neighboring *dessas* had gathered," all eager (reportedly) to receive the *soentik*.

> Deeply impressed by the solemnity of the occasion, the common people came forward when their names were called. Fearful, shy, and timidly they approached the man with the syringe, who administered a light injection above the left collarbone. Visibly relieved, they departed the gallery.[70]

This sketch of the event was copied verbatim across multiple newspapers. It painted a somewhat ambiguous picture of the local population as both eager to submit themselves to vaccination yet "fearful" and "timid" when the moment was there—arriving in multitudes from afar yet "relieved" to depart again. One might think they were entirely unfamiliar with this arcane health practice, even though vaccination for smallpox (and later cholera) had been regularly practiced in Java since the 1820s.[71] While newspapers emphasized how readily the Javanese population cooperated, such tensions do prompt questions about how voluntary their participation in this experiment really was. Newspapers also noted that lists of names were called for people to receive their vaccination, indicating (if anything) the high degree of civilian oversight by the colonial state. In fact, this tight surveillance was imperative. The trial was conducted following an alternating system in which half the inhabitants of a household received the vaccine. Over the next six months, thirty-eight out of 37,000 vaccinated people contracted plague and died. Among the controls, 213 out of 39,000 people died: about five times as many.[72] But even before these results were known, mass vaccination had begun.

On January 23, 1935, a large vaccination campaign with the "Otten vaccine" began across Priangan. By May, 700,000 people had been vaccinated. The practice was expanded to other parts of Java and by the end of the year 2.3 million vaccinations had been given. With a daily rate of 20,000 vaccinations on a population of 2.7 million people living in plague-affected districts, health officials estimated that revaccination could be achieved roughly every four months. Plague mortality was dramatically reduced. The precise impact of vaccination was impossible to determine, but as Offringa told the governor-general:

> the weekly plague figures had at the start of 1935 "reached such a staggering height" that without the support of a vaccine we could anticipate a very high figure of 30,000 deaths.[73]

Instead, the number of plague deaths fell to 12,995 in 1935, to 6,000 in 1936, and to fewer than 4,000 in 1937, the lowest figure since 1919 (introduction, table 1). Otten became something of a national hero. In a meeting of the Volksraad of July 1925, several speakers paid tribute to his breakthrough and representative di Nata stressed how keenly the Indies population had volunteered themselves to receive the vaccine.[74] In 1936, Otten was made a commander in a Dutch chivalric order.[75] In 1938, he received a prestigious medal from the Queen Wilhelmina Jubilee Society at a ceremony attended by the governor-general, the vice-president of the Raad van Indië, and other notables.[76] In parliament, representatives celebrated his vaccine as "a tremendous improvement, unique in all the world."[77] And through the remainder of the Dutch colonial period, Otten shared his research with foreign health workers. In October 1935, the prominent Chinese-Malay physician Wu Lien-teh visited Java to study the vaccine.[78] According to a French source of 1941, "le vaccin Tjiwidej" was tested in other locations that may have included Madagascar, South Africa, Senegal, and the Soviet Union.[79]

Vaccination and Home Improvement

But vaccination was never intended to replace home improvement. Even before Otten embarked on his new research project in 1929, a vaccine was regarded by the Dutch as a "palliative aid"—never a "permanent" form of plague control.[80] Given the short duration of any plague vaccine, it could never lastingly remove the threat of the disease to humans. And as long as rat plague prevailed, there was a chance that human plague would resurge. At best, a plague vaccine would be a powerful ally to the home improvement scheme. Be that as it may, the impact of the Otten vaccine on recorded plague mortality was as dramatic as its impact on the treasury was modest. A special budget of f. 20,000 was submitted to the Volksraad in January 1936 to finance a mass vaccination scheme that covered 2.7 million people. The DVG needed f. 10,800 to employ physicians, f. 5,400 for *mantri* assistants, f. 3,800 for eventualities, with travel expenses coming out of the ordinary budget of the health service.[81] These costs stood in stark contrast with the ordinary budget for plague control, which had totaled f. 2.3 million in 1930 and still consumed f. 1.1 million in 1935.[82] This difference notwithstanding, plague physicians and officials were adamant that home improvement, home inspection, and plague propaganda should continue.

Shortly after putting Otten's vaccine to a field trial, Offringa wrote to the governor-general that "it is of great importance to stress . . . that home improvement remains indispensable, no matter how successful vaccination may be."[83] Likewise, a memorandum on the DVG budget of 1935 submitted by Colijn to parliament maintained:

> Meanwhile, a vaccine may not even in the most positive instance be considered in itself sufficient to rid the Indies, and perhaps other countries too, of the feared disease; without the implementation of other control measures, in particular the home improvement, a recurrence of the epidemic would always remain a possibility.[84]

Otten himself concurred. In October 1935, for instance, he gave a lecture in Batavia that repeatedly stressed the matter. Vaccination was a "repressive" control method, home improvement an "enduring" one. Only the latter addressed the root of the problem: human-rat cohabitation. Vaccination might save many lives, concluded Otten, but:

> I should warn expressly that in this success we should not find reason to slow the pace of home improvement any further: only home improvement can definitively rid us of this pestilence, vaccination offers only

temporary alleviation, it remains a palliative, of which a too frequent use can only tarnish its expected success.[85]

In other words, Otten declared his vaccine a stopgap and in doing so voiced his opposition to the "slowing pace" of home improvement. He repeated this argument frequently. In a reflective essay on twenty-five years of plague control in Java, published in 1936, Otten wrote:

> However great an asset vaccination with a live vaccine might be to plague control, home improvement remains indispensable; only with the help of this preventive system of control might it be possible to hit the rat in its existential requirements and thus eradicate rat plague, the root of the evil.[86]

Even after his return to the Netherlands in the aftermath of World War II, Otten continued to stress the point. In a lecture at physics society Diligentia in 1946, shortly before his death, Otten concluded: "Home improvement . . . is the principal preventive method, that targets the root of all evil . . . and brings about a definitive end of the *plague disease*, of both man and rat."[87]

Other health workers tended to agree. In Amsterdam, the professor of tropical medicine E. P. Snijders extolled Otten's breakthrough but warned that vaccination—"no matter how successful"—would not lastingly address the conditions that allowed plague to spread. Since the sufficient means of plague control (i.e., home improvement) always followed the epidemic "at a distance," however, vaccination offered a way "to bridge this difference in pace."[88] Newspapers in both the Indies and the Netherlands likewise celebrated Otten's breakthrough, even as they too emphasized the enduring need for home improvement for the remainder of the colonial period.

Home improvement was consequently carried forward. The *Indisch Verslag* of 1936 noted that "home improvement continued in the usual manner" and had "not lost anything in value since the introduction of vaccination, since vaccination may not influence the epizootic." "As for durability," it reiterated, "the importance of home improvement is much greater."[89] Nonetheless, a memorandum by the minister of colonies of February 1939 admitted that the pace of home improvement was slowing down, partly as a cost-saving measure. This development was acceptable, argued the Dutch government, because the Otten vaccine allowed the scheme to be rolled out in a more deliberate manner without negatively impacting the health of the population.[90] The average number of houses being improved averaged around 40,000 a year through the 1930s. When plague spread through Priangan after 1928, however, the backlog of houses requiring improvement rose sharply. The scheme was still ongoing in parts of the residencies of Kedoe, Semarang, Solo, and Pekalongan in Central Java and would not be completed there until 1935.[91] The Otten vaccine would consequently save lives and offer a more rapid (and more economical) form of relief in newly affected districts. It created breathing space for the financially embattled plague service: time to act and space to reflect, it would seem, for the introduction of the vaccine belatedly allowed Dutch health officials to address an increasingly worrying side effect of home improvement.

Home Improvement and Malaria

At some point in the 1920s, Dutch physicians and officials began to notice a curious phenomenon. It seemed as though wherever home improvement was implemented, plague declined but another disease gained ground. Frequently, the renovations were followed by veritable "explosions" or "eruptions" of malaria. Given the political, scientific, and financial investments in the home improvement scheme—locally, nationally, and internationally—the existence of a causal relation between these phenomena was a sensitive matter. Consequently, it seems, this "inconstant" occurrence was not discussed in public until much later. The timing was significant. Just months after an international body of health experts at the Bandoeng Rural Hygiene Conference of 1937 had endorsed the Dutch home improvement scheme as a shining example of plague control, the first of two papers on "home improvement and malaria" was published.

Correlation

In December 1937, the head of the plague service first introduced the possibility that a correlation existed between home improvement and outbreaks of malaria to the public.[92] In a paper published in the *Mededeelingen*, Rosier claimed that the oldest observations of this phenomenon dated to "rather recently." Quite: it had been nine years since physicians first reported a curious increase in malaria cases after plague control work in the residencies of Kedoe, Magelang, and Soerakarta in 1928. Two years later, malaria outbreaks in Soerakarta were first "positively ascribed to home improvement."[93] And at the same time, the phenomenon was already observed further west in Central Java. In his diary, the Dutch plague physician and photographer G. M. Versteeg recounted a tour through the residency of Pekalongan with Rosier. On April 17, 1930, he wrote:

Visit to the improved kampongs. Very orderly, but far too airy. Bad open *gedek*, large, unnecessary ventilation holes. . . . In my opinion the unprotected houses are far too open. Rosier pointed at the malaria epidemic, which manifested shortly after home improvement. Saw several individual patients.[94]

His reference to malaria in the wake of home improvement was casual: it was something familiar that required no additional explanation. The fragment demonstrates that Rosier was aware of this phenomenon in multiple districts more than seven years before his paper was published, and that other members of his staff were also informed.

Nor was knowledge of this occurrence reserved to members of the colonial health service. Government officials were also in the loop. In 1932, the outgoing *resident* of Pekalongan wrote to his successor:

Another curious fact is that everywhere were home improvement has been implemented by the plague control service, a malaria explosion occurs soon after, which slowly disappears after the distribution of quinine. It is blamed on the airier building style after home improvement. The real cause is, however, not yet known.[95]

In the meantime, the population of Central and West Java had also started to suspect something. They reportedly spoke of *sakit wonéng* or "house disease" in reference to the fever outbreaks that followed in the wake of home improvement.[96] In fact, a solitary article that was published in the Indies newspaper *Soerabaisch Handelsblad* and copied in the Dutch newspaper *Het Vaderland* had already broached the matter in 1930. It noted that home improvement in Soerakarta had quickly been followed by an outbreak of malaria. "Enquiring after this," the author noted, "we were told that the statistics of the last seven years absolutely confirm" that this was a recurring phenomenon. Two potential causes were identified. First, the habit of local populations to sleep outside during the renovation of their house (exposing them to night-biting mosquitoes). Second, the creation of new breeding sites in the vicinity of villages that were being renovated as a result of local rooftile production (allowing mosquitoes to thrive).[97] These articles effectively claimed that a link between home improvement and malaria had become apparent since 1923. Somehow, they failed to get traction at the time.

Back in 1937, Rosier emphasized that home improvement had generated "excellent" results against plague. But if there was any truth in the "recent" suggestion that the scheme facilitated the spread of malaria then this could "discredit" the entire operation.[98] Other factors such as the global recession and the development of Otten's vaccine also came into play. And when the home improvement scheme moved into West Java, there was the health of Dutch colonials in Batavia, Buitenzorg, and Bandoeng to consider. They were little affected by plague, but malaria did pose a threat. The time had come to review the available evidence.

Malaria in the Indies

To fully grasp the challenge this phenomenon presented to colonial officials, it is important to remember that malaria had long been recognized as the true pathogenic menace of the Indies. Whatever the reputation of plague, malaria was consistently described as the leading endemic disease in the archipelago. In 1908, de Vogel called it "the chief enemy of the population of our colonies."[99] The *Koloniaal Verslag* of 1928 declared that malaria remained "undoubtedly the worst scourge of the population of the Dutch East Indies."[100] And as late as March 1940, the Dutch minister of colonies reiterated the primacy of malaria over other tropical diseases in a parliamentary debate in no uncertain terms:

> I would point out that one can speak of all manner of tropical diseases, but that one must always acknowledge that malaria is in reality the principal disease. In the tropics, malaria is the chief disease and the chief underminer of the strength of the population. All other sorts of illnesses find their ultimate cause in the reduced strength of the population caused by malaria. He who combats malaria combats also tuberculosis and many other diseases. Consequently, a tropical country such as the Indies cannot but emphasize the control of malaria.[101]

None of these sources would provide clear figures on the incidence or death-rate of malaria. In 1954, however, a World Health Organization report on malaria in newly independent Indonesia still listed this disease as the "number one" health threat in the archipelago. In ordinary (as opposed to epidemic) years, it estimated, 20–50 of every 1,000 deaths were caused by malaria.[102] In short, malaria was recognized as the leading disease to erode health, happiness, and prosperity in the Indies.[103] Nevertheless, attempts at malaria control were limited. A few signature drainage projects aside (Sibolga, Tandjong Priok), most interventions were local and short-lived. Often, they relied on species sanitation (i.e., the elimination of mosquitoes) and the distribution of quinine (an antimalarial drug and prophylactic) in the wake of an outbreak. The Dutch East Indies actually produced over 90 percent of the world's supply of quinine at this time, but this did not mean that the drug was widely available to local populations.[104] A dedicated department for malaria control was not created until 1924. There was, in other words, a wide divide between the impact of malaria and its priority to health officials.

Pekalongan

To study if and how there was a relation between home improvement and malaria, Rosier decided to study the available evidence from Pekalongan, on the north coast of Central Java. Plague had entered this residency in two waves in 1921 and 1925. Home improvement began in 1925 and was completed in 1931. Coastal parts of the residency were "malarious," while the more mountainous terrain where plague had established itself was regarded "from experience" as malaria-free. Almost as soon as the renovations began, however, outbreaks of malaria were reported. And worryingly, the previously infrequent disease persisted long after the work had been completed. A correlation quickly became apparent. By overlaying the routes and dates of home improvement on the advance of malaria as arrows on a map, the latter followed the former closely. Both arrows followed a clear route that circled in on itself, revealing how the district at the center—Petoengkriono—was affected by malaria only after the renovation work began in 1930, despite bordering on districts where home improvement and malaria had begun five years earlier. Both the chronological order of events and the unlikely geographical advance of malaria toward this district, Rosier admitted, "plead for the existence of a common factor."[105]

To further strengthen this claim, Rosier presented several more pieces of anecdotal and epidemiological evidence. His use of imagery stands out.[106] Alongside several maps, he compiled two tables that again hinted at a causal relationship. The first listed forty-four out of seventy-one districts where home improvement had been completed since 1928 and where physicians had reported fresh outbreaks of malaria soon after. These were located in the residencies and regencies of Magelang, Wonosobo, Bandjarnegara, Klaten, Bojolali, Batang, Pekalongan, Brebes, Tegal, Koeningan, Tjiamis, and Tasikmalaja; in short, throughout the interior of Central Java. The second table recorded per quarter the occurrence of plague, home improvement, and malaria in eight districts of Pekalongan between 1924 and 1934. In each case, the symbols for malaria outbreaks followed those indicating the start of home improvement almost immediately. In the district Bawang, epidemiological evidence for a correlation dated back to 1926.[107]

But perhaps the most striking image in Rosier's report was a series of eight mortality statistics for each of the improved districts of Pekalongan. They suggested a harrowing possibility: that plague control had *exacerbated* overall mortality. Each graph recorded overall mortality per quarter over the period of a decade. Plague mortality was marked in black. Often, plague was already on the wane by the time that "permanent" control in the form of home improvement (marked with arrows) came along: hinting at the efficacy of the emergency *dessa schoonmaak*. Then, we see how in almost every district overall mortality substantially—and lastingly—increased. In Blado, this pattern was evident from the same quarter as the renovations began. In Blandar, it was noticeable from the second quarter onward. The most poignant evidence came once more from Petoengkriono. This district never hosted plague but was improved for "tactical" reasons. From the second quarter in which home improvement took place onward, we see a dramatic rise in overall mortality that Rosier put down to previously unheard-of outbreaks of malaria. The introduction of this disease in malaria-free regions would indeed have impacted hard on local populations due to a lack of partial acquired immunity. In concluding his paper, Rosier added: "we must remember that the epidemics described were all powerfully combated by the supply of quinine." In other words, these disturbing figures already presented "a mitigated form of the course of [malaria] without such interventions."[108]

The evidence suggested that *woningverbeteringsmalaria* was a real thing, but what caused it? Rosier offered several suggestions. During the renovations, residents lived in temporary sheds. The village grounds were full of rubbish and demolition material. Drainage ditches were blocked by debris. Earth was dug up for tile production. Trees and bamboo were cut down. When the rains came, a village was filled with puddles. These conditions facilitated mosquito breeding and access to humans. Meanwhile, malaria parasites were either already present or introduced by the "invasion of outsiders" involved with home improvement, such as laborers, traders, drivers, porters, inspectors, physicians, and engineers. "In short," concluded Rosier, "the quiet, orderly, remote and often malaria-free dessa is disturbed in her isolation."[109] The "rejuvenated" dwellings themselves were light and airy, qualities that appealed to the sanitary-minded physician but that also opened them up to mosquitoes, as Versteeg had already observed in 1930. Finally, there was a socioeconomic component. Home improvement placed new financial burdens on homeowners that impacted their ability to purchase food. In turn, a lack of protein and vitamins gnawed away at their ability to resist infection. It was evident that in many localities the conditions for a transitory malaria outbreak were consequently enhanced, but what factors caused the disease to persist?

Tasikmalaja

In 1938, the government physician J. W. Grootings published a second paper on home improvement and malaria. His investigation concentrated on the phenomenon in the regencies Tasikmalaja and Tjiamis in East Priangan. Plague had started to spread in earnest after 1930 and home improvement only caught up in 1933. Despite the small scale of the renovation works, Grootings's predecessor in the district, B. K. Zon, had already reported that local populations believed that "the houses now contain many more mosquitoes than before."[110] According to Zon, a quick mosquito survey between two improved villages and one unimproved village had resulted in an average yield of 6.7 and 11.1 mosquitoes per house in the former against 3.75 mosquitoes per house in the latter during one hour of catching. Zon had duly informed his superiors that "improved houses are more attractive to mosquitoes" and that home improvement facilitated contact between *Anopheles* mosquitoes and humans. "The more severe incidence of malaria since home improvement," he concluded, "would partially be explained by this."[111]

The paper by Grootings resembled that of Rosier. First, it praised the efficacy of home improvement against plague. Next, it brushed over more common financial concerns to stress that local populations were not necessarily opposed to the scheme. That was to say, if it had not been for a growing sense that home improvement brought about another health challenge:

> What now is the case? In the aforementioned subdistrict the people are quite unanimously of the opinion that Home Improvement is necessarily followed by malaria. This opinion is not merely that of the dumb masses, but is shared by the more educated among the population and even by Native Officials.[112]

The "dumb masses" had been perceptive "for this turned out to have in fact been the case." Through maps, graphs, and tables, Grootings was able to verify their suspicion that malaria followed hot on the heels of home improvement across these regencies. His survey of mortality statistics for districts being improved led to the following conclusions:

1. All graphs show sometime after home improvement a rise of the mortality rate to a height *never seen before.*
2. This rise of the mortality rate *runs parallel to the progress of home improvement.*
3. The *height* of the mortality curve *in most cases overlaps with the completion of* 90–100 percent *of all houses being improved.*
4. *The rise in mortality is independent of the season.*[113]

This information suggested a direct, quantitative link between the progress of home improvement and the advance of malaria. But the question remained: What caused it?

The suggestions of Rosier went a long way toward explaining the initial outbreaks of malaria, but as in Pekalongan, the disease persisted too long after home improvement in Tasikmalaja to be related to the renovation work alone. A fundamental and permanent change appeared to have taken place. At long last, Grootings dared to ask: Was there was something about the improved dwelling itself that facilitated transmission? "Is the idea so absurd? No, it is the most logical conclusion."[114] After all, if all other conditions in a community remained the same or stabilized once the work was completed, the altered house itself was the only remaining explanation. Grootings recognized that the impact of home improvement on the traditional Javanese house was tremendous. The *atap* roof was replaced with tiles. The bamboo frame was replaced with wood. Dirt floors were now replaced with concrete or tiles. And where the old dwelling was dark and poorly ventilated, the improved dwelling was light and airy. But perhaps the crucial difference, Grootings suggested, was that the old dwelling normally had a cooking area in the main compartment. Instead, the improved structure featured a separate kitchen area with a smoke vent.[115] The improved dwelling was not just more "open," it was simply not as infused with smoke as its predecessor.

From this observation, Grootings arrived at a straightforward hypothesis. Given that the nocturnal *Anopheles* mosquito was generally averse to smoke, the key change that took place was that the simple act of sleeping indoors no longer provided the same protection against malaria as it had before. Several photographs and diagrams in his paper illustrated this suggestion. They were accompanied by unusual captions. Or rather, the captions were familiar, but their meaning was curiously inverted. Terms that normally denoted health and hygiene now suggested risk and disease and vice versa. One photograph of a traditional house was described as "kitchen *inside* on the ground essentially in the sleeping quarters. Pay attention to the black soot on the walls!" The fragment captured a familiar European criticism of "native" dirt and poverty, but were instead put forward as evidence of the protection they offered against mosquitoes. Likewise, a sketch of an improved house ("ventilation present") and a photograph of a traditional house and an improved house (with arrows pointing out "ventilation openings!") now presented "airiness" as a potential health hazard. The photograph was additionally glossed: "important difference between neatness and ventilation!" With regard to malaria, however, airiness had become dangerous. "Soot on the walls" was not dirt but a crucial defense against mosquitoes. And neatness—however important it was in the battle against plague—offered no protection against malaria.[116]

Finally, Grootings returned to Zon's data on mosquito incidence. He organized simultaneous mosquito surveys in communities that featured both improved and unimproved houses. The outcome cemented the relation between home improvement and malaria. A table of the results suggested a nearly five-fold increase in mosquito incidence in renovated structures: with an average of 1.6 and 2.7 mosquitoes per ten unimproved houses in Tjiamis and Tasikmalaja respectively against 9 and 10 mosquitoes per ten improved houses. "Contact between man and mosquito," concluded Grootings, "has become more intimate in an improved dwelling!"[117]

Plague Rat or Anopheles

The remark by Grootings regarding human–mosquito "intimacy" within the improved Javanese dwelling transports us back to the early days of the plague outbreak in 1911. At the time, after all, it had been the unsuspected proximity of humans and rats inside the traditional bamboo house that had suggested home improvement to begin with. While the human-animal relations underpinning health were only just being uncovered, Dutch scientists and physicians were contributing to such research by newly recognizing the traditional bamboo house as a vibrant space of multispecies encounters. Through photographs, maps, tables, and diagrams, they distinguished the environmental conditions that underpinned human-rat interactions and that consequently underpinned plague transmission. In other words, they began to identify a plague ecology that was quite peculiarly Javanese. This newfound complexity, however, was immediately simplified again to draw the house into plague's existing rat-flea-man transmission scheme and articulate it as the key link where this chain might be broken. The identification of "home improvement malaria" demonstrated the dangers of this reductionist approach by underscoring that human-animal relations were not quite as linear as had been imagined: chains of disease transmission did not exist in isolation.

According to Rosier, home improvement malaria was evidence of the fact that Dutch interventions "in established natural conditions . . . can acutely favor malaria transmission." His paper spoke of biological balance, and how it had been disrupted.[118] And likewise, Grootings wrote that, historically, "the specific style of house construction" in Java had helped to "create a sort of balance, a biological balance" that had worked to "protect the population against a close contact with anopheles." This notion of biological balance, he continued, had traditionally been "of the utmost importance" to the hygien-ist. But the home improvement scheme, Grootings admitted, constituted a "one-sided hygienic intervention" that had broken this balance: with fresh out-breaks of malaria as a result. Consequently, home improvement malaria was a form of *"man-made malaria."*[119] How were matters to proceed from here? It is telling of the importance of home improvement that neither Rosier nor Grootings suggested alterations to the scheme. In fact, despite their newfound awareness of the overlapping disease ecologies that centered on the house, both physicians advocated *further* environmental change to tackle the new chal-lenge posed by malaria. A thorough study of malaria was in order, followed by targeted interventions in the immediate vicinity of districts undergoing im-provement. The plague service could screen workmen for malaria infection, for instance, or time the renovations in relation to periods of irrigation of the rice fields. In low-lying regions, wrote Rosier, "typical" mosquito breeding sites could be removed, while in hilly terrain afforestation offered recourse. Groot-ings compiled a list of eight recommendations to address the problem. De-spite his straightforward conclusions as to what caused home improvement malaria, these were surprisingly convoluted. Seven of his suggestions ranged from planting new vegetation, and draining artificially inundated rice fields after the harvest, to releasing new larvivorous fish species in nearby ponds. Only his last recommendation offered a correction for the disruption that Grootings previously identified. "One could conduct a trial with distribut-ing bed nets," he concluded, and thereby deny the nocturnal *Anopheles* mos-quito the opportunity to feed on humans while they slept.

Between 1911 and 1942, plague killed an estimated 7,000 people per year on average. The mortality for malaria over this period was both incalculable and uncalculated. Certainly, it exceeded that for plague by an order of magnitude. The question of how many lives were lost to malaria on account of plague con-trol is impossible to answer. An attempt to extrapolate from the available data, however, is painfully suggestive. In 1991, the engineer W. B. Snellen wrote:

> From Grootings' curves, I have calculated the average of the maximum mortality rates in 17 sub-districts as recorded before house improvement; this was 38 per thousand. The average of the peak mortality rate re-corded after house improvement in 8 sub-districts is twice as high: 77 per thousand.[120]

In other words, the average mortality rate in eight improved districts was twice as high as the average in seventeen districts before (and without) home im-provement. It was a public health disaster with clear roots in human activity— and it is important to recall Rosier's comment that these figures likely presented a "mitigated" picture as these outbreaks had been recognized and were responded to with the distribution of quinine. Earlier and elsewhere, the consequences of home improvement may have been more severe.

At the time, the public response to the studies of Rosier and Grootings was surprisingly mild. No one, at least, seemed to think that Dutch health officials had knowingly facilitated malaria transmission for the better part of a decade— or to have concealed the possibility thereof. One of the first newspapers to pick up the story in January 1938 merely summarized Rosier's findings.[121] The Indies newspaper *Het Nieuws van den Dag* was more critical. It called home improvement malaria "disastrous" and asked after the desirability of the scheme if the lives saved from plague, on the one hand, were lost to malaria, on the other.[122] When Grootings's publication came out, this newspaper again pointed out the painful "dilemma" this phenomenon posed to the DVG. Which health threat was worse, "plague rat or anopheles?"[123] *De Locomotief* linked the good with the bad under the subheading: "new houses are more pleasant not just for the local population, but also for the anopheles."[124] The Dutch newspaper *De Telegraaf* referred to these new insights as "striking" but cautioned against jumping to conclusions.[125] And when toward the end of 1938 it was decided to suspend home improvement on the Bandoeng plateau on account of the threat posed by malaria, the *Algemeen Handelsblad voor Nederlandsch-Indië* went so far as to praise the government for "the timely recognition of this danger."[126] In the Volksraad, di Nata and other representatives raised the question of whether the government accepted that a correlation existed and what it intended to do about it.[127] The government's response was that "an answer to this question cannot currently be given" and that the Malaria Bureau had started an investigation.[128] The question of accountability never came up.

Health actors who had been involved with home improvement were remarkably silent on the matter. Plague experts such as van Loghem, de Vogel, Flu, and Otten appear not to have commented on the matter in public. The issue was brought up in parliament and newspapers occasionally referred to the phenomenon, but no serious threat to the home improvement scheme emerged. Back in the Netherlands, the prominent malariologist Nicholaas H. Swellengrebel (formerly a bacteriologist with the plague service) published a short commentary. He had studied the evidence presented by his colleagues, fielded some general objections to their methods and conclusions, and conceded that the data appeared to point toward a causal link between home improvement and malaria. Further research was necessary to determine the underlying causes. Still, his paper offered an opening for a future shift in policy. "For what," he asked tentatively, "should one do with a control measure for a disease that one suspects to induce a similar if not indeed higher mortality for another disease than the one being suppressed?"[129]

In practice, the answer to this question was simple: nothing. The recognition of *woningverbeteringsmalaria* posed a challenge but did not push home improvement off its pedestal. The phenomenon was troubling but had few direct implications. In 1938, more than 56,000 houses were improved. In 1939, this figure stood at a barely diminished 54,000. And in 1940 (the last full year for which records were available) the tally still exceeded 39,000: pushing the total over the 1.6 million mark (introduction, table 1). For 1942, 50,000 houses were still expected to be improved.[130] Only in the vicinity of Bandoeng was the scheme apparently halted to keep malaria at bay.[131] Starting in January 1940, trials were held in Priangan to see if home improvement could be implemented while simultaneously guarding against an outbreak of malaria—without success.[132] Other than that, the DVG stated that "the districts to be improved must be carefully surveyed in order to prevent further outbreaks of malaria."[133] When such outbreaks did occur, the Malaria Bureau was called in to respond with "quinine distribution, etc."[134] Finally, a three-year long "correlation inquest" began in 1939.[135] In summary, home improvement, cleaning, and inspection continued as before—still accompanied by plague propaganda and newly joined by vaccination—right up until the Japanese invasion in March 1942.

Conclusion

After 1928, health officials in Java were faced with a new series of challenges regarding plague and plague control. First, the disease expanded into new territory in West Java while home improvement lagged behind in Central Java. Second, the global economic downturn after 1930 put further pressure on the plague service as budget cuts across the colonial civil service caused its staff and funding to be slashed in half. As a result, the number of plague cases exploded and reached unprecedented heights. Between 1932 and 1934, more people died of plague in Priangan than did in East Java over the thirty years that plague was endemic. In 1935, the live vaccine by Otten offered a new and highly economical alternative to home improvement and dramatically reduced plague mortality. In 1941, the last full year of Dutch colonial rule in the archipelago, just a few hundred plague deaths were recorded across the island. The signature home improvement scheme, however, was not abandoned.

Shortly after Dutch-style home improvement received a strong international endorsement from the Bandoeng Rural Hygiene Conference in 1937, in fact, it emerged that home improvement had continued despite having been implicated in fresh outbreaks of malaria for at least a decade. Still, this phenomenon did not halt the home improvement scheme or diminish the importance that was attached to it. Plague eclipsed malaria. And home improvement had become so central to Dutch colonial health policy that it could not easily be abandoned, practically or ideologically. It seems fair to stress that health officials had not intended for malaria to spread. The considerable delay in responding to this phenomenon, however, exposes how different and competing interests dictated health policy. Home improvement was about saving lives, certainly, but it was also about saving lives from plague specifically, and about *being seen* to save them too. Home improvement embodied Dutch scientific ingenuity, political ability, and commitment to its colonial project—ethically or otherwise.

Why could this fatal side effect of home improvement not be admitted to until 1937? A cynical reading would be to suggest that the development of the Otten vaccine was instrumental here. It offered an opening for a future shift in policy without loss of face on the colonial and scientific stage. After eliciting a final formal declaration of support from foreign health professionals in 1937, "home improvement malaria" could gradually be brought into the open. It allowed for the disclosure of a potentially fatal flaw in what had become the poster-child health policy of the Dutch reform period, by at the same time pointing to the dramatic reduction in plague deaths that had been achieved since 1935. Perhaps many extra lives had been lost to malaria over the years. But look: no more plague.

Conclusion

In 1941, only about 350 people died of plague in Java.[1] It was the lowest figure on record since the start of the outbreak in 1911 (see chapter 3, table 4). This achievement came after the highest death rates on record just a few years earlier, and was wholly attributable to the introduction of vaccination. The development of a live plague vaccine by Louis Otten offered a cheap and efficient alternative to plague control. Since 1935, small teams of vaccinators managed to distribute approximately two million doses a year at an annual cost of just f. 75,000.[2] Nevertheless, state agents remained committed to the policy they had perfected over the last thirty years: home improvement. After all, they argued, vaccination failed to permanently remove the plague threat. According to discussions in the Volksraad on the Indies budget for 1942, fully half the funds provided for the prevention and control of infectious disease continued to be earmarked to support the home improvement scheme.[3] But home improvement was slow, costly, and reactive. It was unpopular, unable to achieve its stated aim of breaking human-rat cohabitation on its own, and it had become implicated in the production of fresh outbreaks of malaria. On account of home improvement, the full cost of plague control—around f. 1.1 million a year—stood in increasingly sharp contrast to the actual burden of this disease.[4] Why were Dutch colonial scientists, physicians, and officials so intent on pursuing the home improvement scheme and its attendant policies of home inspection and hygiene education under these circumstances?

The answer to this question, as this book has sought to demonstrate, rested in the fact that plague control had long since ceased to be about plague alone. Instead, the development, implementation, and outcomes of plague control had become tied to matters of Dutch scientific and colonial power, prestige, and ambition. Soon, however, this signature health intervention of the Dutch colonial period met with a sudden end.

The Javanese and Plague Control

The Dutch approach to plague control—dominated by home improvement, hygiene education, and latterly vaccination—drastically impacted the lives of millions of Javanese. Their response to these interventions has however gone largely unrecorded: in Dutch sources for certain and in Indonesian sources for as far as I can determine. How did people feel about the intrusions into their homes, environments, practices, beliefs, and indeed bodies? Or about the expansion of government oversight into their communities? Official sources such as the *Mededeelingen* and the *Koloniaal Verslag* are notoriously quiet about opposition toward colonial rule. Instead, they emphasize the assistance of local regents, acquiescence of local populations, or an occasional form of passive resistance.[5] Newspapers toed the line, often citing verbatim from these reports, highlighting the impressive results that colonial officials, physicians, and assistants had achieved in collaboration with local populations, and referring only in passing to cases of disgruntlement that interfered with plague control and that tended to be linked to "superstition."[6] Reading across these and other sources over time, however, a more nuanced image of local responses does emerge. People could comply with Dutch policies, engage with them creatively, or selectively resist only particular facets of plague control for very specific reasons. Plague control was shaped by such responses and was—it should be pointed out—implemented by a corps of hundreds of primarily Javanese staff.[7]

Already in the plague reports of 1912, we learn of local populations who asserted agency in their response to plague and plague control regulations. They would design their own ratproof housing features, for instance, made choices about whether or not they wanted to be vaccinated, to enter quarantine camps or stay with relatives, and would volunteer their assistance to family and neighbors.[8] From published government sources we learn that home improvement was in fact unpopular throughout its existence but that what was truly resented was the forced evacuations from plague-stricken houses and villages. The *dessa schoonmaak* protocol was introduced in 1915 partially to meet this objection by reducing the duration of these evacuations. And the installation of hatches in pneumonic plague huts to allow for rudimentary nursing of patients only began after a Javanese father had remained healthy while nursing his child who suffered from this form of plague through the half-opened door of their house.[9] These sources also inform us of occasional instances of active resistance to the Dutch health interventions. For instance, some populations were critical of having to contribute to plague control in unpaid labor.[10] In 1915, one reads that police capacity in Soerabaja was expanded "in the interest of plague control" but the developments necessitating this remain unclear.[11] Only occasionally do we glimpse a political motive, as in 1920 when "cases of resistance" to plague control were linked to members of the Indies nationalist movement Sarekat-Islam.[12] The creation of the Volksraad in 1918, finally, offered select Indies representatives an official forum to voice concerns over facets of plague control. The financial burden that home improvement placed on local populations was a recurring topic of debate, and the lack of flexibility in implementing plague control interventions to accommodate local practices or religious beliefs was frequently complained about.[13]

Unpublished government sources such as the *Memories van Overgave* are perhaps more revealing of local responses to plague control. These reports were written by the outgoing *resident* of a district for their successor and normally reflected on local political conditions as well as health matters. The local history of plague, plague control, and the repayment of monetary advances for home improvement were normally included. Overall, these reports present plague control as a peaceable affair even when the interventions were admittedly disliked. They discuss local problems in implementing plague control rather than fundamental challenges. Some, however, suggest a more volatile history. In Kedoe, M. B. van der Jagt observed in 1927 that "resistance had to be suppressed several times" when home improvement first began. He blamed local antipathy on "communist propaganda" and noted: "In the dessa Danoeredjo, members of the resistance were convicted to 7 days in prison, and subsequently had to transport the construction materials to the dessa under police escort and renovate their houses under police supervision." Sometime later, "a public disturbance took place on the grounds of the assistant-*wedono*."[14] This was one of the clearest references to local opposition to home improvement. Elsewhere, resistance to plague control would concentrate on one policy in particular: the spleen puncture. This procedure involved the injection of a large needle into the spleen of a suspected plague corpse to extract a sample of fluid that helped bacteriologists to confirm a diagnosis. The practice was resented by Javanese populations, who felt it violated the integrity of the body or thought it hurtful to the soul of the deceased.[15]

Already in 1919, the Dutch physician Feico van Loon observed that performing a spleen puncture correctly at the first attempt was imperative "especially in an Islamic population . . . where there is often a degree of passive resistance." A repeat attempt was sure to cause unrest.[16] After 1930, when plague had spread further west, resistance to the spleen puncture became more pronounced. In Tegal, the *resident* wrote that "the spleen puncture gave rise to difficulty, c.q. [or else] to opposition" in four specific villages. This resistance was ultimately overcome but only after an intervention by both the local regent and the *pengoeloe* (an Islamic village cleric).[17] Later, in West Priangan, a colleague similarly reported that coroner inquests and spleen punctures presented no difficulties in his district, but only "thanks to the personal preventive action by the Regent of Tjiandjoer."[18] In Pekalongan government officials encountered significant resistance. The governor of Central Java, A. H. Neys, blamed this confrontation between colonial medicine and local culture on "the mentality and religious convictions of the population" as well as on "de Inlandsche beweging"—a catchall for various nationalist organizations that caused officials growing concern.[19] A good deal of "tact" was required in order to perform a spleen puncture. Still, tensions would come to a head. In 1931, there had been an attack on a native official in the *dessa* Remboel during which three police officers were hurt. The most traumatic incident occurred in April 1933, when a *mantri* arriving in the *dessa* Kalialang to perform an inquest on a suspected plague corpse was met with an angry crowd and stoned to death as he tried to flee the scene. A few days later, another protest in nearby Djiwoeng allegedly drew 800 people. Newspapers reported that the protests appeared to have an "antiauthority character" and "that home improvement also encounters difficulties in this region."[20] Ultimately, forty-two suspects were charged for the stoning, of whom twenty-two were convicted.[21]

Over the last few years of Dutch colonial rule, reports of resistance to plague control became less pronounced. In 1934, the *resident* of Pekalongan counted only nine "puncture refusals" and noted a significant reduction in "clandestine" burials intended to avert a spleen puncture.[22] The departing governor of Central Java, J. C. de Vos, noted in 1937 that active as well as passive resistance had died down. Vaccination and revaccination had been introduced and went ahead unobstructed, he wrote, while "truants counted for less than 3%."[23] This claim (as well as the absence of reporting on other forms of resistance) might be misleading, however. In a detailed list of vaccination and revaccination rates published in 1938, we note that turnout to receive the Otten vaccine varied considerably between districts. In Bodjongloa and Garoet, for instance, they were as low as 54.0 and 59.7 percent, while in Boeahbatoe and Temanggoeng they reached 92.6 and 93.3 percent.[24] This truancy could certainly be understood as a form of passive resistance to colonial policy. Meanwhile, one notices in these sources that enthusiasm for home improvement and home inspection remained tepid at best, with officials complaining in 1936 that "maintenance of the improved dwellings is largely neglected."[25] A report in the *Mededeelingen* by the Indies physician Soerono on a new experiment with "voluntary" home improvement is quite revealing of the fact that this signature health policy remained unpopular. Local populations in Cheribon were now "persuaded" toward improving their dwelling—in their own time and at their own expense—by means of propaganda for the benefits thereof (as well as by regular intrusions in their domestic life in the form of home inspections). The "otherwise so important factors of force and punishment," noted Soerono cheerfully, were thus absent. It was nevertheless "not unthinkable that a degree of mild pressure" was exerted by overzealous officials to prompt homeowners to participate in the allegedly voluntary scheme.

Overall, these sources (combined with numerical data of houses improved and vaccinations given) appear to suggest that large segments of the Javanese population simply endured the Dutch plague control measures. They were unpopular, accepted, engaged with, enforced, and ignored. There was considerable leeway in how populations engaged with these and other health interventions, in other words, and red lines were certainly articulated as well. Indeed, in the case of the spleen puncture, such lines were crossed by state agents at their peril. It seems curious that such an invasive policy as home improvement would not be linked to political resistance more frequently, though perhaps the omission of references to such an entanglement from official sources carries its own message here. In theory, the Dutch government pursued a uniform and high-handed solution toward countering plague. In practice, however, plague control or facets thereof had to be responsive to the customs and beliefs of local populations—and were reshaped in the process.

War, Plague, and Decolonization

In September 1939, the German invasion of Poland marked the start of World War II. After a brief period of neutrality in the escalating conflict, the Netherlands was likewise invaded and occupied by German forces in May 1940. The Dutch government fled to London. Its colonies in Southeast Asia and the Caribbean now had to fend for themselves. In the Dutch East Indies, the threat of invasion by Japan loomed large as this expansionist power sought to secure access to key resources. In the end, it was the Dutch government-in-exile that declared war following the Japanese attack on Pearl Harbor in December 1941.

After successive defeats of the American, Australian, British, and Dutch forces in the region, Japan invaded Java on March 1, 1942, and quickly overran its defenses. Within a week the governor-general surrendered and a Japanese military administration took charge. The European civilian population as well as Allied prisoners-of-war were placed in internment camps. The Eurasian community (the so-called Indo population) was permitted to live outside the camps but was subject to strict regulations.[26]

The Japanese invasion brought an effective end to Dutch colonial rule in the archipelago. It also marked the start of an exceptionally volatile period in Indonesian history.[27] Over the next three years, food, resources, and millions of laborers were rallied to support the Japanese war effort—with grave consequences. Although no major military operations took place in the region for the remainder of the war, a figure of four million Indonesian deaths due to forced labor, exhaustion, malnutrition, and infectious disease is often cited.[28] The Japanese military administration nevertheless fostered Indonesian nationalist ideals and took steps toward the creation of an independent state. Two days after the Japanese surrender to the Allies, on August 17, 1945, the leaders of the nationalist movement proclaimed Indonesian independence. Shortly after, a period of ethnic violence erupted across Java. The Japanese army that had been tasked with maintaining order until Allied troops were brought in mostly remained in their barracks and retained nominal control over the internment camps. Outside the camps nationalist paramilitary groups began to persecute Indo and Chinese populations as well as native Indonesians suspected of harboring pro-Dutch sentiments. This period—known as the Bersiap—led to the deaths of thousands of people of primarily mixed Dutch and Indies but also Chinese descent (the total tally having recently been revised downward from around 30,000 to some 6,000 deaths).[29] The Dutch government refused to acknowledge the unilateral declaration of independence, furthermore, and began to ship over a large number of conscripts from the Netherlands. When negotiations failed, it launched two violent offensives in 1947 and 1948 that reasserted Dutch control over much of Java and Sumatra. Strong international condemnation and the suspension of Marshall aid from the United States ultimately forced the government to withdraw and a formal transfer of power took place on December 27, 1949. On the Dutch side, the conflict cost the life of 6,177 soldiers. On the Indonesian side, a reported figure of 100,000 military casualties is now regarded as merely the lower limit—to which must be added another 25,000 to 100,000 civilian casualties.[30]

Unsurprisingly, plague briefly surged back over this turbulent period. Wartime conditions naturally favored the incidence of infectious disease and the close system of plague surveillance developed by the Dienst der Volksgezond-heid was disrupted. According to postwar sources, plague deaths climbed to a high of 1,214 in 1943 before falling again to just 190 in 1945.[31] Given the dire health situation in Java toward the end of the war, this figure was certainly underreported. Plague nevertheless failed to regain its former heights. Over the years of war and decolonization, cases would concentrate in Priangan, with only smaller outbreaks in East and Central Java. A testament, perhaps, to the efficacy of home improvement and hygiene education in the long run? An out-break in Djokjakarta (where home improvement had been widely imple-mented) was nonetheless reported by Dutch newspapers to have claimed 2,409 lives in 1946.[32] The fact that this city was also described by one Dutch politi-cian as "de geestelijke pesthaard" (the ideological source of contagion) of the nationalist movement reminds us to treat such sources with caution.[33] Still, the time that plague claimed well over ten thousand lives a year appeared to have come to an end. In 1951, fewer than 3,000 cases were reported across Java. This figure had decreased "thirtyfold" three years later.[34] Afterward, between vaccination, the development of antibiotic medication, and improving socio-economic conditions, plague all but disappeared. The disease persists in ani-mal reservoirs in parts of Java to this day, however, leading to individual cases of human plague at long intervals.[35]

Despite its limited mortality, plague remained a source of official anxiety over this period of war and decolonization. Indeed, the Japanese military ad-ministration would resume plague control almost without missing a beat. For instance, after his initial arrest, the Eurasian *assistent-resident* of Bandoeng was released in April 1942 and placed in charge of plague control in Garoet soon after.[36] At the Pasteur Institute, Otten was for a while allowed to remain in his post to continue to produce vaccines and serums. In a photograph of staff at the institute of September 1942, we see him seated in the front row beside two Japa-nese soldiers.[37] Soon after, he too was sent to an internment camp. A live vaccine produced from Otten's avirulent plague strains would continue to be produced by Japanese scientists for the remainder of the occupation. When Dutch re-searchers took back control of the institute in February 1946, they complained that Otten's plague cultures "had become heavily polluted" and that errors in distributing the vaccine had led to serious side effects.[38] Their disdain aside, these comments inform us that a form of plague control remained in place that was presumably run primarily by Indonesian medical personnel.[39]

The home improvement scheme met with a sudden and inglorious end. There is no evidence to suggest that the Japanese military administration continued it. Instead, sources indicate they concentrated on vaccination alone.

The regular system of six-monthly vaccinations and revaccinations was disrupted and gave way to a more ad hoc program. According to Otten, speaking in 1946, Japanese officials were "scared to death of infectious disease" and wanted to launch a vaccination drive after every plague case they identified. According to records he managed to hold on to, over 417,000 doses were delivered in the second half of 1942.[40] From now on, the European population in the internment camps was an explicit focus of plague control as well, but they did not particularly enjoy it. The Dutch comedian Wim Kan, interned in Tjimahi, noted in his diary that he received a plague vaccine on September 25, 1942. It made him feel unwell and he gloomily reported, "Ik heb de pest in."[41] In November, the officer of health T. Eijden, interned in Malang, reported that he received 6 liters of Otten vaccine to distribute among his campmates. Since he had learned that Otten had been removed from the Pasteur Institute, he was mistrustful of its quality and first injected himself and three other volunteers. The group then switched plans, destroying the material and secretly refilling the bottles with spare vaccine against typhus, cholera, and dysentery. Less than two months later, Eijden received 2.2 liters of "killed" Haffkine vaccine that he distributed without objection.[42] Other interned physicians later recounted boiling the plague vaccine they received before distributing it out of similar concerns.[43] A year later, in October 1943, C. M. Reinders-Folmers, interned in Bandoeng, wrote in her diary: "We are getting injections against the Plague from *mantries*."[44] It has been difficult to uncover much more about plague and plague control over this period, but such statements again appear to suggest that a plague service of sorts was operational outside the camps as well.[45]

Afterward, during the Indonesian National Revolution, home improvement would not be revived. As before, physicians in the Dutch-administered parts of Java had to rely on vaccination. The program was more chaotic than before and could target only specific populations, such as the civilian population of Bandoeng or army personnel. As the Dutch virologist R. Gispen reported in May 1948, "interventions that aim to break contact between humans and the source of infection, such as home improvement, will have to wait until order and prosperity are restored." In practice, this meant that "the role of vaccination will likely be of even greater importance in the coming years than before the war."[46] Newspapers published over this period reported that vaccination drives took place in areas with fresh outbreaks, that plague vaccine was occasionally delivered "by parachute" to Republican areas such as Magelang and Wonosobo, and that plague vaccine began to be produced in Djokjakarta as well.[47] In brief, one of the most invasive health interventions of the Dutch colonial period had come to an unceremonious end.

Medicine and Colonialism in the Indies

This turbulent era of war and decolonization is at present being extensively researched. In the Netherlands and Indonesia, four academic institutes recently completed a five-year government-supported investigation into the nature, causes, and consequences of Dutch violence between 1945 and 1950.[48] This project emerged out of a broad societal call to reassess the darker side of the Dutch colonial past, with slavery as another topic of intense public and scholarly attention.[49] A broader understanding of the physical forms of violence under Dutch colonialism is long overdue, but it is imperative not to lose sight of other (and perhaps less self-evident) facets of the coercive nature of Dutch colonial rule. "While the violent character of the colonial regime can be taken for granted," observed the historian Marieke Bloembergen in 2007, "there is still much that we do not know about the actual practice of implementing state violence in colonial Indonesia."[50] The domain of health, disease, and medicine is certainly worth exploring in this regard—as the history of plague in Java illustrates. Were forced evacuations, mandatory renovations, regular home inspections, forcing people into debt, the alteration of landscapes and art forms, neglecting a phenomenon such as *woningverbeteringsmalaria*, the propagation of a foreign medical cosmology, the documentation and representation of it all in photographs, and all their attendant social, cultural, and environmental consequences not a form of "colonial violence" as well? Scholars have long since demonstrated the complex relation between medicine and empire in other contexts. From cruder arguments of medicine as a "tool of empire" to sophisticated analyses of the ways in which local and colonial medical traditions interacted, they have shown how colonial pasts reverberate into present-day health challenges and shape global health structures and practices.[51] Until very recently, such histories took very little cognizance of the former Dutch empire.[52] If we are indeed to arrive at a better understanding of the impact and afterlives of Dutch colonial rule, however, then the realm of medicine is in urgent need of further scholarly attention.

In this book, I have traced how the introduction of plague in Java in 1911 prompted an unparalleled health intervention by the Dutch colonial state. Despite the relatively modest burden of this disease over the following thirty years, no other disease elicited a comparable health response, nor one that was impressed quite so visibly on the land. Plague control was emphatically "colonial" from the outset. For starters, its implementation was embedded in existing power structures, cultural hierarchies, and racial assumptions. It relied in part on unpaid labor and forced homeowners to assume debts that they were frequently unable to repay. Early plague science that implicated the traditional Javanese house in plague transmission went beyond detailing a rudimentary plague ecology: rather, by effectively labeling Javanese materials, designs, and practices as *pestgevaarlijk* it pathologized entire cultures and environments. The home improvement scheme that ostensibly sought to break human-rat cohabitation at once reshaped Javanese architecture, material culture, landscapes, environments, and indeed social relations. And by replacing *atap* roofs with tiles or metal covers, the renovations literally "revealed" previously obscured villages and populations to colonial administrators. The rapid acknowledgment that no measure of improvement would ever make a house intrinsically rat-proof resulted in an increasingly systematic hygiene education and home inspection scheme that expanded Dutch colonial oversight further still. It also extended Dutch cultural influence by inducing Javanese populations to see their dwellings in new ways, reform domestic and hygienic practices, and lay a foundation for a broader "appreciation" of European scientific medicine.

The fact that plague control was about more than health alone is perhaps most powerfully illustrated by the sizeable archive of plague photography. These images overwhelmingly emphasized the productive response of the Dutch colonial government to this health threat. They present physicians, officials, laborers, and residents hard at work at countering the outbreak. Most of all, they sought to demonstrate the "visible" improvement that the Dutch policy of home improvement wrought in people, houses, and landscapes. In other words, as I have sought to demonstrate throughout, plague control offered a *spectacle* of Dutch colonial rule in the Indies. It offered visual evidence of the need for this intervention as well as the scale on which it was implemented, and in doing so justified existing colonial relations. The tremendous scale and impact of the home improvement scheme were cast as evidence of the Dutch commitment to its new "ethical" course in colonial governance—all the while intimating that continued colonial oversight and control were indispensable for the present moment. Naturally, the more coercive facets of the scheme remained out of sight. The extensive circulation that plague photography enjoyed in the Indies, the Netherlands, and indeed abroad—often alongside other visual materials such as maps, graphs, and models—was proof of Dutch scientific acumen and colonial ability. This propagandistic use of home improvement as a representation of the benign nature of Dutch colonial rule was increasingly evident over the 1910s and 1920s. The overriding importance of this function was starkly illustrated by the fact that home improvement was continued in the 1930s when it had been implicated as the cause behind fresh outbreaks of malaria—and starker still when it persisted when vaccination offered a powerful and cost-effective alternative. In the end, it appears that the esthetics of plague control in Java were simply more important to the Dutch colonial government than its efficacy.

APPENDIX 1

List of Key Government Officials

Below follows a list of key officials in the Dutch East Indies who were involved in the organization of healthcare in the colony between 1911 and 1942, with their dates in office. Between 1925 and 1930, there appears to have been no formal leader of the department of plague control and the organization of this scheme was ambiguously divided between the head of the Public Health Service and the senior plague physician in Central Java (the center of the epidemic at the time). Officials were often appointed on an "acting" basis, for instance to cover extended periods of furlough for their colleagues or in anticipation of a formal appointment.

Governor-General of the Dutch East Indies
Gouverneur-Generaal van Nederlands-Indië

Alexander Idenburg (December 1909–March 1916)
Johan van Limburg Stirum (March 1916–March 1921)
Dirk Fock (March 1921–September 1926)
Andries de Graeff (March 1926–September 1931)
Bonifacius de Jonge (September 1931–September 1936)
Alidius Tjarda van Starkenborgh Stachouwer (September 1936–March 1942)

Director of the Civil Medical Service
Leider van de Burgerlijke Geneeskundige Dienst

acting: Dr. J. Schülein (January 1911–December 1912)
Dr. Willem Thomas de Vogel (January 1913–November 1921)
acting: Dr. J. Noordhoek Hegt (February 1915–August 1915)
acting: Dr. O. D. Ouwehand (August 1915–October 1915)
Dr. Jan Jacobus van Lonkhuyzen (November 1921–December 1924)

Director of the Public Health Service
Leider van de Dienst der Volksgezondheid

Dr. Jan Jacobus van Lonkhuyzen (January 1925–May 1931)
acting: Dr. Louis Otten (December 1926–January 1928)
Dr. Johannes Offringa (May 1931–December 1938)
acting: Dr. W. F. Theunissen (December 1934–November 1935)
Dr. W. F. Theunissen (December 1938–March 1942)

Director of the Plague Service (independent)
Leider van de Dienst der Pestbestrijding

Dr. W. J. van Gorkom (January 1915–November 1915)
Acting–Dr. K. van Roon (November 1915–October 1918)
Dr. Louis Otten (October 1918–February 1924)

Department of Plague Control (reintegrated)
Hoofd van het Departement van Pestbestrijding

Dr. G. M. Versteeg (March 1929–May 1931)
Dr. P. Cool (May 1931–April 1933)
Dr. H. J. Rosier (April 1933–ca. 1942)

Director of the Smallpox Vaccination Institute and Pasteur Institute

Hoofd van de Landskoepokinrichting en het Instituut Pasteur

Dr. A. H. Nijland (January 1899–July 1918)

Dr. J. Noordhoek Hegt (July 1918–May 1924)

Dr. Louis Otten (May 1924–March 1942)

APPENDIX 2

Instructions for Inhabiting
an Improved House

Below is an excerpt from a series of plague control regulations published in 1921, entitled *Requirements for the Improvement of Plague-Dangerous Buildings as well as Their Inhabitation and Use*. This section offered a detailed list of "requirements for the inhabitation and use of buildings and commons" that had been determined by the head of the Dienst der Pestbestrijding in 1919. Similar regulations had existed since 1911 and remained in force until the end of Dutch colonial rule. The regulations formed a basis for both home inspection and hygiene education targeting plague.

Beknopt overzicht betreffende organisatie en uitvoering der pestbestrijdingsmaatregelen (Semarang: A. Bisschop, 1921), 38–44.

C. Requirements for the Inhabitation and Use of Buildings and Commons

1. Sleeping spaces
    (a) Sleeping spaces and *balé-balés* must be on feet, which reach at least one foot above the floor.
    (b) They must be at least one foot away of any of the surrounding walls.
    (c) They must not be placed in rooms or part of the rooms in which goods are stored.
    (d) It is forbidden for *balé-balés* to have *watons* made of bamboo, unless they have been opened up [*trontong*].

(e) It is forbidden for *balé-balé*s to have beams made of bamboo, unless they have been halved.

(f) Should the feet of a *balé-balé* be dug into the ground, the upper part should be able to be removed, so that the whole floor beneath the *balé-balé* can be inspected.

2. Hearths

(a) Hearths must be built of masonry bricks or baked loam mixed with *damèn* or *idjoek*.

3. Household goods

(a) Small household goods should be stored orderly in wardrobes or on racks (of split—halved—bamboo).

(b) On the floors no objects may be stacked in a disorderly way.

(c) Wardrobes, racks, and suitcases [*grobog*] must (if they are placed on an earthen floor) have feet, which reach at least half a foot above the floor.

(d) It is forbidden to use the space beneath wardrobes, racks, sleeping spaces, and other furniture for storing objects.

4. Goods

(a) Goods must be stacked in an orderly way.

(b) They must rest *or* immediately on the floor, *or* on an even piece of the floor connecting to the ground, *or* on a shelf with feet which reach at least one foot above the floor that, if made of bamboo, must be opened up or halved.

(c) Inside, these shall be removed one foot distance from the *gedek* walls, and outside at least two feet.

5. Lighting

(a) *In all parts of a building, including those parts above ceilings and paneling (unless the latter are entirely closed off from the inside of the building), daylight should be able to enter freely.*

(b) In each closure in the façade (*toetoep keong, ampé-ampé*) must be placed light openings amounting to an aggregated surface of at least 1250 cm.

The upside of the ridge beam as well as the inside of the roof . . . must be whitewashed.

All walls on the inside of a building should be whitewashed, walls from unbaked stone also on the outside.

(c) All spaces, in which daylight cannot enter, . . . must be supplied with their own light openings, with either glass rooftiles or windows.

6. Cleanliness
   (a) Dirt and rubbish must be destroyed or buried daily.
   (b) House and commons must be made tidy and clear of rats' nests.

Glossary

adat: customs and practices observed by Muslim communities, in Java mingled with animist traditions

afdeeling; assistent-resident: subdistrict; subdistrict official

Algemeen Soerabaisch Gezondheidscomité: General Health Committee of Soerabaja

atap: palm leaf thatch

balé-balé: Javanese bedstead

Binnenlandsch Bestuur: Interior Government

blandar: main support beams of a traditional Javanese house

blandar woewoeng: part of the roof construction of a traditional Javanese house

bouw: Indies unit of measurement, equal to 7,095.5 m² (76,375.33 square feet)

Burgerlijke Geneeskundige Dienst: Civil Medical Service

Commissie voor de Volkslectuur: Committee for Popular Reading

controleur: local official supporting an *assistent-resident*

Departement voor Medisch-Hygiënische Propaganda: Department for Medical-Hygienic Propaganda

Departement voor Medische Propaganda: Department for Medical Propaganda

dessa: native village (often used interchangeably with *kampong*)

dessa schoonmaak: *dessa* cleaning

Dienst der Volksgezondheid: Public Health Service

doctor djawa: Javanese physician

doekoen: Javanese traditional healer

drüsenfieber: glandular fever

Ethische Politiek: Ethical Policy

gedek: woven bamboo mats

Geneeskundig Laboratorium: Medical Laboratory

gouvernementsarts: government physician

inlands / inlandsche: native

Inlandsche arts / Indische arts: native physician / Indies physician

inspecteur-technical: technical investigator

joglo: Javanese roof style used by aristocracy

kadjang: woven mats of diverse plant fibers (bamboo, cane, palm leaves) *kampong*: native quarter in city

Koloniaal Instituut: Colonial Institute

Koloniaal Verslag; Indies Verslag: *Colonial Report; Indies Report*

Koninklijk Nederlandsch-Indisch Leger: Royal Dutch-Indies Army

Korte Berichten: *Short Notices*

kraton: Javanese royal palace

Landskoepokinrichting: National Smallpox Institute

limasan: Javanese roof style used by more prosperous residents

loerah: village chief

mandoer: native foreman

mantri: assistant

medische propaganda: medical propaganda

modelkampong: model *kampong*, used for instruction

Oosthoek: eastern parts of Java

padi: paddy, unmilled rice

pendopo: Javanese roof style resembling the *joglo* for open, pavilion-style buildings with a religious or official function

pengeret: secondary support beams of a traditional Javanese house

pondok: Hut, shelter

pyan: ceiling in a traditional Javanese house

Raad van Indië: Council of the Indies (government advisory body)

raden (adjeng): Javanese noble titles

rampasan: Javanese shield roof design

regentschap, regent: historic districts often overlapping with a (sub)district/prince

residentie; resident: district; district official

runcing: bamboo spear

sawah: irrigated rice field

School tot Opleiding van Inlandsche Artsen (STOVIA): School for Training Native Physicians

snoezige: cute

soentik: vaccination, jab

soesa: fuss

soko goeroe: main support posts of a traditional Javanese house

tikoes: rat

tiang: part of the roof construction of a traditional Javanese house

trontong: bamboo poles with slits in them

tukung kayu: Javanese traditional carpenter

Volkshuisvestingscongres: Public housing conference

Volksraad: People's Council (semilegislative government body)

wedono: Javanese district chief

woningbrigade: house brigades

woninghygiene: domestic hygiene, hygiene of the house

woningschoonmaak: house cleaning

woningverbeteringsmalaria: home improvement malaria

Notes

Introduction

1. Christos Lynteris, "Introduction: Imaging and Imagining Plague," in *Plague Image and Imagination from Medieval to Modern Times*, ed. Christos Lynteris (Cham: Palgrave Macmillan, 2021), 1–10.

2. WHO, "Fact Sheet: Plague," accessed April 7, 2021, https://www.who.int/news-room/fact-sheets/detail/plague; Christos Lynteris, *Ethnographic Plague: Configuring Disease on the Chinese-Russian Frontier* (London: Palgrave Macmillan, 2018), 5–6.

3. Kirsty Walker, "The Influenza Pandemic of 1918 in Southeast Asia," in *Histories of Health in Southeast Asia: Perspectives on the Long Nineteenth Century*, ed. Tim Harper and Sunil S. Amrith (Bloomington: Indiana University Press, 2014), 61–71. Malaria was consistently described as "the most prevalent and most deadly" disease in the Indies, but figures regarding its incidence were rarely provided. J. G. Overbeek and W. J. Stoker, "Malaria in Nederlandsch-Indië en haar bestrijding," *Mededeelingen van den Dienst der Volksgezondheid in Nederlandsch-Indië* (hereafter *MvdDdV*) 27, no. 1–2 (1938): 183–205.

4. Mary P. Sutphen, "Not What, but Where: Bubonic Plague and the Reception of Germ Theories in Hong Kong and Calcutta, 1894–1897," *Journal of the History of Medicine* 52 (1997): 81–113.

5. Terence H. Hull, "Plague in Java," in *Death and Disease in Southeast Asia: Explorations in Social, Medical and Demographic History*, ed. Norman Owen (Oxford: Oxford University Press, 1987), 210–230; Branwyn Poleykett, "Building out the Rat: Animal Intimacies and Prophylactic Settlement in 1920s South Africa," *Engagement*, February 7, 2017, https://aesengagement.wordpress.com/2017/02/07/building-out-the-rat-animal-intimacies-and-prophylactic-ssettlement-in-1920s-south-africa/.

6. Nicholaas H. Swellengrebel, "Plague in Java," *Journal of Hygiene* 48, no. 2 (1950): 135–145.

7. Eric Tagliacozzo, "Before the Gangrene Set in: The Dutch East Indies in 1910," in *Asia Inside Out: Changing Times*, ed. Eric Tagliacozzo, Helen F. Siu, and Peter C. Perdue (Cambridge, MA: Harvard University Press, 2015), 226–249.

8. Myron Echenberg, *Plague Ports: The Global Urban Impact of Bubonic Plague, 1894–1901* (New York: New York University Press, 2010); Lukas Engelmann, John Henderson, and Christos Lynteris, eds., *Plague and the City* (London: Routledge, 2018).

9. The extensive literature on plague in Hong Kong, for instance, is almost entirely devoted to discussing 1894 while plague's subsequent thirty-year presence in that city is largely neglected.

10. As such, plague control fit into a broader "nationalist" push among Dutch physicians. Leo van Bergen, *Van koloniale geneeskunde tot internationale gezondheidszorg: Een geschiedenis van honderd jaar Nederlandsche Vereniging voor Tropische Geneeskunde* (Amsterdam: KIT Publishers, 2007), 27–32.

11. Carol Benedict, "Bubonic Plague in Nineteenth-Century China," *Modern China* 14, no. 2 (1988): 107–155.

12. The official end of the third plague pandemic is often traced back to a declaration by the World Health Organization in 1959, which to the best of my knowledge was never issued. The earliest reference to such a declaration I have found is in Robert Hendrickson, *More Cunning than Man: A Social History of Rats and Man* (New York: Kensington, 1983), 64; Myron Echenberg, "Pestis Redux: The Initial Years of the Third Bubonic Plague Pandemic, 1894–1901," *Journal of World History* 13, no. 2 (2002): 429–449.

13. Lynteris, *Ethnographic Plague*, 1; Hull, "Plague in Java," 211–212; David Arnold, "Disease, Rumor, and Panic in India's Plague and Influenza Epidemics, 1896–1919," in *Empires of Panic: Epidemics and Colonial Anxieties*, ed. Robert Peckham (Hong Kong: Hong Kong University Press, 2015), 111–129.

14. "The Epidemic of Plague in Hong Kong," *British Medical Journal* 1, no. 1746 (1894): 1326.

15. Christos Lynteris, *Human Extinction and the Pandemic Imaginary* (Abingdon: Routledge, 2020); Christos Lynteris, "The Epidemiologist as Culture Hero: Visualizing Humanity in the Age of 'the Next Pandemic,'" *Visual Anthropology* 29, no. 1 (2016): 36–53; Merle Eisenberg and Lee Mordechai, "The Justinianic Plague and Global Pandemics: The Making of the Plague Concept," *American Historical Review* 125, no. 5 (2020): 1632–1667.

16. Lynteris, *Ethnographic Plague*, 1.

17. Robert Peckham, "Matshed Laboratory: Colonies, Cultures, and Bacteriology," in *Imperial Contagions: Medicine, Hygiene, and Cultures of Planning in Asia*, ed. Robert Peckham and David Pomfret (Hong Kong: Hong Kong University Press, 2013), 123–148.

18. Tom Solomon, "Hong Kong, 1894: The Role of James A. Lowson in the Controversial Discovery of the Plague Bacillus," *Lancet* 350, no. 9070 (1997): 59–62.

19. Alexandre Yersin, "La peste bubonique à Hong-Kong," *Annales de l'Institut Pasteur* 8 (1894): 662–667.

20. Andrew Cunningham, "Transforming Plague: The Laboratory and the Identity of Infectious Disease," in *The Laboratory Revolution in Medicine*, ed. Andrew Cunningham and Percy Williams (Cambridge: Cambridge University Press, 2002), 209–244.

21. Echenberg, *Plague Ports*, 43.

22. Christos Lynteris, "Vagabond Microbes, Leaky Laboratories and Epidemic Mapping: Alexandre Yersin and the 1898 Plague Epidemic in Nha Trang," *Social History of Medicine* 34, no. 1 (2021): 190–213.

23. Lukas Engelmann, "A Plague of Kinyounism: The Caricatures of Bacteriology in 1900 San Francisco," *Social History of Medicine* 33, no. 2 (2020): 489–514.

24. Christos Lynteris, "A 'Suitable Soil': Plague's Urban Breeding Grounds at the Dawn of the Third Pandemic," *Medical History* 62, no. 3 (2017): 343–357.

25. Echenberg, *Plague Ports*, 57–58.

26. Lynteris, "Suitable Soil," 354–355.

27. Robert Peckham, "Hong Kong Junk: Plague and the Economy of Chinese Things," *Bulletin of the History of Medicine* 90, no. 1 (2016): 32–60, 34.

28. James Mohr, *Plague and Fire: Battling Black Death and the 1900 Burning of Honolulu's Chinatown* (Oxford: Oxford University Press, 2005).

29. Echenberg, *Plague Ports*, 304–305.

30. Christos Lynteris, "Introduction: Infectious Animals and Epidemic Blame," in *Framing Animals as Epidemic Villains: Histories of Non-Human Disease Vectors*, ed. Christos Lynteris (Cham: Palgrave Macmillan, 2019), 1–26.

31. Nicholas A. Evans, "Blaming the Rat? Accounting for Plague in Colonial Indian Medicine," *Medicine Anthropology Theory* 5, no. 3 (2018): 16.

32. P.-L. Simond, "La propagation de la peste," *Annales de l'Institut Pasteur* 62 (1898): 625–687.

33. The speed with which this new transmission scheme was subsequently adopted varied considerably between places, as illustrated by the case of I. Groneman, who had already endorsed it in a booklet published in 1899 after a conversation with Yersin. I. Groneman, *Pestbestrijding naar aanleiding van gesprekken met Dr. Yersin* (Jogjakarta: W. A. van der Hucht, 1899), 9–12.

34. Lynteris, *Human Extinction and the Pandemic Imaginary*, 45–54.

35. Evans, "Blaming the Rat?," 35.

36. Tagliacozzo, "Before the Gangrene Set in," 226.

37. Hans Pols, *Nurturing Indonesia: Medicine and Decolonisation in the Dutch East Indies* (Cambridge: Cambridge University Press, 2018), 71–92.

38. *Rapport der Commissie tot Voorbereiding eener Reorganisatie van den Burgerlijken Geneeskundigen Dienst*, 1908, no. 2899, index 2.22.15, NL-HaNA.

39. Liesbeth Quirine Hesselink, *Healers on the Colonial Market: Native Doctors and Midwives in the Dutch East Indies* (Leiden: KITLV Press, 2011), 30–36.

40. Hesselink, *Healers on the Colonial Market*, 36, 283.

41. Leo van Bergen, *Uncertainty, Anxiety, Frugality: Dealing with Leprosy in the Dutch East Indies, 1816–1942* (Singapore: NUS Press, 2018), 14.

42. Pols, *Nurturing Indonesia*, 26.

43. Pols, *Nurturing Indonesia*, 93–94.

44. Hesselink, *Healers on the Colonial Market*, 283.

45. Pols, *Nurturing Indonesia*, 93–115.

46. Marieke Bloembergen and Remco Raben, "Wegen Naar het Nieuwe Indië, 1890–1950," in *Het koloniale beschavingsoffensief: Wegen n aar het Nieuwe Indië*, ed. Marieke Bloembergen and Remco Raben (Leiden: KITLV Press, 2009), 7–24.

47. Susie Protschky, "Camera Ethica: Photography, Modernity and the Governed in Late-Colonial Indonesia," in *Photography, Modernity and the Governed in Late-Colonial Indonesia*, ed. Susie Protschky (Amsterdam: Amsterdam University Press, 2015), 11–40, 11–12.

48. The historian Elsbeth Locher-Scholten's five-part study *Ethiek in fragmenten* has provided a suitably "fragmented" form with which to approach this ill-defined era in Dutch colonial history.

Elsbeth Locher-Scholten, *Ethiek in fragmenten: vijf studies over koloniaal denken en doen van Nederlanders in de Indonesische Archipel 1877–1942* (Utrecht: HES Publishers, 1981).

49. Protschky, "Camera Ethica," 12.

50. On this, see also Van Bergen, *Uncertainty, Anxiety, Frugality.*

51. *Rapport der Commissie tot Voorbereiding eener Reorganisatie*, NL-HaNA.

52. Willem Thomas de Vogel, *Beknopt verslag over den Burgerlijken Geneeskundigen Dienst van 1911 t/m 1918* (Weltevreden: Albrecht, 1920), 7–8.

53. De Vogel, *Beknopt verslag*, 7–8, 18–19.

54. The BGD was later known as the DVG. Sources are ambiguous about when, exactly, the plague service was reintegrated with the DVG: with some indicating its final year of independent operation was 1921 and others saying the service was formally reintegrated only in 1923. *Kort overzicht organisatie DVG*, 1929, in Collection W. Th. de Vogel, D H 1568, no. 214, Leiden University Library Special Collections, Leiden, The Netherlands (hereafter UBL); "De Burgerlijke Geneeskundige Dienst in Nederlandsch Indië," *Nederlands Tijdschrift voor Geneeskunde* (hereafter *NTvG*) 69 (1925): 2595–2597.

55. Hesselink, *Healers on the Colonial Market*, 273; J. Scott-Keltie and M. Epstein, eds., *The Stateman's Year-Book* (London: Macmillan, 1914), 1126.

56. Vivek Neelakantan, "Eradicating Smallpox in Indonesia: The Archipelagic Challenge," *Health and History* 12, no. 1 (2017): 61–87.

57. The institute was initially called the Parc Vaccinogène; *Koloniaal Verslag* (1895), 152.

58. Peter Boomgaard, "Smallpox, Vaccination, and the Pax Neerlandica, Indonesia, 1550–1930," *Bijdragen tot de taal-, land- en volkenkunde* 159, no. 4 (2003): 590–617.

59. Van Bergen, *Uncertainty, Anxiety, Frugality.*

60. Siddharth Chandra, Goran Kuljanin, and Jennifer Wray, "Mortality from the Influenza Pandemic of 1918–19 in Indonesia," *Population Studies* 67, no. 2 (2013): 185–193.

61. De Vogel, *Beknopt verslag*, 22.

62. Andrew Goss, "Building the World's Supply of Quinine: Dutch Colonialism and the Origins of a Global Pharmaceutical Industry," *Endeavour* 38, no. 1 (2014): 8–18; Arjo Roersch van der Hoogte and Toine Pieters, "Quinine, Malaria, and the Cinchona Bureau: Marketing Practices and Knowledge Circulation in a Dutch Transoceanic Cinchona-Quinine Enterprise (1920s–30s)," *Journal of the History of Medicine and Allied Sciences* 71, no. 2 (2016): 197–225.

63. Maurits Bastiaan Meerwijk, "Phantom Menace: Dengue and Yellow Fever in Asia," *Bulletin of the History of Medicine* 94, no. 2 (2020): 215–243.

64. This figure is derived from Frederick Norman White's report on the Indies for the League of Nations in 1922. At that time, he noted, only five ports counted as "first-class ports" (despite the absence of quarantine facilities in three of them) while 188 could provide no medical provisions "of any kind." Norman White, *The Prevalence of Epidemic Disease and Port Health Organisation and Procedure in the Far East* (Geneva: League of Nations, 1923), 69; Hans Pols, "Quarantine in the Dutch East Indies," in *Quarantine: Local and Global Histories*, ed. Alison Bashford (London: Palgrave Macmillan, 2016), 85–102.

65. Susie Protschky, *Images of the Tropics: Environment and Visual Culture in Colonial Indonesia* (Leiden: KITLV Press, 2011), 52–69.

66. M. Neumann van Padang, "History of the Volcanology in the Former Netherlands East Indies," *Scripta Geologica* 71 (1983): 1–76.

67. Pols, "Quarantine in the Dutch East Indies."

68. J. W. Wolff, *De ontwikkeling van de gezondheidszorg op cultuurondernemingen in de Tropen* (Amsterdam: Scheltema & Holkema, 1949), 13–17; Ann Laura Stoler, *Capital-*

ism and Confrontation in Sumatra's Plantation Belt, 1870–1979, 2nd ed. (Ann Arbor: University of Michigan Press, 1985), 2.

69. *Gedenkboek der gemeente semarang 1906–1931* (Semarang: De Locomotief, 1931), 110–111; Pauline K. M. van Roosmalen, "Netherlands Indies Town Planning: An Agent of Modernization (1905–1957)," in *Cars, Conduits, and Kampongs: The Modernization of the Indonesian City, 1920–1960*, ed. Freek Colombijn and Joost Coté (Leiden: Brill, 2015), 87–119.

70. For example, Radjimo Sastro Wijono, "Public Housing in Semarang and the Modernization of Kampongs, 1930–1960," in Colombijn and Coté, *Cars, Conduits, and Kampongs*, 172–192; Rudolf Mrazek, *Engineers of Happy Land: Nationalism and Technology in Indonesia* (Princeton, NJ: Princeton University Press, 2002).

71. Suzanna Jansen, *Het pauperparadijs: Een familiegeschiedenis* (Amsterdam: Balans, 2017); Liesbeth van de Grift, "On New Land a New Society: Internal Colonisation in the Netherlands, 1918–1940," *Contemporary European History* 22, no. 4 (2013): 609–626.

72. David Serlin, "Introduction: Towards a Visual Culture of Public Health," in *Imagining Illness: Public Health and Visual Culture*, ed. David Serlin (Minneapolis: University of Minnesota Press, 2010): xi–ix.

73. Georges Canguilhem, *The Normal and the Pathological*, trans. Carolyn R. Fawcett and Robert S. Cohen (New York: Zone, 1991), 39–40; Lynteris, "Introduction: Infectious Animals."

74. Maurits Bastiaan Meerwijk, "Viral Imagery of Dengue Fever in the Age of Bacteriology," *Isis* 111, no. 2 (2020): 239–263.

75. Christos Lynteris, "The Prophetic Faculty of Epidemic Photography: Chinese Wet Markets and the Imagination of the Next Pandemic," *Visual Anthropology* 29, no. 2 (2016): 118–132.

76. Christos Lynteris, "Tarbagan's Winter Lair: Framing Drivers of Plague Persistence in Inner Asia," in Lynteris, *Framing Animals as Epidemic Villains*, 65–90, 66.

77. Lukas Engelmann, "What Are Medical Photographs of Plague?," *Remedia*, January 31, 2017, https://remedianetwork.net/2017/01/31/what-are-medical-photographs -of-plague/.

78. *Mededeelingen van den Burgerlijken Geneeskundigen Dienst in Nederlandsch-Indië* 1 (1912): 1–267.

79. Protschky, "Camera Ethica," 12.

80. Protschky, "Camera Ethica," 16.

81. Protschky, "Camera Ethica," 19.

82. Protschky, *Images of the Tropics*, 17.

83. Michael C. Jackson, *Critical Systems Thinking and the Management of Complexity* (Hoboken, NJ: Wiley, 2019), 35–40. The terms "ecology" and "ecosystem" were coined in 1866 and 1935, respectively, while the concept of multiple and overlapping human, animal, microbial, and environmental entanglements would gather traction only about the latter date.

1. Plague, Rats, and the House in Java

1. Resident of Pasoeroean, "Verslag omtrent het voorkomen van pest in de Residentie Pasoeroean, May 1911," Manuscript Grote Bundel (hereafter MGB), no. 4674, Arsip Nasional Republik Indonesia, Jakarta (hereafter ANRI); Willem Thomas de Vogel,

"Uittreksel uit het verslag aan de Regeering over de Pest-Epidemie in de Afdeeling Malang, November 1910–Augustus 1911," *MvdBGD* 1 (1912): 34–35.

2. J. de Haan, "De bacteriologische diagnose van pest in de afdeeling Malang," *MvdBGD* 1 (1912): 3–5.

3. I. Snapper, "Medical Contributions from the Netherlands Indies," in *South East Asia, Colonial History*, vol. 3, *High Imperialism (1890s–1930s)*, ed. Paul Kratoska (London: Routledge, 2001), 129–152, 142.

4. *Koloniaal Verslag* (1900), 105.

5. "Petition," 1899, Besluit (hereafter Bt), no. 824, ANRI.

6. *Koloniaal Verslag* (1899), 120.

7. *Koloniaal Verslag* (1900), 105–106.

8. "Handelingen," Tweede Kamer, 70ste Vergadering, April 29, 1914, 1914.

9. Warwick Anderson, *Colonial Pathologies: American Tropical Medicine, Race, and Hygiene in the Philippines* (Durham, NC: Duke University Press, 2006), 61–63.

10. *Koloniaal Verslag* (1906), 38, 171; "Pest in Deli," *Het Nieuws van den Dag voor Nederlandsch-Indië* (hereafter *NvdD*), May 22, 1905; Johannes J. van Loghem, "Het pest-vraagstuk voor Nederlandsch-Indië," *NTvG* 53 (1909): 44–51.

11. "Handelingen," Tweede Kamer, 71ste Vergadering, April 30, 1914, 1924.

12. Resident of Soerabaja, "Rapport omtrent het eerste optreden, de herkenning en de bestryding der pestziekte in het gewest Soerabaja, 11 Mei 1911," MGB, no. 4674, ANRI.

13. Resident of Soerabaja, "Rapport."

14. Resident of Soerabaja, "Rapport."

15. De Haan, "De bacteriologische diagnose van pest," 3–5.

16. "Voorloopig rapport aangaande het onderzoek naar het eventueel voorkomen van pest in de afdeeling Malang, April 1911," MGB, no. 4674, ANRI.

17. "Misschien toch pest," *NvdD*, March 6, 1911.

18. J. Dijkstra, "Het een en ander over de pest in het Malangsche," *Maandblad voor Ziekenverpleging* 21, no. 6 (1911): 444–446, 444.

19. "Voorzorg," *De Preangerbode*, January 29, 1911. Returning *hajjis* were frequently suspected of carrying back disease; see Eric Tagliacozzo, *The Longest Journey: Southeast Asians and the Pilgrimage to Mecca* (Oxford: Oxford University Press, 2013), 133–155.

20. "Van den dag," *De Preangerbode*, February 28, 1911.

21. "Vrees voor pest op Java," *Algemeen Handelsblad*, February 25, 1911.

22. Resident of Soerabaja, "Rapport."

23. De Haan, "De bacteriologische diagnose van pest," 3–5; *Koloniaal Verslag* (1900), 107.

24. De Haan, "De bacteriologische diagnose van pest," 3–5. The bacterium would be renamed *Yersinia pestis* in 1944.

25. A. van Schaik, *Malang: Beeld van een stad* (Purmerend: Asia Maior, 1996), 16–26; Municipal Council Malang, *Malang: De bergstad van Oost-Java* (Malang: 1927), 8–10.

26. Pols, "Quarantine in the Dutch East Indies," 90–91.

27. "De pest," *Bataviaasch Nieuwsblad*, April 6, 1911.

28. "Handelingen," Tweede Kamer, 70ste Vergadering, April 29, 1914, 1914.

29. David Arnold, "Disease, Rumor, and Panic in India's Plague and Influenza Epidemics, 1896–1919," in *Empires of Panic: Epidemics and Colonial Anxieties*, ed. Robert Peckham (Hong Kong: Hong Kong University Press, 2015), 111–129.

30. De Haan, "De bacteriologische diagnose van pest," 6.

31. Suzanna de Vogel to Augusta de Vogel, March 30, 1911, in Collection W. Th. de Vogel, D H 1568, UBL.

32. De Vogel, "Uittreksel," 41–45.

33. "Telegram," March 30, 1911, MGB, no 4674, ANRI.

34. "Telegram," March 30, 1911, MGB, no 4674, ANRI; De Haan, "De bacteriologische diagnose van pest," 6.

35. De Haan, "De bacteriologische diagnose van pest," 6, 22.

36. "Pest op Java," *Nieuwe Rotterdamsche Courant*, April 1, 1911. The reference to plague being imported by a *hajji* linked back to a newspaper article, stating that a case of plague had been detected among pilgrims returning through Soerabaja about January 24, 1911: "Een geval van pest," *Nieuwe Rotterdamsche Courant*, March 10, 1911.

37. Jan Hendrik de Waal Malefijt to Alexander Idenburg, April 2, 1911, in Collection A. W. F. Idenburg, no. 129, Historical Documentation Center for Dutch Protestantism, Amsterdam, The Netherlands (hereafter HDC).

38. "Telegram no. 323," April 2, 1911, HDC.

39. "Telegram no. 336," April 5, 1911, HDC; Resident of Pasoeroean, "Verslag."

40. De Haan, "De bacteriologische diagnose van pest," 18–21.

41. Idenburg to de Waal Malefijt, April 5, 1911, HDC.

42. Idenburg to de Waal Malefijt, May 3, 1911, HDC.

43. Idenburg to de Waal Malefijt, May 3, 1911, HDC.

44. De Vogel, "Uittreksel," 37–38.

45. Arnold, "Disease, Rumor, and Panic," 111–112; Lynteris, *Ethnographic Plague*, 121–122; Idenburg to de Waal Malefijt, April 5, 1911, HDC.

46. J. de Bruijn and G. Puchinger, *Briefwisseling Kuyper-Idenburg* (Franeker: T. Weber, 1985), 238–242, note 2; De Vogel, "Uittreksel," 45–50.

47. De Vogel, "Uittreksel," 72–73, 135, figure 14.

48. De Vogel, "Uittreksel," 58. On the first and second Indian Plague Commissions and the latter's role in establishing the role of rats in plague transmission, see Evans, "Blaming the Rat?," 15–42.

49. Resident of Soerabaja, "Rapport."

50. Resident of Pasoeroean, "Verslag."

51. "Besmet verklaard," *De Preangerbode*, April 6, 1911.

52. "Telegram," April 5, 1911, ANRI.

53. "Telegram," April 7, 1911, ANRI.

54. "Telegrams," April 6, 7, and 9, 1911, ANRI; De Vogel, "Uittreksel," fig. 2.

55. De Vogel, "Uittreksel," 42–43; Resident of Kediri to Director of Government Engineering, May 5, 1911, MGB, no. 4674, ANRI.

56. "Verslagen van vereenigingen," *NTvG* (1912): 720; Johannes J. van Loghem, "De pest op Java," *NTvG* 56 (1912): 217–218.

57. "De pest in het Malangsche," *NvdD*, April 8, 1911.

58. "De pest," *Bataviaasch Nieuwsblad*, April 6, 1911; "De pest," *Bataviaasch Nieuwsblad*, April 11, 1911; "De pest," *Bataviaasch Nieuwsblad*, April 12, 1911.

59. Dijkstra, "Het een en ander over de pest in het Malangsche," 444–446.

60. "Voorloopig rapport."

61. A. A. F. M. Deutmann, "De pest in Karanglo in de maanden Mei, Juni en Juli," *MvdBGD* 1 (1912): 187–267.

62. De Vogel, "Uittreksel," 65.

63. Deutmann, "De pest in Karanglo," 193–194.

64. Deutmann, "De pest in Karanglo," 223–229; O. L. E. de Raadt, "Uittreksels uit de verslagen" *MvdBGD* 1 (1912): 172–182.

65. De Vogel, "Uittreksel," fig. 10.

66. De Vogel, "Uittreksel," fig. 66.

67. According to van Loghem, the floor was regularly disinfected while the patient stayed there, with disinfectant applied from the outside through the house. Van Loghem, "De pest op Java," 227–228; De Vogel, "Uittreksel," fig. 13.

68. De Vogel, "Uittreksel," 72.

69. UBL Digital Collections, Item KITLV 68951, http://hdl.handle.net/1887.1/item:763052; De Vogel, "Uittreksel," 69.

70. Deutmann, "De pest in Karanglo," 190.

71. De Vogel, "Uittreksel," 65.

72. Lynteris, "Suitable Soil," 343–357.

73. Deutmann, "De pest in Karanglo," 191.

74. Resident of Pasoeroean, "Verslag."

75. Nationaal Museum van Wereldculturen (hereafter NMVW)–Collection Database, Item TM-10006670, https://hdl.handle.net/20.500.11840/226981.

76. Deutmann, "De pest in Karanglo," 191–193.

77. Deutmann, "De pest in Karanglo," 246.

78. Resident of Soerabaja to the Department Secretary of the Governor-General, May 14, 1911, MGB, no. 4674, ANRI.

79. Only some, like Deutmann, had limited research experience: A. A. F. M. Deutmann, *De pest: Vaccinatie en sérotherapie, een kritisch-experimenteele studie* (Amsterdam: F. van Rossen, 1900).

80. "Telegram no. 5," May 26, 1911, ANRI.

81. Idenburg to de Waal Malefijt, May 3, 1911, HDC.

82. Suzanna de Vogel to Augusta de Vogel, May 4, 1911, UBL.

83. De Vogel, "Uittreksel," 36.

84. Willem de Vogel to Augusta de Vogel, January 12, 1912, UBL.

85. "Telegram no. 329," April 2, 1911, inventory no. 763, index 2.10.36.50, Nationaal Archief, The Hague, The Netherlands (hereafter NL-HaNA).

86. Johannes J. van Loghem, "Brieven uit Indië: Het pestvraagstuk voor Nederlandsch-Indië," *NTvG* 53 (1909): 44–51; Johannes J. van Loghem Jr. and J. van der Noordaa, "Johannes Jacobus van Loghem (1878–1968), microbioloog-hygiënist," in *Erflaters van de geneeskunde: Beroemde Nederlandse artsen beschreven voor hun (kinds)kinderen*, ed. C. J. E. Kaandorp, J. J. E. van Everdingen, and A. Mooij (Alphen aan den Rijn: Belvédère, 2002): 128–137.

87. Johannes J. van Loghem, "Over pest," *Maandblad voor Ziekenverpleging* 21, no. 3 (1911): 150–155.

88. "Telegram no. 333," April 4, 1911, "Telegram no. 341," April 5, 1911, "Telegram no. 346," April 5, 1911, NL-HaNA.

89. "Telegram no. 355," April 8, 1911, NL-HaNA.

90. Johannes J. van Loghem, "Brieven uit Indië: Het Congres voor Tropische Ziekten te Bombay," *NTvG* 53 (1909): 1702–1707; Johannes J. van Loghem, "Eenige epidemiologische gegevens omtrent de pest op Java," *MvdBGD* 1 (1912): 142.

91. "Dr. Schülein geïnterviewd," *De Sumatra Post*, May 31, 1911. The author notes that inoculations with the plague serum would be a slow process that could be conducted only by European physicians: "Natives cannot be 'broken in' to work with this more dangerous plague vaccine."

92. "Handelingen," Tweede Kamer, 70ste Vergadering, April 29, 1914, 1921.

93. "Handelingen," Tweede Kamer, 70ste Vergadering, April 29, 1914, 1914.

94. For a pertinent study of the notion of sovereignty in public health matters, see Celia Lowe, "Viral Sovereignty Security and Mistrust as Measures of Future Health in the Indonesian H5N1 Influenza Outbreak," *Medicine Anthropology Theory* 6, no. 3 (2019): 109–132.

95. Philipp Teichfischer, "German-Jewish Doctors as Members of the Colonial Health Service in the Dutch East Indies in the First Half of the Nineteenth Century," in *Jewish Medicine and Healthcare in Central Eastern Europe: Shared Identities, Entangled Histories*, ed. Marcin Moskalewicz, Ute Caumanns, and Fritz Dross (Dordrecht: Springer, 2019), 131–153.

96. De Vogel, "Uittreksel," 57–65.

97. De Vogel, "Uittreksel," 45–47.

98. Van Loghem, "Eenige epidemiologische gegevens," 139–157.

99. De Vogel, "Uittreksel," 62–63.

100. Nicholaas H. Swellengrebel, "Mededeeling omtrent onderzoekingen over de biologie van ratten en vlooien en over andere onderwerpen, die betrekking hebben op de epidemiologie der pest op Oost-Java," *MvdBGD* 2, no. 1 (1913): 1–86; Van Loghem, "Eenige epidemiologische gegevens," 157–162.

101. Swellengrebel, "Mededeeling."

102. Photographs of the Third Plague Pandemic, Centre for Research in the Arts, Humanities and Social Sciences, University of Cambridge, Item PhotoID_11671, https://www.repository.cam.ac.uk/handle/1810/285204.

103. Van Loghem, "Eenige epidemiologische gegevens," 134–157.

104. De Vogel, "Uittreksel," 62; Van Loghem, "Eenige epidemiologische gegevens," 120.

105. De Vogel, "Uittreksel," 78.

106. Deutmann, "De pest in Karanglo," 242–244.

107. Carl Mense, ed., *Handbuch der tropenkrankheiten*, vol. 2 (Leipzig: Johan Ambrosius Barth, 1905), 403, as quoted in Willem Thomas de Vogel, "The Connection of Man and Rat in the Plague Epidemic in Malang, Java, in 1911," in *Transactions of the Second Biennial Congress Held at Hongkong 1912*, ed. Francis Clark (Hong Kong: Noronha, 1913), 147–149.

108. Evans, "Blaming the Rat?," 16.

109. Van Loghem, "Eenige epidemiologische gegevens," 120.

110. De Vogel, "Connection of Man and Rat."

111. Deutmann, "De pest in Karanglo," 244.

112. Local Government of Kediri to the Governor-General, May 11, 1911, MGB, no. 4674, ANRI.

113. Van Loghem, "Eenige epidemiologische gegevens," 121–122; Deutmann, "De pest in Karanglo," 243–244.

114. Willem de Vogel to Augusta de Vogel, June 7, 1911, UBL.

115. Peckham, "Hong Kong Junk," 35; Ann H. Kelly and Aldumena Marí Sáez, "Shadowlands and Dark Corners: An Anthropology of Light and Zoonosis," *Medicine Anthropology Theory* 5, no. 3 (2018): 21–49.

116. On this, see for instance the six-volume series *Kromoblanda* self-published between 1915 and 1923 by the philanthropist H. F. Tillema, which proffered a critique of "the question of living" in the colony.

117. This epiphany was widely attributed to van Loghem, but its exact date remains ambiguous.

118. Deutmann, "De pest in Karanglo," 224.

119. Van Loghem, "Eenige epidemiologische gegevens," 122–124.

120. Deutmann, "De pest in Karanglo," 244.

121. De Raadt, "Uittreksels uit de verslagen," 180–182; Van Loghem, "Eenige epidemiologische gegevens," 122–123.

122. De Haan, "De bacteriologische diagnose van pest," 9; Van Loghem, "De Pest op Java," 212.

123. Van Loghem, "Eenige epidemiologische gegevens," 129.

124. Deutmann, "De pest in Karanglo," 245–246.

125. Maurits Bastiaan Meerwijk, "Bamboo Dwellers: Plague, Photography, and the House in Java," in *Plague Image and Imagination from Medieval to Modern Times*, ed. Christos Lynteris (Cham: Palgrave Macmillan, 2021), 205–234.

126. Deutmann, "De pest in Karanglo," 248.

127. Van Loghem, "Eenige epidemiologische gegevens," 126.

128. De Vogel, "Uittreksel," 81.

129. Van Loghem, "Eenige epidemiologische gegevens," 127.

130. Van Loghem, "De pest op Java," 211.

131. Meerwijk, "Bamboo Dwellers."

132. On photography and its truth claims about 1900, see Jennifer Tucker, *Nature Exposed: Photography as Eyewitness in Victorian Science* (Baltimore, MD: Johns Hopkins University Press, 2005), 6–7; Protschky, "Camera Ethica."

133. Shawn Michelle Smith, *At the Edge of Sight: Photography and the Unseen* (Durham, NC: Duke University Press, 2013); Kelly and Sáez, "Shadowlands and Dark Corners." See also Lynteris, "Suitable Soil," 351–352.

134. Canguilhem, *Normal and the Pathological*, 39–40.

135. Van Loghem, "Eenige epidemiologische gegevens," 130–131.

136. Lukas Engelmann, "Configurations of Plague: Spatial Diagrams in Early Epidemiology," *Social Analysis* 63, no. 4 (2019): 89–109.

137. De Vogel, "Connection of Man and Rat," 149.

138. Christos Lynteris, "Suspicious Corpses: Body Dumping and Plague in Colonial Hong Kong," in *Histories of Post-Mortem Contagion: Infectious Corpses and Contested Burials*, ed. Christos Lynteris and Nicholas H. A. Evans (Basingstoke: Palgrave Macmillan, 2018), 109–134; Christos Lynteris and Nicholas H. A. Evans, "Introduction: The Challenge of the Epidemic Corpse," in Lynteris and Evans, *Histories of Post-Mortem Contagion*, 19–22.

139. Van Loghem, "Eenige epidemiologische gegevens," 135.

140. Van Loghem, "Eenige epidemiologische gegevens," 129.

141. Deutmann, "De pest in Karanglo," 250. See also Engelmann, Henderson, and Lynteris, *Plague and the City*; Prashant Kidambi, *The Making of a Modern Metropolis: Colonial Governance and Public Culture in Bombay, 1890–1920* (Aldershot: Routledge, 2007), 71–113.

142. Mrazek, *Engineers of Happy Land*.

143. The focus on the native plague patient or corpse in Hong Kong and Bombay was not evident to the same extent in Java. David Arnold, *Colonizing the Body: State Medicine and Epidemic Disease in Nineteenth-Century India* (Berkeley: University of California Press, 1993), 200–239; Lynteris, "Suspicious Corpses," 109–134.

144. De Vogel, "Connection of Man and Rat," 148.

145. On "trained judgement," "mechanical reproduction," and "objectivity" in scientific imagery, see Lorraine Daston and Peter Galison, *Objectivity* (New York: Zone, 2007).

2. Colonizing the Home with Bamboo, Tiles, and Timber

1. Robert Nieuwenhuys, *Mirror of the Indies: A History of Dutch Colonial Literature* (Hong Kong: Periplus, 1999), 126–127; Karin Peterson, *In het Voetspoor van Louis Couperus: Pasoeroean door de Lens van Salzwedel* (Amsterdam: KIT Publishers, 2009), 15–18.

2. Louis Couperus, *De stille kracht* (Amstelveen: L. J. Veen, 1900), 155.

3. Dienst der Pestbestrijding (hereafter DP), *Verslag over het tweede kwartaal 1915* (Batavia: Javasche Boekhandel & Drukkerij, 1915), 197; Hull, "Plague in Java," 210–230, 212.

4. Arnold, *Colonizing the Body*, 7–10.

5. Geoffrey G. Pope, "Bamboo," in *A History of Physical Anthropology: An Encyclopedia*, ed. Frank Spencer (New York: Garland, 1997), 1:159–161.

6. David Arnold, "India's Place in the Tropical World, 1770–1930," *Journal of Imperial and Commonwealth History* 26, no. 1 (1998): 1–21.

7. J. A. Loebèr, *Bamboe in Nederlandsch-Indië* (Amsterdam: de Bussy, 1909), 5–24; Willem Wolters, "Geographical Explanations for the Distribution of Irrigation Institutions: Cases from Southeast Asia," in *A World of Water: Rain, Rivers and Seas in Southeast Asian Histories*, ed. Peter Boomgaard (Leiden: KITLV Press, 2007), 209–234; Susanne Lucas, *Bamboo* (London: Reaktion, 2013), 30, 63–100; Georges B. Cressey, *Asia's Lands and Peoples: A Geography of One-Third of the Earth and Two-Thirds of Its People* (New York: McGraw-Hill, 1944), 536.

8. Alfred Russell Wallace, *The Malay Archipelago*, vol. 1 (London: Macmillan, 1869), 120–121; Alfred Russell Wallace, "On the Bamboo and Durian of Borneo," *Hooker's Journal of Botany* 8 (1856): 225–230.

9. Timothy J. LeCain, *The Matter of History: How Things Create the Past* (Cambridge: Cambridge University Press, 2017), 134.

10. Loebèr stated that bamboo was "guilty" of having delayed the development of other crafts. Thus, a stagnant bamboo age ran parallel to a progression from stone to bronze to iron ages elsewhere. Loebèr, *Bamboe*, 77–79.

11. Loebèr, *Bamboe*, 43–46; Hesselink, *Healers on the Colonial Market*, 124–125.

12. Gilles Lessard and Amy Chouinard, eds., *Bamboo Research in Asia* (Ottawa: International Development Research Centre, 1980), 63–68.

13. J. J. X. Pfijffer zu Neueck, *Schetsen van het eiland Java* (Amsterdam: J. C. van Kesteren, 1838), 80–81; Neueck, *Skizzen von der insel Java* (Schaffhausen: Franz Hurter, 1829), 28.

14. *Koloniaal Verslag* (1911), 208.

15. Peckham, "Matshed Laboratory," 134.

16. Lisa Drummond, "Colonial Hanoi: Urban Space in Public Discourse," in *Harbin to Hanoi: The Colonial Built Environment in Asia, 1840–1940*, eds Laura Victoir and Victor Zatsepine (Hong Kong: Hong Kong University Press, 2013), 222–223; Danielle Labbé, Caroline Herbelin, and Quang-Vinh Dao, "Domesticating the Suburbs: Architectural Production and Exchanges in Hanoi during the Late French Colonial Era," in Victoir and Zatsepine, *Harbin to Hanoi*, 256; Gerrit Verschuur, *Aux colonies d'Asie et dans l'Océan Indien* (Paris: Hachette, 1900), 116–120.

17. H. F. Tillema, *Kromoblanda*, vol. 1 (The Hague: Electrische Drukkerij, 1915), 106.

18. For example, H. F. Tillema, *Kromoblanda*, vol. 4 (Wassenaar: H. Uden Masman, 1921), 302.

19. Peckham, "Matshed Laboratory," 123.

20. Anderson, *Colonial Pathologies*, 211.

21. Poleykett, "Building out the Rat."

22. O. L. E. de Raadt, *De woningverbetering als middel ter bestrijding en voorkoming van het pestgevaar op Java* (Malang: N. V. Jahn's Drukkerij, 1912).

23. Dienst der Volksgezondheid (hereafter DVG), *Control of Endemic Diseases in the Netherlands Indies* (Weltevreden: Landsdrukkerij, 1929), 36–45.

24. De Vogel, "Uittreksel," 84, fig. 27.

25. De Vogel, "Connection of Man and Rat," 147–149.

26. Van Loghem, "Eenige epidemiologische gegevens," 137–138.

27. "De pest te Toeloengagoeng," *De Sumatra Post*, November 24, 1911.

28. *Koloniaal Verslag* (1912), 5, 133–134.

29. For example, De Raadt, *De woningverbetering*.

30. *Koloniaal Verslag* (1914), 157.

31. *Koloniaal Verslag* (1915), 179, 226.

32. Willem Thomas de Vogel, "Inspectie rapport," November 18, 1912, Terzijde Gelegde Agendas (hereafter TGA), no. 6671, ANRI.

33. Willem Thomas de Vogel to Unknown, November 18, 1912, UBL.

34. De Vogel, "Inspectie rapport."

35. Photographs of the Third Plague Pandemic, Centre for Research in the Arts, Humanities and Social Sciences, University of Cambridge, Item PhotoID_11632, https://www.repository.cam.ac.uk/handle/1810/285303. According to a catalog entry, this photograph was taken by Dr. Otto de Raadt: Rijksmuseum Boerhaave, Leiden, Collection Database, Item P20286.

36. W. Schülein to Alexander Idenburg, December 28, 1912, TGA, no. 6671, ANRI.

37. Assistant-Resident of Malang, "Report," August 11, 1913, TGA, no. 6671, ANRI.

38. Assistant-Resident of Kediri, "Report," August 25, 1913, TGA, no. 6685, ANRI.

39. "De reis van den landvoogd," *Nieuwe Rotterdamsche Courant*, August 4, 1912; "De G. G. in de pest-streek," *NvdD*, February 24, 1914; "Besmettelijke ziekten. Pestgevaarlijke gebouwen," *Staatsblad van Nederlandsch-Indië*, no. 486 (1914): 1–5.

40. "De gouverneur-generaal op reis," *Het Vaderland*, February 9, 1916. This intervention is dated back to December 1915, in G. J. Lammers, *A. W. F. Idenburg: In zijn leven en werken geschetst* (Amsterdam: De Standaard, 1935), 23.

41. De Vogel, "Uittreksel," 91–105.

42. Resident of Soerabaja to the Department Secretary of the Governor-General, May 14, 1911, ANRI.

43. W. Th. de Vogel to Mother, June 7, 1911, UBL.

44. Theodore Thomson, trans., *The International Sanitary Convention of Paris, 1903* (London: Darling and Son, 1904). Some sources suggest the legal basis for this event was a "plague ordinance" of 1902; "De quarantaine te Soerabaja," *NvdD*, May 6, 1911.

45. Marieke Bloembergen, "The Dirty Work of Empire: Modern Policing and Public Order in Surabaya, 1911–1919," *Indonesia* 83 (2007): 119–150.

46. According to a report by Frederick Norman White to the League of Nations of 1922, the value of all combined exports from Soerabaja amounted to *f.* 209 million, which was followed at a distance by the port of Batavia (*f.* 137 million). Frederick Norman White, "Draft Report," 1922, R843, no. 23230, League of Nations Archives, Geneva, Switzerland (hereafter LoN).

47. Resident of Soerabaja to the Secretary of the Governor-General, May 14, 1911, ANRI.

48. "De quarantaine te Soerabaja," *NvdD*, May 6, 1911; "De pestconferentie te Soerabaja," *Bataviaasch Nieuwsblad*, May 10, 1911.

49. Resident of Soerabaja to the Department Secretary of the Governor-General, May 14, 1911, ANRI; "Telegram no. 777," May 10, 1911, ANRI.

50. "Ministerie van Koloniën," *Nederlandsche Staatscourant*, 16 May 1911; *Koloniaal Verslag* (1911), 7.

51. Resident of Soerabaja to the Department Secretary of the Governor-General, May 14, 1911, ANRI.

52. Resident of Soerabaja, "Report," September 1, 1911, TGA, no. 6685, ANRI.

53. "Gezondheidscomité te Soerabaja," *De Sumatra Post*, August 7, 1911.

54. "Voor 't Algemeen Welzijn," *De Sumatra Post*, June 19, 1911.

55. Johannes Terburgh, "Nota omtrent de woningverbetering in de gemeente Soerabaja van Juni 1911 tot ultimo Juni 1913," August 13, 1913, TGA, no. 6685, ANRI.

56. Resident of Soerabaja, "Report."

57. Resident of Soerabaja, "Report."

58. Director of Education and Worship, "Missive," September 9, 1911, TGA, no. 6685, ANRI.

59. Director of Education and Worship, "Missive."

60. "De ASGC en de regeering," *De Telegraaf*, November 27, 1911.

61. Terburgh, "Nota."

62. Terburgh, "Nota."

63. Racism against Chinese populations was prevalent in Southeast Asia, including the Dutch East Indies, and often articulated through concerns for health. See, for example, Anderson, *Colonial Pathologies*, 62–63, 98; Tracy C. Barrett, *The Chinese Diaspora in South-East Asia: The Overseas Chinese in Indochina* (New York: I. B. Tauris, 2012).

64. Terburgh, "Nota."

65. Terburgh, "Nota."

66. *Koloniaal Verslag* (1912), 130n3.

67. Terburgh, "Nota."

68. "Ministerie van koloniën," *Nederlandsche Staatscourant*, December 19, 1912.

69. As cited in "De pest te Soerabaja," *Bataviaasch Nieuwsblad*, October 7, 1912.

70. Norman White, "Draft Report," table inset between 9–10, LoN.

71. White, "Draft Report," 9.

72. White, "Draft Report," 26.

73. De Vogel, *Beknopt verslag*, 7–8.

74. *Koloniaal Verslag* (1914), 7–8.

75. "Handelingen," Tweede Kamer, 70ste Vergadering, April 29, 1914, 1901.

76. *Koloniaal Verslag* (1914), 7–8; De Vogel, *Beknopt verslag*, 18–19.

77. DP, *Verslag over het eerste kwartaal 1915* (Batavia: Javasche Boekhandel, 1915), 127–131, 143–156.

78. "Voorlopige algemeene voorschriften," in DP, *Verslag over het eerste kwartaal 1915*, 189–195, 189 (original emphasis).

79. "Voorlopige algemeene voorschriften," 59–61, 987; DP, *Verslag over het vierde kwartaal 1915* (Batavia: Javasche Boekhandel, 1915), 42.

80. "Toelichting op de voorschriften ter uitvoering van artikel 10 der Ordonantie van 6 Juli 1914 (Staatsblad No. 486)," in DP, *Verslag over het eerste kwartaal 1915*, 179–183.

81. DP, *Verslag over het eerste kwartaal 1916* (Batavia: Javasche Boekhandel 1917), 17.

82. DP, *Verslag over het tweede kwartaal 1916* (Batavia: Javasche Boekhandel 1917), 16.

83. DP, *Verslag over het eerste kwartaal 1915*, 154–156, 196–197.

84. DP, *Verslag over het eerste kwartaal 1915*, 158.

85. DP, *Verslag over het tweede kwartaal 1915*, 197.

86. DP, *Verslag over het eerste kwartaal 1915*, 163.

87. DP, *Verslag over het eerste kwartaal 1915*, 158.

88. DP, *Verslag over het eerste kwartaal 1915*, 66.

89. DP, *Verslag over het eerste kwartaal 1915*, 65–66.

90. For example, *Koloniaal Verslag* (1917), xxvii.

91. Sylvia Gooswit, "Woningverbetering als pestbestrijdingsmaatregel op Java vanaf 1915," *Jambatan* 7, no. 1 (1989): 29–36; Purwanto Hadi, Vincentia Reni Vitasurya, and Eduardus Kevin Pandu, "The Shift of Symbolic Meaning of *Joglo* Houses for People in Brayut Tourism Village," in *Reframing the Vernacular: Politics, Semiotics, and Representation*, ed. Gusti Ayu Made Suartika and Julie Nichols (Cham: Springer, 2020), 65–74.

92. DP, *Verslag over het eerste kwartaal 1915*, 189–195.

93. DP, *Verslag over het jaar 1919* (Batavia: Javasche Boekhandel & Drukkerij, 1920), apps. 11, 12.

94. DP, *Verslag over het eerste kwartaal 1915*, 189–195.

95. Henri Maclaine Pont, "Het Inlandsch bouwambacht, zijn beteekenis en Toekomst?," *Djawa* 3, no. 2 (1923): 79–89.

96. Noto Diningrat, "Grondslagen," *Nederlandsch-Indië Oud en Nieuw* 4, no. 4 (1923): 107–117.

97. Gooswit, "Woningverbetering," 34–35.

98. Louis Otten, "De pest op Java, 1911–1923" *MvdDdV* 13, no. 2 (1924): 119–262, see unnumbered photographs.

99. *Koloniaal Verslag* (1915), 200–201.

100. DP, *Verslag over het eerste kwartaal 1915*, 66–68.

101. Louis Otten to Governor-General, February 13, 1919, MGB, no. 7149, ANRI.

102. DP, *Verslag over het eerste kwartaal 1915*, 66, 189–195; Otten, "De pest op Java, 1911–1923: 234, 246–247; H. Vervoort, "Some Remarks on Rat-Proof Roof-Building," in *Transactions of the Fifth Biennial Congress Held at Singapore, 1923* (London: John Bale, 1924), 348–351.

103. "Note on the Proposal of the Municipal Council of Semarang concerning Home Improvement," December 22, 1916, MGB, no. 2892, ANRI.

104. DP, *Verslag over het jaar 1919*, 126–129.

105. "Note on the Proposal of the Municipal Council of Semarang."

106. Creutzberg to the Governor-General, March 29, 1917, MGB, no. 4892, ANRI.

107. Ministerie van Koloniën: Memories van Overgave, no. 65, index 2.10.39, NL-HaNA.

108. Louis Otten to Governor-General, February 13, 1919, ANRI.

109. Van Loghem, "Eenige epidemiologische gegevens," 130–138.

110. Assistant-Resident of Malang, "Report."

111. Assistant-Resident of Malang, "Toelichting," July 19, 1912, TGA, no. 6671, ANRI.

112. DP, *Verslag over het eerste kwartaal 1915*, 157.

113. DP, *Verslag over het jaar 1919*, 54.

114. Gooswit, "Woningverbetering," 34–35.

115. "Rapport omtrent de voorziening van dakpannen voor de woningverbetering bij de pestbestrijding in de residentie Soerakarta, vervolg no. 10," circa 1916, MGB, no. 4958, ANRI.

116. Louis Otten to Governor-General, February 13, 1919, ANRI; DP, *Verslag over het jaar 1919*, 50–53.

117. See for instance a photograph of a "rooftile storage site near Pakis" containing around two million rooftiles: Het Geheugen van Nederland, Item A101-1-68. https://resolver.kb.nl/resolve?urn=urn:gvn:VKM01:A101-1-68.

118. Otten to Governor-General, February 13, 1919, ANRI.

119. DP, *Verslag over het jaar 1919*, 50–55.

120. See, for example, *Koloniaal Verslag* (1914), 226.

121. "Opmerkingen over de begrooting van Nederlandsch-Indië voor het dienstjaar 1919," *Koloniaal Tijdschrift* 8, no. 1 (1919): 71–72; "Koloniaal tijdschrift," *Algemeen Handelsblad*, December 21, 1919; *Tien begrootingen met den Volksraaad 1919–1928* (Weltevreden: Landsdrukkerij, 1929), 330; *Het tweede tiental begrootingen met den Volksraad, 1929–1938* (Batavia: Landsdrukkerij, 1938).

122. H. J. Rosier, "Verslag betreffende de pestbestrijding op Java over het Jaar 1935," *MvdDdV* 26, no. 3 supplement (1937): 1–100, app. 1; *Het tweede tiental begrootingen*, 474–475.

123. H. J. Rosier, "Verslag betreffende de pestbestrijding op Java over het Jaar 1933," *MvdDdV* 24, no. 3 supplement (1935): 272.

124. "Jaarverslag van den Burgerlijken Geneeskundigen Dienst in Nederlandsch-Indië over 1924," *MvdDdV* 16, no. 2 (1927): 223.

125. Rosier, "Verslag betreffende de pestbestrijding, 1935," 67.

126. H. J. Rosier, "Verslag betreffende de pestbestrijding op Java over het Jaar 1934," *MvdDdV* 25, no. 2 (1936): 160.

127. Ministerie van Koloniën: Memories van Overgave, no. 64, index 2.10.39, NL-HaNA.

128. See for instance: H. J. Rosier, "Verslag betreffende de pestbestrijding op Java over het jaar 1938," *MvdDdV* 28, no. 2–3 (1939): 237.

129. K. van Roon to Governor-General, June 23, 1917, MGS, no. 4892, ANRI.

130. Otten to Governor-General, February 13, 1919, TGA, no. 7149, ANRI.

131. *Koloniaal Verslag* (1921), 46.

132. H. J. Rosier, "Woningverbetering en Malaria," *MvdDdV* 26, no. 4 (1937): 360.

133. *Koloniaal Verslag* (1920), 62.

134. Elise van Nederveen Meerkerk, *Women, Work and Colonialism in the Netherlands and Java: Comparisons, Contrasts, and Connections, 1830–1940* (Cham: Palgrave Macmillan, 2019), 61–63.

135. DP, "Verslag over het eerste kwartaal 1915," *Mededeelingen* 7, no. 5 (1918): 1–71, 41–42; *Koloniaal Verslag* (1920), 63.

136. De Vogel, "Uittreksel," 84, figs. 31–32. See also Rijksmuseum Boerhaave, Leiden, Collection Database, Objects P20269 and P20213, https://boerhaave.adlibhosting.com/Details/collect/69931, https://boerhaave.adlibhosting.com/Details/collect/69875.

137. Rijksmuseum Boerhaave, Leiden, Collection Database, Object P20206, https://boerhaave.adlibhosting.com/Details/collect/69868.

138. De Raadt, *De woningverbetering*, 16.

139. Marin Gerard van Heel, *Gedenkboek van de koloniale tentoonstelling Semarang, 20 Augustus–22 November 1914*, vol. 2 (Batavia: Mercurius, 1916), 17–18.

140. DP, *Verslag over het eerste kwartaal 1915*, 69–70.

141. "Handelingen," Tweede Kamer, 70ste Vergadering, April 29, 1914, 1919.

142. BGD to the Governor-General, January 20, 1918, Bt, no. 2478, ANRI.

143. Director of Public Works to the Governor General, August 10, 1918, Bt, no. 2478, ANRI.

144. Public works was over this period itself involved in a broader policy of *kampong* improvement that focused on paving roads and constructing cement sewers. Freek Colombijn, *Under Construction: The Politics of Urban Space and Housing during the Decolonization of Indonesia, 1930–1960* (Leiden: Brill, 2014), 114, 191.

145. J. C. van Reigersberg Versluys, "Mededeeling omtrent het Ingenieurs-Congres in 1919 op Java te Houden," *De Ingenieur* 33, no. 31 (1918): 577–582.

146. Willem Thomas de Vogel to Governor-General, February 6, 1919, Bt, no. 2478, ANRI.

147. Ben F. van Leerdam, *Architect Henri Maclaine Pont: Een speurtocht naar het wezenlijke van de Javaanse architectuur* (Delft: Eburon, 1995), 36, 99–100.

148. Pauline K. M. van Roosmalen, "Ontwerpen aan de stad: Stedenbouw in Nederlands-Indië en Indonesië (1905–1950)," PhD diss., TU Delft, 2008, 69–71.

149. Henri Maclaine Pont, "Javaansche architectuur," *Djawa* 3, no. 4 (1923): 159–170, caption below fig. 8.

150. Henri Maclaine Pont, "Anti-Plague Bamboo Constructions," in *Transactions of the Fourth Congress held at Weltevreden, Batavia* (Weltevreden: Javasche Boekhandel en Drukkerij, 1922), 609–616, figs. 1–2.

151. Van Roosmalen, "Ontwerpen aan de stad," 70–71.

152. Sociaal-Technische Vereeniging, *Verslag volkshuisvestingscongres 1922* (Semarang: Stoomdrukkerij Misset, 1922), 39–40, 117–123.

153. Van Roosmalen, "Ontwerpen aan de stad," 69–71.

154. Maclaine Pont, "Anti-Plague Bamboo Constructions"; Hendrik Petrus Berlage, *Mijn Indische reis* (Rotterdam: W. L. & J. Brusse's, 1931), 43–44.

155. Gerrit de Vries and Dorothee Segaar-Höweler, *Henri Maclaine Pont: Architect, constructeur, archeoloog* (Rotterdam: Stiching Bonas, 2009), 89. "De electrische tram te Soerabaja," *De Ingenieur* 40, no. 11 (1925): 216–223.

156. Vervoort, "Some Remarks on Rat-Proof Roof-Building."

157. Het Geheugen van Nederland, Item A101-1-127, https://resolver.kb.nl/resolve?urn=urn:gvn:VKM01:A101-1-127; Sociaal-Technische Vereeniging, *Verslag Volkshuis-vestingscongres 1922*, figs. I–X.

158. P. A. J. Moojen, *Catalogus van de houtsnijwerk tentoonstelling* ([Bandoeng]: 1921), 8.

159. *Koloniaal Verslag* (1917), xx.

160. Gooswit, "Woningverbetering," 29–36.

3. The Spectacle of Home Improvement

1. Anton Versteeg, *Dagboek van mijn grootvader G. M. Versteeg*, vols 3–6 (self-pub., Pumbo, 2016).

2. Lynteris, "Prophetic Faculty of Epidemic Photography," 118–132; Lynteris, "Tarbagan's Winter Lair," 66.

3. Engelmann, "What Are Medical Photographs of Plague?"

4. Protschky, "Camera Ethica," 11–40.

5. Ruth Rogaski, *Hygienic Modernity: Meanings of Health and Disease in Treaty-Port China* (Berkeley: University of California Press, 2004).

6. John M. MacKenzie and John McAleer, "Introduction: Cultures of Display and the British Empire," in *Exhibiting the Empire: Cultures of Display and the British Empire*, ed. John M. MacKenzie and John McAleer (Manchester: Manchester University Press, 2017), 1–17; Anne Maxwell, *Colonial Photography and Exhibitions* (London: Leicester University Press, 2000); Peter H. Hoffenberg, *An Empire on Display* (Berkeley: University of California Press, 2001).

7. Marieke Bloembergen, *De koloniale vertoning: Nederland en Indië op de wereldten-toonstellingen (1880–1931)* (Amsterdam: Wereldbibliotheek, 2002); Marieke Bloembergen, *Colonial Spectacles: The Netherlands and the Dutch East Indies at the World Exhibitions, 1880–1931* (Singapore: NUS Press, 2006).

8. Guy Debord, *The Society of the Spectacle* (Canberra: Treason, 2002), 6; Pascal Blanchard, Nicolas Bancel, Gilles Boëtsch, Eric Deroo, Sandrine Lemaire, and Charles Forsdick, eds., *Human Zoos: Science and Spectacle in the Age of Colonial Empires*, trans. Teresa Bridgeman (Liverpool: Liverpool University Press, 2008); Bloembergen, *Colonial Spectacles*, 327–333; Ben Timmerman, "Zoos Humains: Meer dan een Spektakel?," MA thesis, University of Ghent, 2017, 18–19; Katelyn E. Knox, *Race on Display in 20th-and 21st-Century France* (Liverpool: Liverpool University Press, 2016); Pramod K. Nayar, *Colonial Voices: The Discourses of Empire* (Malden, MA: Wiley-Blackwell, 2012), 104–106, 145–155.

9. Timothy Mitchell, *Colonising Egypt* (Berkeley: University of California Press, 1988), 5–7.

10. Richard Vokes, "Photography, Exhibitions and Embodied Futures in Colonial Uganda, 1908–1960," *Visual Studies* 33, no. 1 (2018): 11–27; Roslyn Poignant, *Professional Savages: Captive Lives and Western Spectacle* (New Haven, CT: Yale University Press, 2004), 77–88.

11. Guido Carlo Pigliasco, "Colonial Spectacle, Staged Authenticity and Other Heritage Paradoxes on a Fijian Island," paper presented at the conference Europe and the Pacific, Brussels, June 25, 2015; Donna McCormac, *Queer Postcolonial Narratives and the Ethics of Witnessing* (New York: Bloomsbury Academic, 2014), 136.

12. Tucker, *Nature Exposed*, 6–7.

13. Poignant, *Professional Savages*, 161–171.

14. Not unlike Javanese middle-class visitors to the colonial fairs, where photographs of home improvement were often displayed: Arnout H. C. van der Meer, "Performing Colonial Modernity: Fairs, Consumerism, and the Emergence of the Indonesian Middle Class," *Bijdragen tot de Taal-, Land- en Volkenkunde* 173 (2017): 503–538.

15. H. W. van den Doel, *De stille macht: Het Europese binnenlands bestuur op Java en Madoera, 1808–1942* (Amsterdam: Bert Bakker, 1994), 161–214.

16. Photographs of the Third Plague Pandemic, Centre for Research in the Arts, Humanities and Social Sciences, University of Cambridge, Item PhotoID_11564, https://www.repository.cam.ac.uk/handle/1810/285231.

17. De Vogel, "Uittreksel," 72–73, fig. 14.

18. Ari Larissa Heinrich, *The Afterlife of Images: Translating the Pathological Body between China and the West* (Durham, NC: Duke University Press, 2003).

19. Heinrich, *Afterlife of Images*, 96–111. See also Susan Sidlauskas, "Before and After: The Aesthetic as Evidence in Nineteenth-Century Medical Photography," in *Before-and-After Photography: Histories and Contexts*, ed. Jordan Bear and Kate Palmer Albers (London: Bloomsbury Academic, 2017), 15–42.

20. Heinrich, *Afterlife of Images*, 95–111.

21. UBL Digital Collections, Items KITLV 69086 and KITLV69087, http://hdl.handle.net/1887.1/item:763140, http://hdl.handle.net/1887.1/item:762735.

22. Seth Koven, *Slumming: Sexual and Social Politics in Victorian London* (Princeton, NJ: Princeton University Press, 2006), 114–117.

23. H. F. Tillema, *Kromoblanda*, vol. 2 (The Hague: Electrische Drukkerij, 1916), 35–37.

24. Peckham, "Hong Kong Junk," 35, 44.

25. Jason E. Hill, "'Noise Abatement Zone': John Divola's Photographic Fulcrum," in Bear and Albers, *Before-and-After Photography*, 59–78.

26. NMVW–Collection Database, Item A101-1-97, https://hdl.handle.net/20.500.11840/906205.

27. NMVW–Collection Database, Item RV-A101-1-97a, https://hdl.handle.net/20.500.11840/915767.

28. NMVW–Collection Database, Item TM-alb-0346-27, https://hdl.handle.net/20.500.11840/108221.

29. Paul Christiaan Flu, "Catalogue," entry for drawer 22, slide 33, UBL.

30. Lewis W. Hine, *Men at Work: Photographic Studies of Modern Men and Machines* (New York: Dover, 1977).

31. NMVW–Collection Database, Item TM-60017529, https://hdl.handle.net/20.500.11840/21709.

32. "Het Epidemiologisch Bureau van den Volkenbond," *De Locomotief*, February 20, 1930.

33. F. Norman White, "Final Report Dutch East Indies," 13, LoN.

34. See for instance the photographs contained between pages 76 and 77 in Ministerie van Koloniën: Memories van Overgave, no. 65, index 2.10.39, NL-HaNA; NMVW–Collection Database, Item TM-60048078, https://hdl.handle.net/20.500.11840/303395.

35. Ch. W. F. Winckel, as cited in Van Bergen, *Van koloniale geneeskunde tot internationale gezondheidszorg*, 22.

36. Van Loghem, "Over pest," 153.

37. For example, "Uit het Malangsche," *Algemeen Handelsblad*, October 11, 1911.

38. "De pest op Java," *De Telegraaf*, January 26, 1912; "Het een en ander over de pest op Java," *Algemeen Handelsblad*, January 26, 1912.

39. "De pest op Java," *De Telegraaf*, January 26, 1912.

40. "De pest op Java," *NvdD: Kleine Courant*, January 26, 1912; Van Loghem, "Eenige epidemiologische gegevens," 14.

41. "Dr van Loghem over de pest op Java," *Algemeen Handelsblad*, February 12, 1912.

42. "Het Hamburgsche Tropencongres," *Nieuwe Rotterdamsche Courant*, April 7, 1912.

43. Johannes J. van Loghem, "Pestbestrijding op Java," *NTvG* 58 (1914): 1306–1308.

44. "Over het wezen en de verbreiding van eenige besmettelijke ziekten in de Tropen," in *Natuurkundige Voordrachten* (The Hague: W. P. van Stockum, 1915), 42–49.

45. "De organisatie der pestbestrijding op Java," *De Maasbode*, January 26, 1915.

46. "Vraagstukken der Indische Hygiëne," *Algemeen Handelsblad*, November 24, 1920.

47. Van Loghem, "De pestbestrijding op Java," *Het Vaderland*, December 17, 1937; Van Loghem, "De pestbestrijding op Java," *Tijdschrift van het Aardrijkskundig Genootschap* 12, no. 55 (Leiden: Brill, 1938): 157.

48. Tjipto Mangoenkoesoemo, *De pest op Java en hare bestrijding* (Delft: W. D. Meinema, 1914), 151–152.

49. "Woningtoestanden en woningverbetering," *Het Vaderland*, April 13, 1915.

50. "Hygiënisch Genootschap," *Dagblad van Zuid-Holland en 's-Gravenhage*, February 10, 1916.

51. M. Hijmans, "Een en ander over de pest op Java en hare bestrijding," *Nederlandsch-Indië: Oud & Nieuw* 2, no. 5 (1917): 153–169; Hijmans, "Een en ander over de pest op Java en hare bestrijding," *Nederlandsch Indië: Oud & Nieuw* 2, no. 6 (1917): 191–197.

52. H. F. Lumentut, "Iets over de pestbestrijding op Java," *Verslagen der Vergaderingen Indisch Genootschap* (1921): 105–133.

53. Bloembergen, *Colonial Spectacles*, 10–16; Eike Reichardt, *Health, "Race" and Empire: Popular-Scientific Spectacles and National Identity in Imperial Germany, 1871–1914* (Morrisville: Lulu.com 2008), 171–203.

54. "Internationale Tentoonstelling op Hygiënisch Gebied," 1921, in Collection Tentoonstellingen, folder 248, no. 30578, Stadsarchief Amsterdam, The Netherlands.

55. P. Muntendam, "Internationale Hygiëne-Tentoonstelling Amsterdam," *NTvG* 65 (1921): 1953–1956.

56. "De IHTA VIII: Tropische Ziekten," *Algemeen Handelsblad*, October 16, 1921.

57. "De Hygiënische Tentoonstelling: Tropische Hygiëne," *Het Centrum*, October 14, 1921.

58. "Internationale Hygiëne-Tentoonstelling," *Nieuwe Rotterdamsche Courant*, October 9, 1921; "De Hygiënische Tentoonstelling," *De Courant*, October 12, 1921.

59. "De Koningin-Moeder op de IHTA," *Algemeen Handelsblad*, October 17, 1921.

60. "Een Reizende Hygiëne-Tentoonstelling," *De Telegraaf*, March 13, 1922.

61. "Nederlandsche Roode Kruis," *Algemeen Handelsblad*, Juni 16, 1923; "Advertentie," *Leidsch Dagblad*, December 14, 1922; "Tentoonstelling voor Volksgezondheid," *Dagblad van Zuid-Holland en 's-Gravenhage*, April 15, 1922; "Reizende Tentoonstelling van Volksgezondheid," *Nieuwe Rotterdamsche Courant*, April 16, 1922; "Nat. Ver. Voor Vrouwenarbeid," *Algemeen Handelsblad*, April 30, 1922; "Reizende Hygiëne Tentoonstelling," *Nieuwe Tilburgsche Courant*, April 3, 1922; "Hygiëne-Tentoonstelling," *Leeuwarder Courant*, April 9, 1923; "De Reizende Hygiëne-Tentoonstelling," *De Telegraaf*, May 8, 1923.

62. Koninklijke Vereeniging Koloniaal Instituut, *Dertiende jaarverslag* (Amsterdam: de Bussy, 1923), 6, 7, 39.

63. *Catalogus van de Jubileum-Tentoonstelling 1923* (Amsterdam: Holkema en Warendof, 1923), 52–55.

64. Joost van Genabeek and Louise Rietbergen, *De S.D.A.P. en de volkshuisvesting: Inhoud en resultaten van het sociaaldemocratische volkshuisvestingsbeleid in Nederland (1894–1940)* (Utrecht: 1991); *Catalogus*, 24.

65. *Catalogus*, 52–55.

66. Joost Coté, Hugh O'Neill, Pauline K. M. van Roosmalen, and Helen Ibbitson Jessup, *The Life and Work of Thomas Karsten* (Amsterdam: Architecture & Natura, 2017).

67. *Catalogus*, 52–55.

68. "'t einde van de Jubileum-Tentoonstelling," *De Telegraaf*, November 1, 1923.

69. "In het Koloniaal Instituut," *De Telegraaf*, September 8, 1923.

70. "Indische Tentoonstelling Arnhem," Photograph, 1928, number 1523-123-0021, Gelders Archief, Arnhem, The Netherlands; Gelders Archief–Beeldbank, Item 1523-123-0021. https://permalink.geldersarchief.nl/C575DBCFA48E46359B05085BAF1978C5.

71. "Archief van het Koninklijk Instituut voor de Tropen, 1910–1992," No. 6492, index 2.20.69, NL-HaNA.

72. "De Indische Tentoonstelling," *Leeuwarder Courant*, May 28, 1932.

73. "Tropische Geneeskunde te Leiden," *De Locomotief*, January 16, 1931.

74. Photograph, 1936, inventory no. 1379, index 2.24.25, NL-HaNA; NMVW–Collection Database, Item TM-10000063, https://hdl.handle.net/20.500.11840/12023.

75. NMVW–Collection Database, Item TM-60052033, https://hdl.handle.net/20.500.11840/454710.

76. The VR3PP project has catalogued just two other contemporary plague films: a newsreel-style clip on the pneumonic plague outbreak in Manchuria in 1911 and a documentary of plague control in Iran in 1961. *De pest op Java*, dir. Willy Muellens (1927), FLM52319, EYE.

77. "Pest en haar bestrijding in Oost-Indië," *Het Vaderland*, June 3,1927.

78. "De pest op Java," *De Tijd*, February 1, 1927.

79. Johannes J. van Loghem, "Film der pestbestrijding op Java," *NTvG* 71 (1927): 209–210.

80. "Pest en haar bestrijding in Oost-Indië," *Het Vaderland*, June 3,1927.

81. "Een film in dienst der volksgezondheid," *Nieuwe Rotterdamsche Courant*, March 8, 1927.

82. "Onderwijs," *Het Vaderland*, November 15, 1928.

83. "De pestziekte: Lezingen met filmvertooning van dr. E. H. Hermans te Keulen en te Aken," *Nieuwe Rotterdamsche Courant*, March 4, 1929.

84. "De pest op Java," *De Tijd*, February 1, 1930.

85. "Bestrijding van de pest op Java," *De Tijd*, August 6, 1930.

86. Director of Education and Worship to the Commissary for Indies Affairs at the Department of Colonies, August 12, 1933, inventory no. 2383, index 2.10.49, NL-HaNA.

87. Poster, 1928, FR ANOM 0009Fi766, ANOM.

88. "De Nederlandsche Tentoonstelling te Kopenhagen," *Twentsch Dagblad*, August 26, 1922; "Het Holland-Huis te Brussel," *Haarlem's Dagblad*, April 21, 1923; "Ned.-Indische Tentoonstelling in het Holland-Huis te Brussel," *Algemeen Handelsblad*, April 22, 1923; "Nederlandsch-Indië op de Koloniale Tentoonstelling te Parijs in 1931," *Het Centrum*, December 12, 1929.

89. "Naar New York," *De Sumatra Post*, July 14, 1938. On the *mooi Indië* genre, see Protschky, *Images of the Tropics*, 83–92.

90. "De pest en de doktors," *De Tribune*, March 28, 1914.

91. Tomoko Akami, "A Quest to be Global: The League of Nations Health Organization and Inter-Colonial Regional Governing Agendas of the Far Eastern Association of Tropical Medicine 1910–25," *International History Review* 38, no. 1 (2016): 1–23.

92. "Führer des 4. Kongresses der Far Eastern Association of Tropical Medicine vom 6–13 August 1921 in Weltevrden" (Weltevreden: G. Kolff, 1921), 28–32.

93. Louis Otten, "Lecture on Plague," in *Transactions of the Fourth Congress Held at Weltevreden, Batavia* (Weltevreden: Javasche Boekhandel en Drukkerij, 1922), 617–628; "Het Medisch Congres," *Bataviaasch Nieuwsblad*, August 13, 1921.

94. Marta Aleksandra Balińska, "Assistance and Not Mere Relief: The Epidemic Commission of the League of Nations, 1920–1923," in *International Health Organisations and Movements 1918–1939*, ed. Paul Weindling (Cambridge: Cambridge University Press, 1995), 102; Lenore Manderson, "Wireless Wars in the Eastern Arena: Epidemiological Surveillance, Disease Prevention, and the Work of the Eastern Bureau of the League of Nations Health Organisation, 1925–1942," in Weindling, *International Health Organisations*, 109–133.

95. Darwin H. Stapleton, "Malaria Eradication and the Technological Model: The Rockefeller Foundation and Public Health in East Asia," in *Disease, Colonialism, and the State: Malaria in Modern East Asian History*, ed. Ka-che Yip (Hong Kong: Hong Kong University Press, 2009), 71–84.

96. Meerwijk, "Phantom Menace," 215–243.

97. Frederick Norman White, "Diary," R843, no. 23230, LoN.

98. White, "Diary."

99. White, "Diary."

100. White, "Diary"; White, "Draft Report," 9.

101. White, "Draft Report," 5.

102. White, "Draft Report," 13.

103. White, "Draft Report," 14.

104. Dienst der Volksgezondheid (hereafter DVG), *Control of Endemic Diseases in the Netherlands Indies* (Weltevreden: Landsdrukkerij, 1929), 45.

105. F. Norman White, "Presidential Address," *Transactions of the Royal Society of Tropical Medicine and Hygiene* 47, no. 6 (1953): 441–450.

106. Victor G. Heiser, "Diary," 1916, vol. 1, 203–258, Record Group (RG) 12 (Officers' Diaries), Rockefeller Archive Center, Tarrytown, NY (hereafter RAC).

107. John Farley, *To Cast out Disease: A History of the International Health Division of the Rockefeller Foundation (1913–1951)* (Oxford: Oxford University Press, 2004).

108. Terence H. Hull, "Conflict and Collaboration in Public Health: The Rockefeller Foundation and the Dutch Colonial Government in Indonesia," in *Public Health in Asia and the Pacific: Historical and Comparative Perspectives*, ed. Milton J. Lewis and Kerrie L. MacPherson (Abingdon: Routledge 2008), 139–152.

109. *Koloniaal Verslag* (1927), 212.

110. Heiser, "Diary," 1925–1926, 277–278, RG 12, RAC.

111. Heiser, "Diary," 1925–1926, 266–289.

112. "Hygienische zorgen in het Oosten," *Bataviaasch Nieuwsblad*, February 19, 1930.

113. "Onze geleerde gasten," *Bataviaasch Nieuwsblad*, March 5, 1930; "Gunstig medisch oordeel," *Soerabaijsch Handelsblad*, March 4, 1930.

114. Tomoko Akami, "Imperial Polities, Intercolonialism, and the Shaping of Global Governing Norms: Public Health Expert Networks in Asia and the League of Nations Health Organization, 1908–37," *Journal of Global History* 12 (2017): 4–25.

115. Halfden Mahler, "Promotion of Primary Health Care in Member Countries of WHO," *Public Health Reports* 93, no. 2 (1978): 107–113.

116. "Bezoek 'Rural Hygiene Commission,'" *NvdD*, July 10, 1936; "Het Bezoek aan Java," *Algemeen Handelsblad voor Nederlandsch-Indië*, May 20, 1936.

117. *Report of the Intergovernmental Conference of Far-Eastern Countries on Rural Hygiene* (Geneva, 1937), 97.

118. *Report of the Intergovernmental Conference*, 97–98.

119. "De Tentoonstelling," *Bataviaasch Nieuwsblad*, August 3, 1937.

120. "De Volkenbondsconferentie te Bandoeng," *De Indische Courant*, August 4, 1937.

4. Plague Propaganda

1. *Oxford English Dictionary*, s.v. "propaganda, n.," December 2021, https://www.oed.com/view/Entry/152605?rskey=YMEJCR&result=1&isAdvanced=false#eid; F. E. Wynne, "Health Propaganda: I. The Administrative Point of View," *British Medical Journal* 10, no. 2 (1929): 242–243.

2. For discussions of this facet of health propaganda in other contexts, see Liping Bu, *Public Health and the Modernization of China, 1865–2015* (London: Routledge, 2017), 16–19; Paula A. Michaels, "Medical Propaganda and Cultural Revolution in Soviet Kazakhstan, 1928–41," *Russian Review* 59 (2000): 159–178. On the "conversion narratives" inherent to much colonial visual health messaging, see Ruth J. Prince, "The Diseased Body and the Global Subject: The Circulation and Consumption of an Iconic AIDS Photograph in East Africa," *Visual Anthropology* 29 (2016): 159–186.

3. Swellengrebel, "Plague in Java"; DP, *Verslag over het eerste kwartaal 1915*, 197.

4. De Vogel, "Uittreksel," maps for the weeks November 1910 to August 1911.

5. Deutmann, "De pest in Karanglo," 59; De Vogel, "Uittreksel," 39–40.

6. NMVW–Collection Database, Item TM-10024178, https://hdl.handle.net/20.500 .11840/320780.

7. Arnout H. C. van der Meer, *Performing Power: Cultural Hegemony, Identity, and Resistance in Colonial Indonesia* (Ithaca, NY: Cornell University Press, 2020), 19–47.

8. De Vogel, "Uittreksel," fig. 5.

9. De Vogel, "Uittreksel," 55–56.

10. De Vogel, "Uittreksel," 56.

11. *De Preangerbode*, April 12, 1911.

12. De Vogel, "Uittreksel," 59. He is presumably referring here to Frank Morten Todd, *Eradicating Plague from San Francisco* (San Francisco, CA: C. A. Murdoch, 1909). This volume would have contained plenty of examples of handbills, posters, and announcements for the Dutch to copy.

13. Van Loghem, "Eenige epidemiologische gegevens," 138.

14. Suzanna de Vogel to Augusta de Vogel, October 18, 1911, UBL.

15. Van Loghem, "Eenige epidemiologische gegevens," 138; On this vitality of "dark spaces," see also Kelly and Sáez, "Shadowlands and Dark Corners."

16. Van Loghem, "Eenige epidemiologische gegevens," 138. On the recurring association between the Chinese, "things," and plague, see Peckham, "Hong Kong Junk."

17. De Raadt, *De woningverbetering*, 13–16.

18. De Vogel, "Uittreksel," fig. 29.

19. De Vogel, "Uittreksel," fig. 30.

20. De Vogel, "Uittreksel," 65; Deutman, "De pest in Karanglo," 190. See also G. A. Jansen Hendriks, "Een voorbeeldige kolonie: Nederlands-Indië in 50 jaar overheidsfilms, 1912–1962," PhD diss., University of Amsterdam, 2014, 52.

21. For example, "Van inlanders en pest," *De Preangerbode*, May 16, 1911.

22. Joshua Barker, "Surveillance and Territoriality in Bandung," in *Figures of Criminality in Indonesia, the Philippines, and Colonial Vietnam*, ed. Vicente L. Rafael (Ithaca, NY: Cornell Southeast Asia Program, 1999), 95–127.

23. DP, *Verslag over het eerste kwartaal 1916*, 5–6.

24. De Vogel, "Inspectie rapport," ANRI.

25. DP, *Verslag over het eerste kwartaal 1915*, 69–70.

26. DP, *Verslag over het vierde kwartaal 1915*, 43.

27. DP, *Verslag over het eerste kwartaal 1915*, 69–70.

28. DP, *Verslag over het eerste kwartaal 1915*, 73.

29. DP, *Verslag over het eerste kwartaal 1915*, 73–74.

30. DP, *Verslag over het tweede kwartaal 1915*, 196–197.

31. DP, *Verslag over het vierde kwartaal 1915*, 40–44.

32. "Besmettelijke ziekten. Pestgevaarlijke gebouwen," *Staatsblad van Nederlandsch-Indië*, no. 486, July 6, 1914.

33. Lumentut, "Iets over de pestbestrijding op Java," 123.

34. DP, *Verslag over het eerste kwartaal 1916*, 15.

35. DP, *Verslag over het tweede kwartaal 1916*, 48.

36. DP, *Verslag over het tweede kwartaal 1916*, 47–48.

37. DP, *Verslag over het jaar 1920* (Batavia: Javasche Boekhandel & Drukkerij, 1921), 6–7.

38. DP, *Verslag over het jaar 1920, 35.*

39. Van Heel, *Gedenkboek van de Koloniale Tentoonstelling Semarang,* 17–18.

40. Willem Thomas de Vogel, *De taak van den Burgerlijken Geneeskundigen Dienst in Nederlandsch-Indië* (Amsterdam: Ellerman, Harms, 1917), 8–9.

41. E. P. Snijders, "Dr W. Th. de Vogel 90 jaar terugblik op een rijk leven," *NTvG* 97, 1, no. 12 (1953): 714–716.

42. De Vogel, *Beknopt verslag,* 30.

43. Topics included birthing and malaria. Collection Familie von Römer, nos. 51–53, index 2.21.143, NL-HaNA; Lisa Kuitert, *Met een drukpers de oceaan over: Koloniale boekcultuur in Nederlands-Indië 1816–1920* (Amsterdam: Prometheus, 2020), 234–247.

44. De Vogel, *Beknopt verslag,* 39.

45. Jansen Hendriks, "Een voorbeeldige kolonie," 40–41; Openbaar Verbaal, inventory no. 2273, index 2.10.36.04, NL-HaNA.

46. *Koloniaal Verslag* (1920), 213–216; *Korte Berichten,* no. 28 (1931), B 2028, Perpustakaan Nasional Republik Indonesia, Jakarta, Indonesia (hereafter PNRI).

47. Willem Thomas de Vogel, "Report," 1921, TGA, no. 7306, ANRI.

48. L. S. A. M. von Römer, "About the Exhibition in Connection with the Fourth Congress of the Far Eastern Association of Tropical Medicine held at Batavia from 6th–13th August 1921," in *Transactions of the Fourth Congress Held at Weltevreden, Batavia* (Weltevreden: Javasche Boekhandel en Drukkerij, 1922), 381–393.

49. *Korte Berichten,* no. 30 (1931), PNRI.

50. O. L. E. de Raadt, *Penjakit pest Ditanah Djawa* (Batavia: Commissie voor de Volkslectuur, 1915).

51. O. L. E. de Raadt, *Rangsa Ni Sahit Pest, Na Masa Di Poelo Djawa* (1915).

52. *Dari Hal Penjakit Pest (Sampar) Dan Pendjaganja* (Batavia: Landsdrukkerij, 1919).

53. *Kasakit pest Djeung Piken Panoelaksa* (Batavia: Landsdrukkerij, 1919).

54. K. van Roon, *De pest* (Weltevreden: Landsdrukkerij, 1920).

55. Louis Otten, *Beknopt overzicht betreffende organisatie en uitvoering der pestbestrijdingsmaatregelen* (Semarang: A. Bisschop, 1921), 42–44.

56. Dafna Ruppin, *The Komedi Bioscoop: The Emergence of Movie-Going in Colonial Indonesia, 1896–1914* (Bloomington, IN: John Libbey, 2016), 270.

57. "De pest-film," *NvdD,* June 28, 1911.

58. *Koloniaal Verslag* (1915), 9–10; *Bataviaasch Nieuwsblad,* February 17, 1915.

59. *De Sumatra Post,* March 15, 1918.

60. Oscar Gelderblom and Bas van Bavel, "The Economic Origins of Cleanliness in the Dutch Golden Age," *Past & Present* 205, no. 1 (2009): 41–69.

61. *De Sumatra Post,* March 15, 1918.

62. The Rockefeller Foundation, "Charter," May 14, 1913.

63. Heiser, "Diary," 1916, vol. 1, 224–228, RAC.

64. John Hydrick to Victor Heiser, April 21, 1924, RF 5 1 1.02 204 2601, RAC; Pols, *Nurturing Indonesia,* 142–143.

65. Tillema, *Kromoblanda,* 1:45.

66. Tillema, *Kromoblanda,* 2:74.

67. H. M. Neeb, *Korte wenken* (Bandoeng: N. V. Drukkerij, 1927), 15–16.

68. L. Kirschner, M. L. A. Cordesius,, and W. Hoogerbeets, *De Tien Geboden voor Hygiëne in de Tropen*, no. 6 (Bandoeng: N. V. Drukkerij, 1927).

69. Sebastian Weinert, *Der Körper im Blick: Gesundheitsausstellungen vom späten Kaiserreich bis zum Nationalsozialismus* (Oldenbourg: Walter de Gruyter, 2017), 184–186.

70. "De jaarbeurs-trein," *Bataviaasch Nieuwsblad*, July 8, 1927.

71. *Vox Medicorum*, 46–47; *Verslag der Eerste Hygiëne-Tentoonstelling in Nederlandsch-Indië* (Vereeniging tot Bevordering der Hygiëne in Nederlandsch-Indië).

72. *Verslag der Eerste Hygiëne-Tentoonstelling*, 9,.

73. Weinert, *Der Körper im Blick*, 186.

74. *EHTINI: Tweede overzicht der inzendingen* (Bandoeng: N. V. Drukkerij, 1927), 30–31.

75. Ch. W. F. Winckel, "De Eerste Hygiëne-Tentoonstelling in Nederlandsch-Indië te Bandoeng," *NTvG* 71 (1927): 759–763.

76. NMVW–Collection Database, Item TM-60046535, and Photographs of the Third Plague Pandemic, Centre for Research in the Arts, Humanities and Social Sciences, University of Cambridge, Item PhotoID_11689, https://www.repository.cam.ac.uk/handle/1810/285222.

77. UBL Digital Collections, Items KITLV 78094 and KITLV 78095. http://hdl.handle.net/1887.1/item:904927, http://hdl.handle.net/1887.1/item:906750.

78. The Pasar Gambir as a whole allowed the Dutch to emphasize Western modernity alongside "indigenous entertainments and exhibitions rooted in Java's past." Arnout van der Meer, "Ambivalent Hegemony: Culture and Power in Colonial Java, 1808–1927," PhD diss., Rutgers University, 2014, 341–342.

79. *NvdD*, August 30, 1929.

80. "Pamphlet," 1929, RG 5, series 5, subseries 655, box 228, folder 2830, RAC.

81. *Friesch Dagblad*, September 11, 1937.

82. Hull, "Conflict and Collaboration in Public Health," 139–152.

83. John Hydrick to Victor Heiser, July 7, 1925, RG 5, 1.02, 236, 3017, RAC.

84. John Hydrick to Victor Heiser, December 11, 1926, RG 5, 1.02, 270, 3412, RAC.

85. *Bataviaasch Nieuwsblad*, September 28, 1926.

86. Correspondence and invitation card from John Hydrick to Victor Heiser, July 21, 1928, RG 5, 1.02, 309, 3934, RAC.

87. "Een Pest-Film," *Bataviaasch Nieuwsblad*, September 11, 1926.

88. *De pest op Java*, dir. Willy Muellens (1927), FLM52319, EYE.

89. J. J. van Loghem, "Film der Pestbestrijding op Java," *NTvG* 71 (1927), 209–210; "De Indische Pestbestrijding in Beeld," *Haagsche Courant*, April 7, 1927.

90. NMVW–Collection Database, Item TM-60012955, and Photographs of the Third Plague Pandemic, Centre for Research in the Arts, Humanities and Social Sciences, University of Cambridge, Item PhotoID_11645, https://www.repository.cam.ac.uk/handle/1810/285317.

91. Hydrick, "Report for the Third Quarter, 1929," 1, RG 5, 3.655, 228, 2830, RAC.

92. "Note on the Program for 1932," RG 1.1, 655.1, 3, 7, RAC.

93. *De Gezondheidsbrigade* 7, no. 2 (1935).

94. "Sidin en Tikoes," *De Gezondheids-Brigade* 6, no. 9 (1935): 1–6.

95. *De Gezondheidsbrigade* 9, no. 5 (1938).

96. "Enkele vijanden van ons lichaam," *De Gezondheidsbrigade* 9, no. 6 (1938): 45–48; P. Peverelli, *Blijf Gezond!* (Groningen: J. B. Wolters, 1933).

97. "Enkele vijanden van ons lichaam."

5. Plague, Malaria, and Vaccination

1. *Verslag van Bestuur en Staat van Nederlandsch-Indië, Suriname en Curaçao* (1928), 47.

2. "Het dilemma: Pestrat of malaria-muskiet," *De Locomotief,* October 20, 1938.

3. Shailendra Kumar Verma and Urmil Tuteja, "Plague Vaccine Development: Current Research and Future Trends," *Frontiers in Immunology* 7 (2016): 1–8.

4. Echenberg, *Plague Ports,* 59–62.

5. Thomas C. Butler, "Plague History," *Clinical Microbiology and Infection* 20, no. 3 (2014): 202–209; "A Cure for the Plague," *Hong Kong Daily Press,* July 1, 1896.

6. Hong Kong Museum of Medical Sciences Society, *Plague, SARS, and the Story of Medicine in Hong Kong* (Hong Kong: Hong Kong University Press, 2006), 36–37; Matheus Alves Duarte da Silva, "From Bombay to Rio de Janeiro: The Circulation of Knowledge and the Establishment of the Manguinhos Laboratory, 1894–1902," *História, Ciências, Saúde* 25, no. 3 (2017): 1–19.

7. Mark Harrison, *Public Health in British India: Anglo-Indian Preventive Medicine, 1859–1914* (Cambridge: Cambridge University Press, 1994), 144.

8. Harrison, *Public Health in British India,* 87; Arnold, *Colonizing the Body,* 116–158.

9. Arnold, *Colonizing the Body,* 200–239.

10. *Arbeiten aus dem Kaiserlichen Gesundheitsamte* 16 (Berlin: Springer, 1899): 1–356.

11. Sydney Rowland, "XXXVIII. First Report on Investigations into Plague Vaccines," *Epidemiology and Infection* 10, no. 3 (1910): 536–565.

12. Duarte da Silva, "From Bombay to Rio de Janeiro."

13. Kristine A. Campbell, "Knots in the Fabric: Richard Pearson Strong and the Bilibid Prison Vaccine Trials, 1905–1906," *Bulletin of the History of Medicine* 68, no. 4 (1994): 600–638.

14. Wade H. Frost, "Active and Passive Immunization against Plague," *Public Health Reports* 27, no. 34 (1912): 1361–1371.

15. "De pest," *Bataviaasch Nieuwsblad,* April 6, 1911.

16. Deutmann, "De pest in Karanglo," 221–222; A. A. F. M. Deutmann, "De pest in Karanglo in de maanden Mei, Juni, en Juli 1911," *GTNI* 52 (1912): 431–511, 465–466.

17. De Haan, "De bacteriologische diagnose van pest," 24.

18. Photographs of the Third Plague Pandemic, Centre for Research in the Arts, Humanities and Social Sciences, University of Cambridge, Item PhotoID_11635, https://www.repository.cam.ac.uk/handle/1810/285306.

19. J. G. Sleeswijk, "Pest en pestbestrijding op Java," in *Berichten uit Oost-Indië voor de Leden van den Sint-Claverbond* 1 (1915): 3–17.

20. Sleeswijk, "Pest en pestbestrijding op Java," 4.

21. Deutmann, "De pest in Karanglo," 472.

22. Deutmann, "De pest in Karanglo," 223.

23. NMVW–Collection Database, Item TM-10006672, https://hdl.handle.net/20.500.11840/226983.

24. Deutmann, "De pest in Karanglo," 251.

25. "Handelingen," Tweede Kamer, 70ste Vergadering, April 29, 1914: 1897–1901; "Handelingen," Tweede Kamer, 71ste Vergadering, April 30, 1914: 1923–1932; "Pest en pestbestrijding," *Het Vaderland*, April 10, 1914.

26. J. G. Sleeswijk, "De pest op Java," *Tijdschrift voor Sociale Hygiëne* 17 (1914): 75–78; J. G. Sleeswijk, "De pest op Java," *NTvG* 58 (1914): 1060–1062; "De pest en de doktoren," *De Tribune*, March 28, 1914; "Handelingen," Tweede Kamer, 70ste Vergadering, April 29, 1914: 1897–1921; "Uitzendingen voor den Nederlandsch-Indische Staatsdienst," *Nederlandsche Staatscourant*, November 1, 1915.

27. J. J. van Loghem, "Drie jaren pest op Java," *NTvG* 58 (1914): 876–879; van Loghem, "Pestbestrijding op Java."

28. W. A. Borger, "Vaccinatie tegen pest," *MvdBGD* 5, no. 1 (1916): 5–25.

29. P. C. Flu, "Proeven ter immuniseering tegen pest," *MvdBGD* 8 (1920): 18–60.

30. Louis Otten, "De pestbestrijding op Java, 1911–1936," in *Feestbundel 1936* (Batavia: G. Kolf, 1936), 98–99.

31. *Koloniaal Verslag* (1920), 61–62.

32. Otten, "De pest op Java, 1911–1923," 225.

33. Otten, "De pest op Java, 1911–1923," 228–229; M. B. van der Jagt, *Memorie van overgave*, 35–36, inventory no. 64, index 2.10.39, NL-HaNA; J. Pelt, *Memorie van overgave*, 68–77, inventory no. 543, index 2.10.39, NL-HaNA.

34. "Oproeping," *De Nederlandsche Staatscourant*, February 27, 1914.

35. "Pestbestrijding op Java," *Het Vaderland*, March 29, 1914.

36. "Pestbestrijding op Java," *Algemeen Handelsblad*, March 21, 1914; "De pest en de dokters," *De Tribune*, March 28, 1914.

37. "Oproeping," *De Nederlandsche Staatscourant*, March 27, 1914.

38. Letter, Minister of Colonies to Governor-General, February 2, 1914; Letter, de Vogel to Governor-General, March 2, 1914; Memo, de Vogel to Governor-General, April 4, 1914; Letter, de Vogel to Governor-General, May 12, 1914: inv. 1975, Bt, ANRI.

39. "Nederlandsche brieven," *Deli Courant*, May 2, 1914; "Pestbestrijding," *Het Nieuws van den Dag*, July 2, 1914.

40. "De pest op Java," *De Indische Mercuur* 37, no. 17 (1914): 368; "Mededeeling naar aanleiding van de motie in zake pestbestrijding," *Koloniaal Tijdschrift* 3, no. 1 (1914): 577–583.

41. "Voor de pestbestrijding," *De Preangerbode*, July 14, 1914; "Nederlandsch-Indië," *De Java-post*, 12, no. 18 (1914): 281.

42. Nederlandsche Roode Kruis, *Onze pestambulances* (Den Haag: 1914), 4.

43. "De derde Roode Kruis-ambulance te Toeren," *Leeuwarder Courant*, September 25, 1915.

44. *De Mens achter de Medaille: 100 jaar Rode Kruis-onderscheidingen* (Den Haag: Het Nederlandse Rode Kruis, 2014), 21–23.

45. A large part of this set has been digitized and is available on the website of Nationaal Museum van Wereldculturen (https://collectie.wereldculturen.nl/) under inventory numbers RV-A440-y-121 through RV-A440-y-162.

46. "De Roode Kruis Zusters," *Bataviaasch Nieuwsblad*, August 10, 1915.

47. "De derde Roode Kruis-ambulance te toeren," *Leeuwarder Courant*, September 25, 1915.

48. See the section "admissions and deaths" contained in part two of the *Indisch Verslag* from 1939 to 1941.

49. Jan Breman, *Koloniaal profijt van onvrije arbeid: Het Preanger stelsel van gedwongen koffieteelt op Java* (Amsterdam: Amsterdam University Press, 2010).

50. Otten, "De pestbestrijding op Java, 1911–1936," 94, 99–100.

51. Petition of the DVG to the Governor-General, October 1933, Bt, no. 3088, ANRI.

52. Rosier, "Verslag betreffende de pestbestrijding op Java over het jaar 1933," 195.

53. Rosier, "Verslag betreffende de pestbestrijding op Java over het jaar 1934," 115.

54. Hull, "Plague in Java," 225.

55. Report by the Head of the DVG to the Governor-General, August 1934, MGB, no. 4958, ANRI, original emphasis.

56. "Jaarverslag van den Dienst der Volksgezondheid over 1934," *MvdDdV* 24, no. 4 (1935): 404–460.

57. *Handelingen van den Volksraad* (July 13, 1935), 202.

58. "Handelingen," Tweede Kamer, 42ste Vergadering, February 28, 1934: 1400; "Handelingen," Tweede Kamer, 39ste Vergadering, February 21, 1935: 1437–1439.

59. Director of the Cabinet of the Queen to the Minister of Colonies, April 30, 1934, Bt, no. 3088, ANRI.

60. "Persoonlijke belangstelling van H. M. de Koningin," *De Locomotief*, September 18, 1934; "De toeneming van de pest in West-Java," *De Telegraaf*, October 6, 1934.

61. Minister of Colonies to the Governor-General, May 17, 1934, Bt, no. 3088, ANRI.

62. Minister of Colonies to the Governor-General, May 17, 1934, Bt, no. 3088, ANRI.

63. The residency Priangan was separated into three separate residencies (East, Central, and West Priangan) in 1925. In 1931, East and Central Priangan were merged again into one residency (Priangan).

64. Louis Otten, "Experimental Vaccination in Plague: I. Dead Vaccine," *MvdDdV* 22, no. 2 (1933): 131–149.

65. "Nederlandsche Vereeniging voor Tropische Geneeskunde," *NTvG* 78, 2, 25 (1934): 2945–2985.

66. Office of the DVG to the Governor-General, November 17, 1934, Bt, no. 3088, ANRI.

67. "Nieuwe proeven met het pest-serum van Dr. L. Otten," *De Locomotief*, October 13, 1934.

68. Office of the DVG to the Governor-General, November 17, 1934, Bt, no. 3088, ANRI; "Jaarverslag van den Dienst der Volksgezondheid over 1934," *MvdDdV* 24, no. 4 (1935): 417.

69. "De Eerste Inentingen," *De Locomotief*, November 3, 1934; Mary Pos, "Indië strijdt tegen de pest," *De Telegraaf*, July 2, 1939.

70. "De eerste inentingen," *De Indische Courant*, November 7, 1934; "De eerste inentingen," *De Locomotief*, November 3, 1934.

71. Boomgaard, "Smallpox, Vaccination, and the Pax Neerlandica," 603–604.

72. E. P. Snijders, "De resultaten der pestvaccinatie op Java met het vaccin van Otten," *NTvG* 80, no. 1 (1936): 82–83.

73. "Beschouwingen en Raad van het Hoofd van den Dienst der Volksgezondheid," October 30, 1936, Bt, no. 2088, ANRI.

74. *Handelingen van den Volksraad* (July 22, 1935), 5, 333, 351, 868.

75. "Onderscheidingen," *Nederlandsche Staatscourant*, August 29, 1936.

76. "Plechtigheid in Geneeskundige Hoogeschool," *Algemeen Handelsblad*, September 16, 1938.

77. I. H. J. de Vos, in "Handelingen," Tweede Kamer, 48ste Vergadering, March 5, 1940: 1276–1277.

78. "De Strijd tegen den Zwarten Dood," *NvdD*, October 9, 1935.

79. G. Girard, "Note au sujet de la vaccination antipesteuse," 1963, Archives de l'Institut Pasteur (hereafter FR AIP PST); G. Girard, "Renseignements relatifs au vaccin antipesteux," 1941, FR AIP PST.

80. Otten, "De Pest op Java," 229.

81. "20,000 Voor inenting met Dr. Otten's pest-Vaccin," *De Locomotief*, January 14, 1935.

82. Rosier, "Verslag betreffende de pestbestrijding op Java over het jaar 1935," 68.

83. Office of the DVG to the Governor-General, November 17, 1934, Bt, no. 3088, ANRI.

84. "Kamerstuk 4.60," Tweede Kamer, February 1, 1935: 194.

85. Louis Otten, "Pest-vaccinatie op Java," *GTNI* 75, no. 22 (1935): 1850–1864.

86. Otten, "De pestbestrijding op Java," 108.

87. Louis Otten, "Pestbestrijding op Java: Woningverbetering en vaccinatie," in *Natuurkundige voordrachten*, vol. 25 (The Hague: W. P. van Stockum, 1948), 44–62.

88. Snijders, "De resultaten der pestvaccinatie," 82–83.

89. *Indisch Verslag* (1936), 306–307.

90. "Kamerstuk 4.69," Tweede Kamer, February 7, 1939: 201.

91. Otten, "De pestbestrijding op Java," 88–89.

92. Rosier, "Woningverbetering en malaria," 343–344.

93. Rosier, "Woningverbetering en malaria," 343–344.

94. Versteeg, *Dagboek*, 5:137–138.

95. J. J. M. A. Popelier, "Memorie van overgave," 16–17, inventory no. 46, index 2.10.39, NL-HaNA.

96. The term appears to be a Malay-Dutch hybrid: *sakit* (disease) and *wonéng* (from the Dutch *woning*, meaning "house"). Rosier and Grootings (see below) are the only direct source I found for the use of this term—with others paraphrasing them.

97. "Solo," *Soerabaisch Handelsblad*, September 2, 1930; "Malaria-epidemie," *Het Vaderland*, October 11, 1930.

98. Rosier, "Woningverbetering en malaria," 343.

99. W. Th. de Vogel, *Malaria-bestrijding en Hygiëne in Tropische Gewesten* (Amsterdam: J. H. de Bussy, 1908), 6.

100. *Verslag van Bestuur en Staat van Nederlandsch-Indië, Suriname en Curaçao* (1928), 47.

101. "Handelingen," Tweede Kamer, 48ste Vergadering, March 5, 1940, 1281.

102. H. T. Soeparmo and R. L. Laird, "Anopheles Sundaicus and Its Control by DDT Residual House Spraying in Indonesia," WHO/Mal/118, December 2, 1954, World Health Organization.

103. De Vogel, *Beknopt Verslag*, 22.

104. Van der Hoogte and Pieters, "Quinine, Malaria, and the Cinchona Bureau."

105. Rosier, "Woningverbetering en malaria," 343–363.

106. Maurits Bastiaan Meerwijk, "Plague Rat or Anopheles: Health Disasters and Home Improvement in Late-Colonial Java," *Indonesia* (forthcoming).

107. Rosier, "Woningverbetering en malaria," 357.

108. Rosier, "Woningverbetering en malaria," 362.

109. Rosier, "Woningverbetering en malaria," 359.

110. J. W. Grootings, "Woningverbetering en malaria," *MvdDdV* 27, no. 3 (1938): 397–416.

111. Grootings, "Woningverbetering en malaria," 410.

112. Grootings, "Woningverbetering en malaria," 397.

113. Grootings, "Woningverbetering en malaria," 401, original emphasis.

114. Grootings, "Woningverbetering en malaria," 409.

115. UBL Digital Collections, Item KITLV 78094, http://hdl.handle.net/1887.1/item:904927.

116. Grootings, "Woningverbetering en malaria," images between 410–411.

117. Grootings, "Woningverbetering en malaria," 413.

118. Rosier, "Woningverbetering en malaria," 359–360.

119. Grootings, "Woningverbetering en malaria," 413.

120. W. Takken et al., *Environmental Measures for Malaria Control in Indonesia: An Historical Review on Species Sanitation* (Wageningen: Agricultural University, 1991), 124.

121. "Woningverbetering en het optreden van malaria," *De Sumatra Post*, January 13, 1938.

122. "Een bedenkelijk nevenverschijnsel," *NvdD*, January 22, 1938.

123. "Het dilemma: Pestrat of Anopheles," *NvdD*, October 18, 1938.

124. "Het dilemma: Pestrat of Malaria-Muskiet," *De Locomotief*, October 20, 1938.

125. "Malaria en huisvesting," *De Telegraaf*, January 4, 1939.

126. "Vreemde malaria-explosies," *Algemeen Handelsblad voor Nederlandsch-Indië*, October 19, 1938.

127. *Handelingen van den Volksraad* (July 26, 1939): 437.

128. *Volksraad: Memorie van Antwoord, Dienst der Volksgezondheid* (July 17, 1939): 10–11.

129. Nicholaas H. Swellengrebel, "Woningverbetering en malaria op Java," *NTvG* 83 (1939): 105–107.

130. *Volksraad. Memorie van Toelichting, Dienst der Volksgezondheid* (1942): 2.

131. "Waarom elders wel," *De Locomotief*, October 18, 1938.

132. "Malaria-bestrijding en woningverbetering," *Algemeen Handelsblad voor Nederlandsch-Indië*, January 4, 1940; "Malaria-epidemie," *Bataviaasch Nieuwsblad*, September 10, 1940.

133. Rosier, "Verslag betreffende de pestbestrijding op Java over het jaar 1938," 238.

134. "Malaria-epidemie," *Bataviaasch Nieuwsblad*, September 10, 1940.

135. "Woning en malaria," *NvdD*, January 5, 1939; "Pest en malaria," *De Locomotief*, February 24, 1939.

Conclusion

1. There is no official figure provided for this year. I calculated this number by comparing newspaper reports from 1941 with postwar sources.

2. "Ontwerp begrooting van Nederlandsch-Indië voor 1941," *Bijlagen van den Volksraad* (1940), afdeling V A–stuk 4, 12.

3. *Handelingen van den Volksraad* (July 28, 1941): 490–494.

4. *Indisch Verslag* (1941), 499.

5. For example, *Koloniaal Verslag* (1916), 3.

6. For example, "De pest te Temanggoeng," *De Preangerbode*, November 15, 1919.

7. In the years around 1920 the DP employed about 800 staff.

8. De Vogel, "Inspectie rapport"; Deutmann, "De pest in Karanglo," 214.

9. De Vogel, "Beknopt verslag," 72.

10. *Koloniaal Verslag* (1917), 5.

11. *Koloniaal Verslag* (1915), 90.

12. *Koloniaal Verslag* (1920), 102.

13. Oetoyo, *Handelingen van den Volksraad, eerste gewone zitting 1919*, 649; Soejono, *Handelingen van den Volksraad, tweede gewone zitting 1920*, 256; Iskandar Dinata and Wiwoho, *Handelingen van den Volksraad, zittingsjaar 1933–1934*, 179, 262–263.

14. Ministerie van Koloniën: Memories van Overgave, no. 64, index 2.10.39, NL-HaNA.

15. H. J. Rosier, "Verslag betreffende de pestbestrijding op Java over het jaar 1933," *MvdDdV* 24, no. 3 supplement (1935): 214.

16. Feico Herman van Loon, "Pest en Pestbestrijding," PhD diss., University of Amsterdam, 1919, 7–10.

17. Ministerie van Koloniën: Memories van Overgave, no. 48, index 2.10.39, NL-HaNA.

18. Ministerie van Koloniën: Memories van Overgave, no. 27, index 2.10.39, NL-HaNA.

19. Pols, *Nurturing Indonesia*, 107–114; Hendrik Colijn, *Koloniale vraagstukken van heden en morgen* (Amsterdam: De Standaard, 1928), 11–44; J. H. F. Kohlbrugge, *De inlandsche beweging en de onrust in Indië* (Utrecht: A. Oosthoek, 1927).

20. "Tegen de Westersche Geneeskunde," *De Tijd*, 9 April 1933.

21. "De steenigingszaak," *De Locomotief*, 23 October 1933.

22. Ministerie van Koloniën: Memories van Overgave, no. 47, index 2.10.39, NL-HaNA.

23. Ministerie van Koloniën: Memories van Overgave, no. 42, index 2.10.39, NL-HaNA.

24. "Jaarverslag betreffende de pestbestrijding op Java over het jaar 1938," *MvdDdV* 28, no. 2–3 (1939): 264–270.

25. Ministerie van Koloniën: Memories van Overgave, no. 47, index 2.10.39, NL-HaNA.

26. On the state of medical conditions, practice, policy, and education in the Indies under Japanese rule, see Pols, *Nurturing Indonesia*, 161–182.

27. KITLV, NIMH, and NIOD, *Beyond the Pale: Dutch Extreme Violence in the Indonesian War of Independence, 1945–1949* (Amsterdam: Amsterdam University Press, 2022).

28. V. Lieberman and M. C. Ricklefs, eds., *The Encyclopedia of Indonesia in the Pacific War* (Leiden: Brill 2010), 197–199; Gert Oostindië, "The Netherlands and Indonesia 1945–1949: The Political-Historical Context," in KITLV, NIMH, and NIOD, *Beyond the Pale*, 35–68, 44.

29. To the new, lower estimate must also be added an unknown number of Chinese civilian casualties. Harry A. Poeze, "Walking the Tightrope: Internal Indonesian Conflict, 1945–49," in *Colonial Counterinsurgency and Mass Violence: The Dutch Empire in Indonesia*, eds Bart Luttikhuis and A. Dirk Moses (Abingdon: Routledge, 2014), 176–197; Esther Captain and Onno Sinke, "Hatred of Foreign Elements and their "Accomplices": Extreme Violence in the First Phase of the Indonesian Revolution (17 August 1945 to 31 March 1946), in KITLV, NIMH, and NIOD, *Beyond the Pale*, 141–176, 165–168.

30. These figures were provided on the website of the NIOD Institute for War, Holocaust and Genocide Studies and have been retrieved from a range of sources. NIOD, "Indonesische onafhankelijkheid (cijfers)," https://www.niod.nl/nl/veelgestelde-vragen/indonesische-onafhankelijkheidsstrijd-cijfers.

31. Tables listing infectious disease incidence in Java and Madoera for 1942–1945, 400 Indische Collectie, no. 733, NIOD.

32. "In Djokjasche heerscht pest, 2409 Slachtoffers in 1946," *Het Dagblad*, February 1, 1947.

33. F. J. F. M. Duynstee, *De Kabinetsformaties 1946–1965* (Deventer: Kluwer, 1966), 9.

34. Vivek Neelakantan, *Science, Public Health and Nation-Building in Soekarno-Era Indonesia* (Newcastle: Cambridge Scholars, 2017), 206.

35. M. Anker and D. Schaaf, *Report on Global Surveillance of Epidemic-prone Infectious Diseases* (WHO, 2000), 32–37; WHO, *Operational Guidelines on Plague Surveillance, Diagnosis, Prevention and Control* (New Delhi: WHO Regional Office for South-East Asia, 2010), 3–5; J. E. Williams et al., "Plague in Central Java, Indonesia," *Bulletin of the World Health Organization* 58, no. 3 (1980): 459–468.

36. Lou de Jong, *Het Koninkrijk der Nederlanden in de Tweede Wereldoorlog, 1939–1945*, vol. 11b (Leiden: Martinus Nijhof, 1985), 320.

37. J. Kevin Baird and Sangkot Marzuki, *War Crimes in Japan-Occupied Indonesia* (Lincoln, NE: Potomac, 2013); Photograph, no. 3036, index 2.210.62, NL-HaNA.

38. "Verenigingsverslagen," *NTvG* 92, ii, no. 21 (1948): 1566–1580.

39. Pols, *Nurturing Indonesia*, 164–171.

40. Otten, "Pestbestrijding op Java: Woningverbetering en vaccinatie," 60–61.

41. Wim Kan, *Burmadagboek 1942–1945* (Amsterdam: De Arbeiderspers, 1986), 70–71. "To have the plague / the disease inside of you" is a Dutch idiom meaning that one is angry. Kan used the phrase "literally and figuratively."

42. T. Eijden, "Medische aangelegenheden," 400 Indische Collectie, no. 2609, NIOD.

43. "Verenigingsverslagen," *NTvG* 92, ii, no. 21 (1948): 1566–1580.

44. C. M. Reinders-Folmers, "Dagboek," 401, Nederlands-Indische Dagboeken en Egodocumenten, no. 157, NIOD.

45. In the chapter on the Japanese occupation in the Indonesian state history of medicine, *Sejarah Kesehatan Nasional Indonesia*, there is no specific mention of plague or plague control. *Serajah Kesehatan Nasional Indonesia*, vol. 1 (Jakarta: Departement Kesehatan RI, 2009), 71–76.

46. "Verenigingsverslagen," *NTvG* 92, ii, no. 21 (1948): 1566–1580.

47. "Pestserum per parachute," *De Locomotief*, March 25, 1949; "Vliegtuig-actie tegen pest," *Java-bode*, November 4, 1949; "Pest in Djokja," *Indische Courant voor Nederland*, November 5, 1949.

48. These are the Royal Netherlands Institute of Southeast Asian and Caribbean Studies (KITLV), the Netherlands Institute for Military History (NIMH), the NIOD Institute for War, Holocaust, and Genocide Studies (NIOD), and the Department of History at Universitas Gadjah Mada (UGM). They published a final project report in February 2022: KITLV, NIMH, and NIOD, *Beyond the Pale*.

49. The municipal councils of Utrecht, Amsterdam, Rotterdam, and The Hague have each announced research initiatives into the historical involvement of these cities in the slave trade, for instance, while the National Archives are working on an extensive digitization project to make slavery records publicly available. Furthermore, large museums such as the Rijksmuseum in Amsterdam are looking more closely into the origin of items in their collection and are organizing exhibitions on slavery.

50. Bloembergen, "Dirty Work of Empire," 120.

51. See for instance: Daniel R. Headrick, *The Tools of Empire: Technology and European Imperialism in the Nineteenth Century* (New York: Oxford University Press, 1981); Laurence Monnais, *The Colonial Life of Pharmaceuticals: Medicines and Modernity in Vietnam* (Cambridge: Cambridge University Press, 2019).

52. For colonial Indonesia, the major studies in this field are van Bergen, *Uncertainty, Anxiety, Frugality*; Hesselink, *Healers on the Colonial Market*; and Pols, *Nurturing Indonesia*. For the Dutch colonies in the Caribbean, just one book stands out: Stephen Snelders, *Leprosy and Colonialism: Suriname under Dutch Rule, 1750–1950* (Manchester: Manchester University Press, 2017).

Bibliography

Archival Collections

Archives Nationales d'Outre-Mer, Aix-en-Provence, France (ANOM)
  FR ANOM
Archives de l'Institut Pasteur, Paris, France
  FR AIP PST
Arsip Nasional Republik Indonesia, Jakarta, Indonesia (ANRI)
  Manuscript Grote Bundel (MGB)
  Besluit (Bt)
  Terzijde Gelegde Agendas (TGA)
Gelders Archief, Arnhem, The Netherlands
  Collection 1523, Fotoalbums
Historical Documentation Center for Dutch Protestantism, Amsterdam, The
      Netherlands (HDC)
  Collection A. W. F. Idenburg, inventory no. 129
League of Nations Archives, Geneva, Switzerland (LoN)
  12B, Health, 1919–1927
Leiden University Library Special Collections, Leiden, The Netherlands (UBL)
  Collection KITLV
  Collection Paul Christiaan Flu
  Collection Willem Thomas de Vogel, D H 1568
Nationaal Archief, The Hague, The Netherlands (NL-HaNA)
  Collectie Drukwerk, index 2.22.15.
  Commissariaat voor Indische Zaken, 1927–1949, index 2.10.49.
  Family von Römer, 16e–20e eeuw, index 2.21.143.
  Fotoarchief gevormd door het Bureau van de Rijksinspecteur voor Roerende
      Monumenten, 1949–1975, index 2.24.25.
  Koninklijk Instituut voor de Tropen, 1910–1995, index 2.20.69.
  Ministerie van Koloniën: Memories van Overgave, 1852–1962, index 2.10.39.
  Ministerie van Koloniën: Openbaar Verbaal, 1901–1953, index 2.10.36.04.
  Ministerie van Koloniën: Toegangen Geheim Archief, 1901–1958, index
      2.10.36.50.
NIOD Institute for War, Holocaust and Genocide Studies
  400 Indische Collectie
  401 Nederlands-Indische Dagboeken en Egodocumenten
  402 International Military Tribunal for the Far East

Perpustakaan Nasional Republik Indonesia, Jakarta, Indonesia (PNRI)
Rockefeller Archive Center, Tarrytown, New York (RAC)
    Record Group 1.1, Projects
    Record Group 5, International Health Board/Division records
    Record Group 12, Officers' Diaries
Stadsarchief Amsterdam, Amsterdam, The Netherlands.
    Collection Tentoonstellingen

Newspapers and Periodicals

Algemeen Handelsblad
Algemeen Handelsblad voor Nederlandsch-Indië
Bataviaasch Nieuwsblad
Dagblad van Zuid-Holland en 's-Gravenhage
De Courant
De Gids
De Indiër
De Indische Courant
De Indische Mercuur
De Locomotief
De Maasbode
De Preangerbode
De Sumatra Post
De Telegraaf
De Tijd
De Tribune
Friesch Dagblad
Geneeskundige Tijdschrift voor Nederlandsch-Indië (GTNI)
Haagsche Courant
Haarlem's Dagblad
Het Centrum
Het Dagblad
Het Nieuws van den Dag voor Nederlandsch-Indië (NvdD)
Het Vaderland
Hong Kong Daily Press
Indische Courant voor Nederland
Koloniaal Tijdschrift
Leeuwarder Courant
Leidsch Dagblad
Mededeelingen van den Burgerlijken Geneeskundigen Dienst in Nederlandsch-Indië (MvdBGD)
Mededeelingen van den Dienst der Volksgezondheid in Nederlandsch-Indië (MvdDdV)
Nederlands Tijdschrift voor Geneeskunde (NTvG)
Nederlandsche Staatscourant
Nieuwe Rotterdamsche Courant
Nieuwe Tilburgsche Courant

Soerabaijsch Handelsblad
Staatsblad van Nederlandsch-Indië
Twentsch Dagblad
Vox Medicorum

Published Primary Sources

Arbeiten aus dem Kaiserlichen Gesundheitsamte 16. Berlin: Springer, 1899.

Berlage, Hendrik Petrus. Mijn Indische reis. Rotterdam: W. L. & J. Brusse's, 1931.

Borger, W. A. "Vaccinatie tegen pest." Mededeelingen van den Burgerlijken Geneeskundigen Dienst in Nederlandsch-Indië 5, no. 1 (1916): 5–25.

Catalogus van de Jubileum-Tentoonstelling 1923. Amsterdam: Holkema en Warendof, 1923.

Clark, Francis, ed. Transactions of the Second Biennial Congress Held at Hongkong, 1912. Hong Kong: Noronha, 1913.

Couperus, Louis. De stille kracht. Amstelveen: L. J. Veen, 1900.

Cressey, Georges B. Asia's Lands and Peoples: A Geography of One-Third of the Earth and Two-Thirds of Its People. New York: McGraw-I Iill, 1944.

Dari Hal Penjakit Pest (Sampar) Dan Pendjaganja. Batavia: Landsdrukkerij, 1919.

"De Burgerlijken Geneeskundigen Dienst in Nederlandsch Indië." Nederlands Tijdschrift voor Geneeskunde 69 (1925): 2595–2597.

"De electrische tram te Soerabaja." De Ingenieur 40, no. 11 (1925): 216–223.

Deutmann, A. A. F. M. "De pest in Karanglo in de maanden Mei, Juni en Juli." Mededeelingen van den Burgerlijken Geneeskundigen Dienst in Nederlandsch-Indië 1b (1912): 58–138.

——. "De pest te Karanglo in de maanden Mei, Juni, en Juli 1911." Geneeskundige Tijdschrift voor Nederlandsch-Indië 52 (1912): 431–511.

——. De Pest: Vaccinatie en sérotherapie, een kritsch-experimenteele studie. Amsterdam: F. van Rossen, 1900.

Dienst der Pestbestrijding (DP). Verslag over het eerste kwartaal 1915. Batavia: Javasche Boekhandel, 1915.

——. Verslag over het eerste kwartaal 1916. Batavia: Javasche Boekhandel, 1917.

——. Verslag over het jaar 1919. Batavia: Javasche Boekhandel & Drukkerij, 1920.

——. Verslag over het jaar 1920. Batavia: Javasche Boekhandel & Drukkerij, 1921.

——. Verslag over het tweede kwartaal 1915. Batavia: Javasche Boekhandel & Drukkerij, 1915.

——. Verslag over het tweede kwartaal 1916. Batavia: Javasche Boekhandel 1917.

——. Verslag over het vierde kwartaal 1915. Batavia: Javasche Boekhandel, 1915.

Dienst der Volksgezondheid (DVG). Control of Endemic Diseases in the Netherlands Indies. Weltevreden: Landsdrukkerij, 1929.

Dijkstra, J. "Het een en ander over de pest in het Malangsche." Maandblad voor Ziekenverpleging 21, no. 6 (1911): 444–446.

Diningrat, Noto. "Grondslagen." Nederlandsch-Indië Oud en Nieuw 4, no. 4 (1923): 107–117.

"The Epidemic of Plague in Hong Kong." British Medical Journal 1, no. 1746 (1894): 1326.

Feestbundel 1936. Batavia: G. Kolf, 1936.

Flu, Paul Christian. "Proeven ter immuniseering tegen pest." *Mededeelingen van den Burgerlijken Geneeskundigen Dienst in Nederlandsch-Indië* 8 (1920): 18–60.

Gedenkboek der Gemeente Semarang, 1906–1931. Semarang: De Locomotief, 1931.

Groneman, I. *Pestbestrijding naar aanleiding van gsprekken met Dr. Yersin.* Jogjakarta: W. A. van der Hucht, 1899.

Grootings, J. W. "Woningverbetering en malaria." *Mededeelingen van den Dienst der Volksgezondheid* 27, no. 3 (1938): 397–416.

Haan, J. de. "De bacteriologische diagnose van pest in de afdeeling Malang." *Mededeelingen van den Burgerlijken Geneeskundigen Dienst in Nederlandsch-Indië* 1a (1912): 1–28.

Handelingen van den Volksraad, 1918–1942.

Heel, Marin Gerard van. *Gedenkboek van de Koloniale Tentoonstelling Semarang, 20 Augustus–22 November 1914.* Vol. 2. Batavia: Mercurius, 1916.

Het Tweede tiental begrootingen met den Volksraad, 1929–1938. Batavia: Landsdrukkerij, 1938.

Hijmans, M. "Een en ander over de pest op Java en hare bestrijding." *Nederlandsch-Indië: Oud & Nieuw* 2, no. 5 (1917): 153–169.

——. "Een en ander over de pest op Java en hare bestrijding." *Nederlandsch Indië: Oud & Nieuw* 2, no. 6 (1917): 191–197.

"Jaarverslag betreffende de pestbestrijding op Java over het jaar 1938," *Mededeelingen van den Dienst der Volksgezondheid* 28, no. 2–3 (1939): 208–281.

"Jaarverslag van den Burgerlijken Geneeskundigen Dienst in Nederlandsch-Indië over 1924." *Mededeelingen van den Dienst der Volksgezondheid* 16, no. 2 (1927): 205–265.

"Jaarverslag van den Dienst der Volksgezondheid over 1934." *Mededeelingen* 24, no. 4 (1935): 404–460.

Kasakit pest Djeung Piken Panoelaksa. Batavia: Landsdrukkerij, 1919.

Koloniaal Verslag; Verslag van Bestuur en Staat van Nederlandsch-Indië, Suriname en Curaçao; Indisch Verslag.

Koninklijke Vereeniging Koloniaal Instituut. *Dertiende jaarverslag.* Amsterdam: de Bussy, 1923.

Lammers, G. J. A. *W. F. Idenburg: In zijn leven en werken geschetst.* Amsterdam: De Standaard, 1935.

Loebèr, J. A. *Bamboe in Nederlandsch-Indië.* Amsterdam: de Bussy, 1909.

Loghem, Johannes J. van. "Brieven uit Indië: Het Congres voor Tropische Ziekten te Bombay." *Nederlands Tijdschrift voor Geneeskunde* 53 (1909): 1702–1707.

——. "Brieven uit Indië: Het pestvraagstuk voor Nederlandsch-Indië." *Nederlands Tijdschrift voor Geneeskunde* 53 (1909): 44–51.

——. "De pest op Java." *Nederlands Tijdschrift voor Geneeskunde* 56 (1912): 200–234.

——. "Drie jaren pest op Java," *Nederlands Tijdschrift voor Geneeskunde* 58 (1914): 876–879.

——. "Eenige epidemiologische gegevens omtrent de pest op Java." *Mededeelingen van den Burgerlijken Geneeskundigen Dienst in Nederlandsch-Indië* 1b (1912): 2–56.

——. "Film der pestbestrijding op Java." *Nederlands Tijdschrift voor Geneeskunde* 71 (1927): 209–210.

——. "Het pestvraagstuk voor Nederlandsch-Indië." *Nederlands Tijdschrift voor Geneeskunde* 53 (1909): 44–51.

——. "Over pest." *Maandblad voor Ziekenverpleging* 21, no. 3 (1911): 150–155.

——. "Pestbestrijding op Java." *Nederlands Tijdschrift voor Geneeskunde* 58 (1914): 1306–1308.

Loon, Feico Herman van. "Pest en Pestbestrijding," PhD diss., University of Amsterdam, 1919.

Lumentut, H. F. "Iets over de pestbestrijding op Java." *Verslagen der Vergaderingen Indisch Genootschap* (1921): 105–133.

Maclaine Pont, Henri. "Anti-Plague Bamboo Constructions." In *Transactions of the Fourth Congress Held at Weltevreden, Batavia,* 609–616. Weltevreden: Javasche Boekhandel en Drukkerij, 1922.

——. "Het Inlandsch bouwambacht, zijn beteekenis en toekomst?" *Djawa* 3, no. 2 (1923): 79–89.

——. "Javaansche Architectuur." *Djawa* 3, no. 4 (1923): 159–170.

Mangoenkoesoemo, Tjipto. *De pest op Java en hare bestrijding.* Delft: W. D. Meinema, 1914.

Mededeelingen van den Burgerlijken Geneeskundigen Dienst in Nederlandsch-Indië 1 (1912): 1–267.

Mense, Carl, ed. *Handbuch der Tropenkrankheiten.* Vol. 2. Leipzig: Johan Ambrosius Barth, 1905.

Moojen, P. A. J. *Catalogus van de Houtsnijwerk Tentoonstelling.* [Bandoeng]: 1921.

Muntendam, P. "Internationale Hygiëne-Tentoonstelling Amsterdam." *Nederlands Tijdschrift voor Geneeskunde* 65 (1921): 1953–1956.

Natuurkundige Voordrachten. Vol. 25. The Hague: W. P. van Stockum, 1948.

"Nederlandsche Vereeniging voor Tropische Geneeskunde." *Nederlands Tijdschrift voor Geneeskunde* 78, ii, 25 (1934): 2945–2985.

Netherlands Indies Medical and Sanitary Service, ed. *Control of Endemic Diseases in the Netherlands Indies.* Weltevreden: Landsdrukkerij, 1929.

Neueck, J. J. X. Pfijffer zu. *Schetsen van het eiland Java.* Amsterdam: J. C. van Kesteren, 1838.

——. *Skizzen von der insel Java.* Schaffhausen: Franz Hurter, 1829.

"Opmerkingen over de begrooting van Nederlandsch-Indië voor het dienstjaar 1919." *Koloniaal Tijdschrift* 8, no. 1 (1919): 68–82.

Otten, Louis. *Beknopt overzicht betreffende organisatie en uitvoering der pestbestrijdings-maatregelen.* Semarang: A. Bisschop, 1921.

——. "De pestbestrijding op Java, 1911–1936." In *Feestbundel 1936,* 84–108. Batavia: G. Kolf, 1936.

——. "De pest op Java, 1911–1923." *Mededeelingen van den Dienst der Volksgezondheid* 13, no. 2 (1924): 119–260.

——. "Experimental Vaccination in Plague: I. Dead Vaccine." *Mededeelingen van den Dienst der Volksgezondheid* 22, no. 2 (1933): 131–149.

——. "Lecture on plague." In *Transactions of the Fourth Congress held at Weltevreden, Batavia,* 617–628. Weltevreden: Javasche Boekhandel en Drukkerij, 1922.

——. "Pestbestrijding op Java: Woningverbetering en vaccinatie." In *Natuurkundige Voordrachten.* Vol. 25, 44–62. The Hague: W. P. van Stockum, 1948.

——. "Pest-vaccinatie op Java." *Geneeskundige Tijdschrift voor Nederlandsch-Indië* 75, no. 22 (1935): 1850–1864.

Overbeek, J. G., and W. J. Stoker. "Malaria in Nederlandsch-Indië en haar bestrijding." *Mededeelingen van den Dienst der Volksgezondheid* 27, no. 1–2 (1938): 183–205.

"Over het wezen en de verbreiding van eenige besmettelijke ziekten in de Tropen."
   In *Natuurkundige Voordrachten*. The Hague: W. P. van Stockum, 1915.
Peverelli, P. *Blijf Gezond!*. Groningen: J. B. Wolters, 1933.
Raadt, O. L. E. de. *De Woningverbetering als middel ter bestrijding en voorkoming van het
   pestgevaar op Java*. Malang: N. V. Jahn's Drukkerij, 1912.
——. *Penjakit pest Ditanah Djawa*. Batavia: Commissie voor de Volkslectuur, 1915.
——. *Rangsa Ni Sahit Pest, Na Masa Di Poelo Djawa*. 1915.
——. "Uittreksels uit de verslagen." *Mededeelingen van den Burgerlijken Geneeskundigen
   Dienst in Nederlandsch-Indië* 1b (1912): 140–151.
Reigersberg Versluys, J. C. van. "Mededeeling omtrent het Ingenieurs-Congres in
   1919 op Java te Houden." *De Ingenieur* 33, no. 31 (1918): 577–582.
Report of the Intergovernmental Conference of Far-Eastern Countries on Rural Hygiene.
   Geneva, 1937.
Römer, L. S. A. M. von. "About the Exhibition in Connection with the Fourth Congress
   of the Far Eastern Association of Tropical Medicine held at Batavia from
   6th–13th August 1921." In *Transactions of the Fourth Congress Held at Weltevreden,
   Batavia*, 381–393. Weltevreden: Javasche Boekhandel en Drukkerij, 1922.
Rosier, H. J. "Verslag betreffende de pestbestrijding op Java over het jaar 1933."
   Mededeelingen van den Dienst der Volksgezondheid 24, no. 3 supplement (1935):
   191–348.
——. "Verslag betreffende de pestbestrijding op Java over het jaar 1934." *Mededeelin-
   gen van den Dienst der Volksgezondheid* 25, no. 2 (1936): 112–209.
——. "Verslag betreffende de pestbestrijding op Java over het jaar 1935." *Mededeelin-
   gen van den Dienst der Volksgezondheid* 26, supplement (1937): 1–100.
——. "Verslag betreffende de pestbestrijding op Java over het jaar 1938." *Mededeelin-
   gen van den Dienst der Volksgezondheid* 28, no. 2–3 (1939): 208–281.
——. "Woningverbetering en Malaria." in *Mededeelingen van den Dienst der Volksge-
   zondheid* 26, no. 4 (1937): 343–363.
Scott-Keltie, J., and M. Epstein, eds. *The Stateman's Year-Book*. London: Macmillan,
   1914.
Simond, P.-L. "La propagation de la peste." *Annales de l'Institut Pasteur* 62 (1898):
   625–687.
Sleeswijk, J. G. "De pest op Java." *Nederlands Tijdschrift voor Geneeskunde* 58 (1914):
   1060–1062.
——. "De pest op Java." *Tijdschrift voor Sociale Hygiëne* 17 (1914): 75–78.
——. "Pest en pestbestrijding op Java." In *Berichten uit Oost-Indië voor de Leden van den
   Sint-Claverbond* 1 (1915): 3–17.
Snijders, E. P. "De resultaten der pestvaccinatie op Java met het vaccin van Otten."
   Nederlands Tijdschrift voor Geneeskunde 80, no. 1 (1936): 82–83.
——. "Dr W. Th. de Vogel 90 Jaar terugblik op een rijk leven." *Nederlands Tijdschrift
   voor Geneeskunde* 97, 1, no. 12 (1953): 714–716.
Sociaal-Technische Vereeniging. *Verslag Volkshuisvestingscongres 1922*. Semarang:
   Stoomdrukkerij Misset, 1922.
Soerono. "Vrijwillige woningverbetering in het onderdistrict Madja (Regentschap
   Madjalengka), Residentie Cheribon." *Mededeelingen van den Dienst der
   Volksgezondheid* 28, no. 4 (1939): 283–305.

Swellengrebel, Nicholaas H. "Mededeeling omtrent onderzoekingen over de biologie van ratten en vlooien en over andere onderwerpen, die betrekking hebben op de epidemiologie der pest op Oost-Java." *Mededeelingen van den Burgerlijken Geneeskundigen Dienst in Nederlandsch-Indië* 2, no. 1 (1913): 1–86.

——. "Plague in Java." *Journal of Hygiene* 48, no. 2 (1950): 135–145.

——. "Woningverbetering en malaria op Java." *Nederlands Tijdschrift voor Geneeskunde* 83 (1939): 105–107.

Thomson, Theodore, trans. *The International Sanitary Convention of Paris, 1903.* London: Darling and Son, 1904.

Tien Begrootingen met den Volksraaad, 1919–1928. Weltevreden: Landsdrukkerij, 1929.

Tillema, H. F. *Kromoblanda.* Vol. 1. The Hague: Electrische Drukkerij, 1915.

——. *Kromoblanda.* Vol. 2. The Hague: Electrische Drukkerij, 1916.

——. *Kromoblanda.* Vol. 4. Wassenaar: H. Uden Masman, 1921.

Todd, Frank Morten. *Eradicating Plague from San Francisco.* San Francisco, CA: C. A. Murdoch, 1909.

Transactions of the Fifth Biennial Congress Held at Singapore, 1923. London: John Bale, 1924.

Transactions of the Fourth Congress Held at Weltevreden, Batavia. Weltevreden: Javasche Boekhandel en Drukkerij, 1922.

Verschuur, Gerrit. *Aux colonies d'Asie et dans l'Océan Indien.* Paris: Hachette, 1900.

"Verslagen van Vereenigingen." *Nederlands Tijdschrift voor Geneeskunde* (1912): 718–732.

Vervoort, H. "Some Remarks on Rat-Proof Roof-Building." In *Transactions of the Fifth Biennial Congress Held at Singapore, 1923,* 348–351. London: John Bale, 1924.

Vogel, Willem Thomas de. *Beknopt verslag over den Burgerlijken Geneeskundigen Dienst van 1911 t/m 1918.* Weltevreden: Albrecht, 1920.

——. "The Connection of Man and Rat in the Plague Epidemic in Malang, Java, in 1911." In *Transactions of the Second Biennial Congress Held at Hongkong, 1912,* edited by Francis Clark, 147–149. Hong Kong: Noronha, 1913.

——. *De taak van den Burgerlijken Geneeskundigen Dienst in Nederlandsch-Indië.* Amsterdam: Ellerman, Harms, 1917.

——. *Malaria-bestrijding en hygiëne in Tropische Gewesten.* Amsterdam: J. H. de Bussy, 1908.

——. "Uittreksel uit het verslag aan de Regeering over de Pest-Epidemie in de Afdeeling Malang, November 1910–Augustus 1911." *Mededeelingen van den Burgerlijken Geneeskundigen Dienst in Nederlandsch-Indië* 1a (1912): 30–111.

Wallace, Alfred Russell. "On the Bamboo and Durian of Borneo." *Hooker's Journal of Botany* 8 (1856): 225–230.

——. *The Malay Archipelago.* Vol. 1. London: Macmillan, 1869.

White, Frederick Norman. "Presidential Address." *Transactions of the Royal Society of Tropical Medicine and Hygiene* 47, no. 6 (1953): 441–450.

——. *The Prevalence of Epidemic Disease and Port Health Organisation and Procedure in the Far East.* Geneva: League of Nations, 1923.

Winckel, Ch. W. F. "De Eerste Hygiëne-Tentoonstelling in Nederlandsch-Indië te Bandoeng." *Nederlands Tijdschrift voor Geneeskunde* 71 (1927): 759–763.

Wynne, F. E. "Health Propaganda: I. The Administrative Point of View." *British Medical Journal* 10, no. 2 (1929): 242–243.

Yersin, Alexandre. "La peste bubonique à Hong-Kong." *Annales de l'Institut Pasteur* 8 (1894): 662–667.

Published Secondary Sources

Akami, Tomoko. "A Quest to be Global: The League of Nations Health Organization and Inter-Colonial Regional Governing Agendas of the Far Eastern Association of Tropical Medicine 1910–25." *International History Review* 38, no. 1 (2016): 1–23.

——. "Imperial Polities, Intercolonialism, and the Shaping of Global Governing Norms: Public Health Expert Networks in Asia and the League of Nations Health Organization, 1908–37." *Journal of Global History* 12 (2017): 4–25.

Anderson, Warwick. *Colonial Pathologies: American Tropical Medicine, Race, and Hygiene in the Philippines*. Durham, NC: Duke University Press, 2006.

Anker, M., and D. Schaaf. *Report on Global Surveillance of Epidemic-prone Infectious Diseases*. WHO, 2000, 32–37.

Arnold, David. *Colonizing the Body: State Medicine and Epidemic Disease in Nineteenth-Century India*. Berkeley: University of California Press, 1993.

——. "Disease, Rumor, and Panic in India's Plague and Influenza Epidemics, 1896–1919." In *Empires of Panic: Epidemics and Colonial Anxieties*, edited by Robert Peckham, 111–129. Hong Kong: Hong Kong University Press, 2015.

——. "India's Place in the Tropical World, 1770–1930." *Journal of Imperial and Commonwealth History* 26, no. 1 (1998): 1–21.

Baird, J. Keven, and Sangkot Marzuki. *War Crimes in Japan-Occupied Indonesia*. Lincoln, NE: Potomac, 2013.

Balińska, Marta Aleksandra. "Assistance and Not Mere Relief: The Epidemic Commission of the League of Nations, 1920–1923." In *International Health Organisations and Movements, 1918–1939*, edited by Paul Weindling, 81–108. Cambridge: Cambridge University Press, 1995.

Barker, Joshua. "Surveillance and Territoriality in Bandung." In *Figures of Criminality in Indonesia, the Philippines, and Colonial Vietnam*, edited by Vicente L. Rafael, 95–127. Ithaca, NY: Cornell Southeast Asia Program, 1999.

Barrett, Tracy C. *The Chinese Diaspora in South-East Asia: The Overseas Chinese in Indochina*. New York: I. B. Tauris, 2012.

Bashford, Alison, ed. *Quarantine: Local and Global Histories*. London: Palgrave Macmillan, 2016.

Bear, Jordan, and Kate Palmer Albers, eds. *Before-and-After Photography: Histories and Contexts*. London: Bloomsbury Academic, 2017.

Benedict, Carol. "Bubonic Plague in Nineteenth-Century China." *Modern China* 14, no. 2 (1988): 107–155.

Bergen, Leo van. *Uncertainty, Anxiety, Frugality: Dealing with Leprosy in the Dutch East Indies, 1816–1942*. Singapore: NUS Press, 2018.

——. *Van koloniale geneeskunde tot internationale gezondheidszorg: Een geschiedenis van honderd jaar Nederlandsche vereniging voor Tropische geneeskunde*. Amsterdam: KIT Publishers, 2007.

Blanchard, Pascal, Nicolas Bancel, Gilles Boëtsch, Eric Deroo, Sandrine Lemaire, and Charles Forsdick, eds. *Human Zoos: Science and Spectacle in the Age of Colonial Empires*. Translated by Teresa Bridgeman. Liverpool: Liverpool University Press, 2008.

Bloembergen, Marieke. *Colonial Spectacles: The Netherlands and the Dutch East Indies at the World Exhibitions, 1880–1931*. Singapore: NUS Press, 2006.

——. *De koloniale vertoning: Nederland en Indië op de wereldtentoonstellingen (1880–1931)*. Amsterdam: Wereldbibliotheek, 2002.

——. "The Dirty Work of Empire: Modern Policing and Public Order in Surabaya, 1911–1919." *Indonesia* 83 (2007): 119–150.

Bloembergen, Marieke, and Remco Raben, eds. *Het koloniale beschavingsoffensief: Wegen naar het Nieuwe Indië*. Leiden: KITLV Press, 2009.

——. "Wegen naar het Nieuwe Indië, 1890–1950." In *Het koloniale beschavingsoffensief: Wegen naar het Nieuwe Indië*, edited by Marieke Bloembergen and Remco Raben, 7–24. Leiden: KITLV Press, 2009.

Boomgaard, Peter. "Smallpox, Vaccination, and the Pax Neerlandica, Indonesia, 1550–1930." *Bijdragen tot de Taal , Land en Volkenkunde* 159, no. 4 (2003). 590–617.

——, ed. *A World of Water: Rain, Rivers and Seas in Southeast Asian Histories*. Leiden: KITLV Press, 2007.

Breman, Jan. *Koloniaal profijt van onvrije arbeid: Het preanger stelsel van gedwongen koffieteelt op Java*. Amsterdam: Amsterdam University Press, 2010.

Bruijn, J. de, and G. Puchinger. *Briefwisseling Kuyper-Idenburg*. Franeker: T. Weber, 1985.

Bu, Liping. *Public Health and the Modernization of China, 1865–2015*. London: Routledge, 2017.

Butler, Thomas C. "Plague History." *Clinical Microbiology and Infection* 20, no. 3 (2014): 202–209.

Campbell, Kristine A. "Knots in the Fabric: Richard Pearson Strong and the Bilibid Prison Vaccine Trials, 1905–1906." *Bulletin of the History of Medicine* 68, no. 4 (1994): 600–638.

Canguilhem, Georges. *The Normal and the Pathological*. Translated by Carolyn R. Fawcett and Robert S. Cohen. New York: Zone, 1991.

Chandra, Siddharth, Goran Kuljanin, and Jennifer Wray. "Mortality from the Influenza Pandemic of 1918–19 in Indonesia." *Population Studies* 67, no. 2 (2013): 185–193.

Colijn, Hendrik. *Koloniale Vraagstukken van Heden en Morgen*. Amsterdam: De Standaard, 1928.

Colombijn, Freek. *Under Construction: The Politics of Urban Space and Housing during the Decolonization of Indonesia, 1930–1960*. Leiden: Brill, 2014.

Colombijn, Freek, and Joost Coté, eds. *Cars, Conduits, and Kampongs: The Modernization of the Indonesian City, 1920–1960*. Leiden: Brill, 2015.

Coté, Joost, Hugh O'Neill, Pauline K. M. van Roosmalen, and Helen Ibbitson, Jessup. *The Life and Work of Thomas Karsten*. Amsterdam: Architecture & Natura, 2017.

Cunningham, Andrew. "Transforming Plague: The Laboratory and the Identity of Infectious Disease." In *The Laboratory Revolution in Medicine*, edited by Andrew Cunningham and Percy Williams, 209–244. Cambridge: Cambridge University Press, 2002.

Cunningham, Andrew, and Percy Williams, eds. *The Laboratory Revolution in Medicine*. Cambridge: Cambridge University Press, 2002.

Daston, Lorraine, and Peter Galison. *Objectivity*. New York: Zone, 2007.

Debord, Guy. *The Society of the Spectacle*. Canberra: Treason, 2002.

Doel, H. W. van den. *De stille macht: Het Europese binnenlands bestuur op Java en Madoera, 1808–1942*. Amsterdam: Bert Bakker, 1994.

Drummond, Lisa. "Colonial Hanoi: Urban Space in Public Discourse." In *Harbin to Hanoi: The Colonial Built Environment in Asia, 1840–1940*, edited by Laura Victoir and Victor Zatsepine, 207–230. Hong Kong: Hong Kong University Press, 2013.

Duarte da Silva, Matheus Alves. "From Bombay to Rio de Janeiro: The Circulation of Knowledge and the Establishment of the Manguinhos Laboratory, 1894–1902." *História, Ciências, Saúde* 25, no. 3 (2017): 1–19.

Duynstee, F. J. F. M. *De Kabinetsformaties 1946–1965*. Deventer: Kluwer, 1966.

Echenberg, Myron. "Pestis Redux: The Initial Years of the Third Bubonic Plague Pandemic, 1894–1901." *Journal of World History* 13, no. 2 (2002): 429–449.

——. *Plague Ports: The Global Urban Impact of Bubonic Plague, 1894–1901*. New York: New York University Press, 2010.

Engelmann, Lukas. "A Plague of Kinyounism: The Caricatures of Bacteriology in 1900 San Francisco." *Social History of Medicine* 33, no. 2 (2020): 489–514.

——. "Configurations of Plague: Spatial Diagrams in Early Epidemiology." *Social Analysis* 63, no. 4 (2019): 89–109.

——. "What Are Medical Photographs of Plague?" *Remedia*, January 31, 2017. https://remedianetwork.net/2017/01/31/what-are-medical-photographs-of-plague/.

Engelmann, Lukas, John Henderson, and Christos Lynteris, eds. *Plague and the City*. London: Routledge, 2018.

Evans, Nicholas A. "Blaming the Rat? Accounting for Plague in Colonial Indian Medicine." *Medicine Anthropology Theory* 5, no. 3 (2018): 15–42.

Farley, John. *To Cast out Disease: A History of the International Health Division of the Rockefeller Foundation (1913–1951)*. Oxford: Oxford University Press, 2004.

Frost, Wade H. "Active and Passive Immunization against Plague." *Public Health Reports* 27, no. 34 (1912): 1361–1371.

Gelderblom, Oscar, and Bas van Bavel. "The Economic Origins of Cleanliness in the Dutch Golden Age." *Past & Present* 205, no. 1 (2009): 41–69.

Genabeek, Joost van, and Louise Rietbergen. *De S.D.A.P. en de volkshuisvesting: Inhoud en resultaten van het sociaaldemocratische volkshuisvestingsbeleid in Nederland (1894–1940)*. S.I.: S.N., 1991.

Gooswit, Sylvia. "Woningverbetering als pestbestrijdingsmaatregel op Java vanaf 1915." *Jambatan* 7, no. 1 (1989): 29–36.

Goss, Andrew. "Building the World's Supply of Quinine: Dutch Colonialism and the Origins of a Global Pharmaceutical Industry." *Endeavour* 38, no. 1 (2014): 8–18.

Grift, Liesbeth van de. "On New Land a New Society: Internal Colonisation in the Netherlands, 1918–1940." *Contemporary European History* 22, no. 4 (2013): 609–626.

Hadi, Purwanto, Vincentia Reni Vitasurya, and Eduardus Kevin Pandu. "The Shift of Symbolic Meaning of *Joglo* Houses for People in Brayut Tourism Village." In

Reframing the Vernacular: Politics, Semiotics, and Representation, edited by Gusti Ayu Made Suartika and Julie Nichols, 65–74. Cham: Springer, 2020.

Harper, Tim, and Sunil S. Amrith eds. *Histories of Health in Southeast Asia: Perspectives on the Long Nineteenth Century*. Bloomington: Indiana University Press, 2014.

Harrison, Mark. *Public Health in British India: Anglo-Indian Preventive Medicine, 1859–1914*. Cambridge: Cambridge University Press, 1994.

Headrick, Daniel R. *The Tools of Empire: Technology and European Imperialism in the Nineteenth Century*. New York: Oxford University Press, 1981.

Heinrich, Ari Larissa. *The Afterlife of Images: Translating the Pathological Body between China and the West*. Durham, NC: Duke University Press, 2003.

Hendrickson, Robert. *More Cunning than Man: A Social History of Rats and Man*. New York: Kensington, 1983.

Hesselink, Liesbeth Quirine. *Healers on the Colonial Market: Native Doctors and Midwives in the Dutch East Indies*. Leiden: KITLV Press, 2011.

Hill, Jason E. "'Noise Abatement Zone': John Divola's Photographic Fulcrum." In *Before-and-After Photography: Histories and Contexts*, edited by Jordan Bear and Kate Palmer Albers, 59–78. London: Bloomsbury Academic, 2017.

Hine, Lewis W. *Men at Work: Photographic Studies of Modern Men and Machines*. New York: Dover, 1977.

Hoffenberg, Peter H. *An Empire on Display*. Berkeley: University of California Press, 2001.

Hong Kong Museum of Medical Sciences Society. *Plague, SARS, and the Story of Medicine in Hong Kong*. Hong Kong: Hong Kong University Press, 2006.

Hoogte, Arjo Roersch van der, and Toine Pieters. "Quinine, Malaria, and the Cinchona Bureau: Marketing Practices and Knowledge Circulation in a Dutch Transoceanic Cinchona-Quinine Enterprise (1920s–30s)." *Journal of the History of Medicine and Allied Sciences* 71, no. 2 (2016): 197–225.

Hull, Terence H. "Conflict and Collaboration in Public Health: The Rockefeller Foundation and the Dutch Colonial Government in Indonesia." In *Public Health in Asia and the Pacific: Historical and Comparative Perspectives*, edited by Milton J. Lewis and Kerrie L. MacPherson, 139–152. Abingdon: Routledge, 2008.

——. "Plague in Java." In *Death and Disease in Southeast Asia: Explorations in Social, Medical and Demographic History*, edited by Norman Owen, 210–230. Oxford: Oxford University Press, 1987.

Jackson, Michael C. *Critical Systems Thinking and the Management of Complexity*. Hoboken, NJ: Wiley, 2019.

Jansen Hendriks, G. A. "Een voorbeeldige kolonie: Nederlands-Indië in 50 jaar overheidsfilms, 1912–1962." PhD diss., University of Amsterdam, 2014.

Jansen, Suzanna. *Het pauperparadijs: Een familiegeschiedenis*. Amsterdam: Balans, 2017.

Jong, Lou de. *Het Koninkrijk der Nederlanden in de Tweede Wereldoorlog, 1939–1945*. Vol. 11b. Leiden: Martinus Nijhof, 1985.

Kan, Wim. *Burmadagboek 1942–1945*. Amsterdam: De Arbeiderspers, 1986.

Kelly, Ann H., and Aldumena Marí Sáez. "Shadowlands and Dark Corners: An Anthropology of Light and Zoonosis." *Medicine Anthropology Theory* 5, no. 3 (2018): 21–49.

Kidambi, Prashant. *The Making of a Modern Metropolis: Colonial Governance and Public Culture in Bombay, 1890–1920*. Aldershot: Routledge, 2007.

Knox, Katelyn E. *Race on Display in 20th- and 21st-Century France.* Liverpool: Liverpool University Press, 2016.

Kohlbrugge, J. H. F. *De Inlandsche beweging en de onrust in Indië.* Utrecht: A. Oosthoek, 1927.

Koven, Seth. *Slumming: Sexual and Social Politics in Victorian London.* Princeton, NJ: Princeton University Press, 2006.

Kratoska, Paul, ed. *South East Asia, Colonial History.* Vol. 3, *High Imperialism (1890s–1930s).* London: Routledge, 2001.

Kuitert, Lisa. *Met een drukpers de oceaan over: Koloniale boekcultuur in Nederlands-Indië 1816–1920.* Amsterdam: Prometheus, 2020.

Labbé, Danielle, Caroline Herbelin, and Quang-Vinh Dao. "Domesticating the Suburbs: Architectural Production and Exchanges in Hanoi during the Late French Colonial Era." In *Harbin to Hanoi: The Colonial Built Environment in Asia, 1840–1940,* edited by Laura Victoir and Victor Zatsepine, 251–272. Hong Kong: Hong Kong University Press, 2013.

LeCain, Timothy J. *The Matter of History: How Things Create the Past.* Cambridge: Cambridge University Press, 2017.

Leerdam, Ben F. van *Architect Henri Maclaine Pont: Een speurtocht naar het wezenlijke van de Javaanse architectuur.* Delft: Eburon, 1995.

Lessard, Gilles, and Amy Chouinard, eds. *Bamboo Research in Asia.* Ottawa: International Development Research Centre, 1980.

Lewis, Milton J., and Kerrie L. MacPherson. *Public Health in Asia and the Pacific: Historical and Comparative Perspectives.* Abingdon: Routledge 2008.

Lieberman, V., and M. C. Ricklefs, eds. *The Encyclopedia of Indonesia in the Pacific War.* Leiden: Brill 2010.

Locher-Scholten, Elsbeth. *Ethiek in fragmenten: vijf studies over koloniaal denken en doen van Nederlanders in de Indonesische Archipel 1877–1942.* Utrecht: HES Publishers, 1981.

Loghem Jr., Johannes J. van, and J. van der Noordaa "Johannes Jacobus van Loghem (1878–1968), microbioloog-hygiënist." In *Erflaters van de Geneeskunde: Beroemde Nederlandse Artsen beschreven voor hun (kinds)kinderen,* edited by C. J. E. Kaandorp, J. J. E. van Everdingen, and A. Mooij, 128–137. Alphen aan den Rijn: Belvédère, 2002.

Lowe, Celia. "Viral Sovereignty Security and Mistrust as Measures of Future Health in the Indonesian H5N1 Influenza Outbreak." *Medicine Anthropology Theory* 6, no. 3 (2019): 109–132.

Lucas, Susanne. *Bamboo.* London: Reaktion, 2013.

Luttikhuis, Bart, and A. Dirk Moses. *Colonial Counterinsurgency and Mass Violence: The Dutch Empire in Indonesia.* Abingdon: Routledge, 2014.

Lynteris, Christos. "The Epidemiologist as Culture Hero: Visualizing Humanity in the Age of 'the Next Pandemic.'" *Visual Anthropology* 29, no. 1 (2016): 36–53.

——. *Ethnographic Plague: Configuring Disease on the Chinese-Russian Frontier.* London: Palgrave Macmillan, 2018.

——, ed. *Framing Animals as Epidemic Villains: Histories of Non-Human Disease Vectors.* Cham: Palgrave Macmillan, 2019.

——. *Human Extinction and the Pandemic Imaginary.* Abingdon: Routledge, 2020.

——. "Introduction: Imaging and Imagining Plague." In *Plague Image and Imagination from Medieval to Modern Times*, edited by Christos Lynteris, 1–10. Cham: Palgrave Macmillan, 2021.

——. "Introduction: Infectious Animals and Epidemic Blame." In *Framing Animals as Epidemic Villains: Histories of Non-Human Disease Vectors*, edited by Christos Lynteris, 1–26. Cham: Palgrave Macmillan, 2019.

——, ed. *Plague Image and Imagination from Medieval to Modern Times*. Cham: Palgrave Macmillan, 2021.

——. "The Prophetic Faculty of Epidemic Photography: Chinese Wet Markets and the Imagination of the Next Pandemic." *Visual Anthropology* 29, no. 2 (2016): 118–132.

——. "A 'Suitable Soil': Plague's Urban Breeding Grounds at the Dawn of the Third Pandemic." *Medical History* 62, no. 3 (2017): 343–357.

——. "Suspicious Corpses: Body Dumping and Plague in Colonial Hong Kong." In *Histories of Post-Mortem Contagion: Infectious Corpses and Contested Burials*, edited by Christos Lynteris and Nicholas H. A. Evans, 109–134. Basingstoke: Palgrave Macmillan, 2018.

——. "Tarbagan's Winter Lair: Framing Drivers of Plague Persistence in Inner Asia." In *Framing Animals as Epidemic Villains: Histories of Non-Human Disease Vectors*, edited by Christos Lynteris, 65–90. Cham: Palgrave Macmillan, 2019.

——. "Vagabond Microbes, Leaky Laboratories and Epidemic Mapping: Alexandre Yersin and the 1898 Plague Epidemic in Nha Trang." *Social History of Medicine* 34, no. 1 (2021): 190–213.

Lynteris, Christos, and Nicholas H. A. Evans, eds. *Histories of Post-Mortem Contagion: Infectious Corpses and Contested Burials*. Basingstoke: Palgrave Macmillan, 2018.

MacKenzie, John M., and John McAleer, *Exhibiting the Empire: Cultures of Display and the British Empire*. Manchester: Manchester University Press, 2017.

Mahler, Halfden. "Promotion of Primary Health Care in Member Countries of WHO." *Public Health Reports* 93, no. 2 (1978): 107–113.

Manderson, Lenore. "Wireless Wars in the Eastern Arena: Epidemiological Surveillance, Disease Prevention, and the Work of the Eastern Bureau of the League of Nations Health Organisation, 1925–1942." In *International Health Organisations and Movements, 1918–1939*, edited by Paul Weindling, 109–133. Cambridge: Cambridge University Press, 1995.

Maxwell, Anne. *Colonial Photography and Exhibitions*. London: Leicester University Press, 2000.

McCormac, Donna. *Queer Postcolonial Narratives and the Ethics of Witnessing*. New York: Bloomsbury Academic, 2014.

Meer, Arnout H. C. van der. "Ambivalent Hegemony: Culture and Power in Colonial Java, 1808–1927." PhD diss., Rutgers University, 2014.

——. "Performing Colonial Modernity: Fairs, Consumerism, and the Emergence of the Indonesian Middle Class." *Bijdragen tot de Taal-, Land- en Volkenkunde* 173 (2017): 503–538.

——. *Performing Power: Cultural Hegemony, Identity, and Resistance in Colonial Indonesia*. Ithaca, NY: Cornell University Press, 2020.

Meerwijk, Maurits Bastiaan. "Bamboo Dwellers: Plague, Photography, and the House in Java." In *Plague Image and Imagination from Medieval to Modern Times*, edited by Christos Lynteris, 205–234. Cham: Palgrave Macmillan, 2021.

——. "Phantom Menace: Dengue and Yellow Fever in Asia." *Bulletin of the History of Medicine* 94, no. 2 (2020): 215–243.

——. "Plague Rat or Anopheles: Health Disasters and Home Improvement in Late-Colonial Java." *Indonesia* (forthcoming).

——. "Viral Imagery of Dengue Fever in the Age of Bacteriology." *Isis* 111, no. 2 (2020): 239–263.

Michaels, Paula A. "Medical Propaganda and Cultural Revolution in Soviet Kazakhstan, 1928–41." *Russian Review* 59 (2000): 159–178.

Mitchell, Timothy. *Colonising Egypt*. Berkeley: University of California Press, 1988.

Mohr, James. *Plague and Fire: Battling Black Death and the 1900 Burning of Honolulu's Chinatown*. Oxford: Oxford University Press, 2005.

Monnais, Laurence. *The Colonial Life of Pharmaceuticals: Medicines and Modernity in Vietnam*. Cambridge: Cambridge University Press, 2019.

Moskalewicz, Marcin, Ute Caumanns, and Fritz Dross, eds. *Jewish Medicine and Healthcare in Central Eastern Europe: Shared Identities, Entangled Histories*. Dordrecht: Springer, 2019.

Mrazek, Rudolf. *Engineers of Happy Land: Nationalism and Technology in Indonesia*. Princeton, NJ: Princeton University Press, 2002.

Municipal Council Malang. *Malang: De Bergstad van Oost-Java*. Malang: 1927.

Nayar, Pramod K. *Colonial Voices: The Discourses of Empire*. Malden, MA: Wiley-Blackwell, 2012.

Nederveen Meerkerk, Elise van. *Women, Work and Colonialism in the Netherlands and Java: Comparisons, Contrasts, and Connections, 1830–1940*. Cham: Palgrave Macmillan, 2019.

Neelakantan, Vivek. "Eradicating Smallpox in Indonesia: The Archipelagic Challenge." *Health and History* 12, no. 1 (2017): 61–87.

——. *Science, Public Health and Nation-Building in Soekarno-Era Indonesia*. Newcastle: Cambridge Scholars, 2017.

Nieuwenhuys, Robert. *Mirror of the Indies: A History of Dutch Colonial Literature*. Hong Kong: Periplus, 1999.

Owen, Norman, ed. *Death and Disease in Southeast Asia: Explorations in Social, Medical and Demographic History*. Oxford: Oxford University Press, 1987.

Padang, M. Neumann van. "History of the Volcanology in the Former Netherlands East Indies." *Scripta Geologica* 71 (1983): 1–76.

Peckham, Robert, ed. *Empires of Panic: Epidemics and Colonial Anxieties*. Hong Kong: Hong Kong University Press, 2015.

——. "Hong Kong Junk: Plague and the Economy of Chinese Things." *Bulletin of the History of Medicine* 90, no. 1 (2016): 32–60.

——. "Matshed Laboratory: Colonies, Cultures, and Bacteriology." In *Imperial Contagions: Medicine, Hygiene, and Cultures of Planning in Asia*, edited by Robert Peckham and David Pomfret, 123–148. Hong Kong: Hong Kong University Press, 2013.

Peckham, Robert, and David Pomfret, eds. *Imperial Contagions: Medicine, Hygiene, and Cultures of Planning in Asia*. Hong Kong: Hong Kong University Press, 2013.

Peterson, Karin. *In het Voetspoor van Louis Couperus: Pasoeroean door de Lens van Salzwedel*. Amsterdam: KIT Publishers, 2009.

Pigliasco, Guido Carlo. "Colonial Spectacle, Staged Authenticity and Other Heritage Paradoxes on a Fijian Island." Paper presented at the conference Europe and the Pacific, Brussels, June 25, 2015.

Poeze, Harry A. "Walking the Tightrope: Internal Indonesian Conflict, 1945–49." In *Colonial Counterinsurgency and Mass Violence: The Dutch Empire in Indonesia*, edited by Bart Luttikhuis and A. Dirk Moses, 176–197. Abingdon: Routledge, 2014.

Poignant, Roslyn. *Professional Savages: Captive Lives and Western Spectacle*. New Haven, CT: Yale University Press, 2004.

Poleykett, Branwyn. "Building out the Rat: Animal Intimacies and Prophylactic Settlement in 1920s South Africa." *Engagement*, February 7, 2017. https:// aesengagement.wordpress.com/2017/02/07/building-out-the-rat-animal -intimacies-and-prophylactic-ssettlement-in-1920s-south-africa/.

Pols, Hans. *Nurturing Indonesia: Medicine and Decolonisation in the Dutch East Indies*. Cambridge: Cambridge University Press, 2018.

——. "Quarantine in the Dutch East Indies." In *Quarantine: Local and Global Histories*, edited by Alison Bashford, 85–102. London: Palgrave Macmillan, 2016.

Pope, Geoffrey G. "Bamboo." In *A History of Physical Anthropology: An Encyclopedia*, edited by Frank Spencer, 1:159–161. New York: Garland, 1997.

Prince, Ruth J. "The Diseased Body and the Global Subject: The Circulation and Consumption of an Iconic AIDS Photograph in East Africa." *Visual Anthropology* 29 (2016): 159–186.

Protschky, Susie. "Camera Ethica: Photography, Modernity and the Governed in Late-Colonial Indonesia." In *Photography, Modernity and the Governed in Late-Colonial Indonesia*, edited by Susie Protschky, 11–40. Amsterdam: Amsterdam University Press, 2015.

——. *Images of the Tropics: Environment and Visual Culture in Colonial Indonesia*. Leiden: KITLV Press, 2011.

——, ed. *Photography, Modernity and the Governed in Late-Colonial Indonesia*. Amsterdam: Amsterdam University Press, 2015.

Rafael, Vicente L., ed. *Figures of Criminality in Indonesia, the Philippines, and Colonial Vietnam*. Ithaca, NY: Cornell Southeast Asia Program, 1999.

Reichardt, Eike. *Health, "Race" and Empire: Popular-Scientific Spectacles and National Identity in Imperial Germany, 1871–1914*. Morrisville: Lulu.com, 2008.

Rogaski, Ruth. *Hygienic Modernity: Meanings of Health and Disease in Treaty-Port China*. Berkeley: University of California Press, 2004.

Roosmalen, Pauline K. M. van. "Netherlands Indies Town Planning: An Agent of Modernization (1905–1957)." In *Cars, Conduits, and Kampongs: The Modernization of the Indonesian City, 1920–1960*, edited by Freek Colombijn and Joost Coté, 87–119. Leiden: Brill, 2015.

——. "Ontwerpen aan de Stad: Stedenbouw in Nederlands-Indië en Indonesië (1905–1950)." PhD diss., TU Delft, 2008.

Rowland, Sydney. "XXXVIII. First Report on Investigations into Plague Vaccines." *Epidemiology and Infection* 10, no. 3 (1910): 536–565.

Ruppin, Dafna. *The Komedi Bioscoop: The Emergence of Movie-going in Colonial Indonesia, 1896–1914.* Bloomington, IN: John Libbey, 2016.

Schaik, A. van. *Malang: Beeld van een stad.* Purmerend: Asia Maior, 1996.

Serajah Kesehatan Nasional Indonesia. Vol. 1. Jakarta: Departement Kesehatan RI, 2009.

Serlin, David, ed. *Imagining Illness: Public Health and Visual Culture.* Minneapolis: University of Minnesota Press, 2010.

Sidlauskas, Susan. "Before and After: The Aesthetic as Evidence in Nineteenth-Century Medical Photography." In *Before-and-After Photography: Histories and Contexts*, edited by Jordan Bear and Kate Palmer Albers, 15–42. London: Bloomsbury Academic, 2017.

Smith, Shawn Michelle. *At the Edge of Sight: Photography and the Unseen.* Durham, NC: Duke University Press, 2013.

Snapper, I. "Medical Contributions from the Netherlands Indies." In *South East Asia, Colonial History.* Vol. 3, *High Imperialism (1890s–1930s)*, edited by Paul Kratoska, 129–152. London: Routledge, 2001.

Snelders, Stephen. *Leprosy and Colonialism: Suriname under Dutch Rule, 1750–1950.* Manchester: Manchester University Press, 2017.

Soeparmo, H. T., and R. L. Laird. "Anopheles Sundaicus and Its Control by DDT Residual House Spraying in Indonesia." WHO/Mal/118, December 2, 1954. World Health Organization.

Solomon, Tom. "Hong Kong, 1894: The Role of James A. Lowson in the Controversial Discovery of the Plague Bacillus." *Lancet* 350, no. 9070 (1997): 59–62.

Spencer, Frank, ed. *A History of Physical Anthropology: An Encyclopedia.* New York: Garland, 1997.

Stapleton, Darwin H. "Malaria Eradication and the Technological Model: The Rockefeller Foundation and Public Health in East Asia." In *Disease, Colonialism, and the State: Malaria in Modern East Asian History*, edited by Ka-che Yip, 71–84. Hong Kong: Hong Kong University Press, 2009.

Stoler, Ann Laura. *Capitalism and Confrontation in Sumatra's Plantation Belt, 1870–1979.* 2nd ed. Ann Arbor: University of Michigan Press, 1985.

Suartika, Gusti Ayu Made, and Julie Nichols, eds. *Reframing the Vernacular: Politics, Semiotics, and Representation.* Cham: Springer, 2020.

Sutphen, Mary P. "Not What, but Where: Bubonic Plague and the Reception of Germ Theories in Hong Kong and Calcutta, 1894–1897." *Journal of the History of Medicine* 52 (1997): 81–113.

Tagliacozzo, Eric. "Before the Gangrene Set in: The Dutch East Indies in 1910." In *Asia Inside Out: Changing Times*, edited by Eric Tagliacozzo, Helen F. Siu, and Peter C. Perdue, 226–249. Cambridge, MA: Harvard University Press, 2015.

——. *The Longest Journey: Southeast Asians and the Pilgrimage to Mecca.* Oxford: Oxford University Press, 2013.

Tagliacozzo, Eric, Helen F. Siu, and Peter C. Perdue, eds. *Asia Inside Out: Changing Times.* Cambridge MA: Harvard University Press, 2015.

Takken, W., W. B. Snellen, J. P. Verhave, B. G. J. Knols, and S. Atmosoedjono. *Environmental Measures for Malaria Control in Indonesia: An Historical Review on Species Sanitation.* Wageningen: Agricultural University, 1991.

Teichfischer, Philipp. "German-Jewish Doctors as Members of the Colonial Health Service in the Dutch East Indies in the First Half of the Nineteenth Century." In *Jewish Medicine and Healthcare in Central Eastern Europe: Shared Identities, Entangled Histories*, edited by Marcin Moskalewicz, Ute Caumanns, and Fritz Dross, 131–153. Dordrecht: Springer, 2019.

Timmerman, Ben. "Zoos Humains: Meer dan een Spektakel?" MA thesis, University of Ghent, 2017.

Tucker, Jennifer. *Nature Exposed: Photography as Eyewitness in Victorian Science.* Baltimore, MD: Johns Hopkins University Press, 2005.

Verma, Shailendra Kumar, and Urmil Tuteja. "Plague Vaccine Development: Current Research and Future Trends." *Frontiers in Immunology* 7 (2016): 1–8.

Versteeg, Anton. *Dagboek van mijn grootvader G. M. Versteeg.* Vols 3–6. Self-published, Pumbo, 2016.

Victoir, Laura, and Victor Zatsepine, eds. *Harbin to Hanoi: The Colonial Built Environment in Asia, 1840–1940.* Hong Kong: Hong Kong University Press, 2013.

Vokes, Richard. "Photography, Exhibitions and Embodied Futures in Colonial Uganda, 1908–1960." *Visual Studies* 33, no. 1 (2018): 11–27.

Vries, Gerrit de, and Dorothee Segaar-Höweler. *Henri Maclaine Pont: Architect, constructeur, archeoloog.* Rotterdam: Stiching Bonas, 2009.

Walker, Kirsty. "The Influenza Pandemic of 1918 in Southeast Asia." In *Histories of Health in Southeast Asia: Perspectives on the Long Nineteenth Century*, edited by Tim Harper and Sunil S. Amrith, 61–71. Bloomington: Indiana University Press, 2014.

Weindling, Paul, ed. *International Health Organisations and Movements, 1918–1939.* Cambridge: Cambridge University Press, 1995.

Weinert, Sebastian. *Der Körper im Blick: Gesundheitsausstellungen vom späten Kaiserreich bis zum Nationalsozialismus.* Oldenbourg: Walter de Gruyter, 2017.

Williams, J. E., B. W. Hudson, R. W. Turner, J. Sulianti Saroso, and D. C. Cavanaugh. "Plague in Central Java, Indonesia." *Bulletin of the World Health Organization* 58, no. 3 (1980): 459–468.

Wolff, J. W. *De ontwikkeling van de gezondheidszorg op cultuurondernemingen in de Tropen.* Amsterdam: Scheltema & Holkema, 1949.

Wolters, Willem. "Geographical Explanations for the Distribution of Irrigation Institutions: Cases from Southeast Asia." In *A World of Water: Rain, Rivers and Seas in Southeast Asian Histories*, edited by Peter Boomgaard, 209–234. Leiden: KITLV Press, 2007.

World Health Organization (WHO). "Fact Sheet: Plague." Accessed April 7, 2021. https://www.who.int/news-room/fact-sheets/detail/plague.

——. *Operational Guidelines on Plague Surveillance, Diagnosis, Prevention and Control.* New Delhi: WHO Regional Office for South-East Asia, 2010.

Yip, Ka-che, ed. *Disease, Colonialism, and the State: Malaria in Modern East Asian History.* Hong Kong: Hong Kong University Press, 2009.

INDEX

Note: Page numbers in *italics* indicate illustrations.

Lightning Source UK Ltd.
Milton Keynes UK
UKHW041425051122
411698UK00001B/1